Radiologic Atlas of Pulmonary Abnormalities in Children

Second Edition

Edward B. Singleton, M.D.

Director of Radiology, St. Luke's Episcopal Hospital
Professor of Radiology, Baylor College of Medicine
Clinical Professor of Radiology, University of Texas Medical Branch

Milton L. Wagner, M.D.

Associate Radiologist, St. Luke's Episcopal Hospital
Clinical Professor of Radiology, Baylor College of Medicine

Robert V. Dutton, M.D.

Associate Radiologist, St. Luke's Episcopal Hospital
Clinical Associate Professor of Pediatrics and Radiology,
    Baylor College of Medicine

All are associated with the
St. Luke's Episcopal Hospital,
Texas Children's Hospital, and the
Texas Heart Institute,
Baylor College of Medicine
Houston, Texas

1988

W. B. SAUNDERS COMPANY
Harcourt Brace Jovanovich, Inc.

Philadelphia / London / Toronto / Montreal / Sydney / Tokyo

W. B. SAUNDERS COMPANY
Harcourt Brace Jovanovich, Inc.

West Washington Square
Philadelphia, PA 19105

Library of Congress Cataloging-in-Publication Data

Singleton, Edward B., 1920–

Radiologic atlas of pulmonary abnormalities in children.

Includes bibliographies and index.

1. Pediatric respiratory diseases—Diagnosis—Atlases.
2. Diagnosis, Radioscopic—Atlases.   I. Wagner, Milton
L., 1931–   II. Dutton, Robert V. [DNLM: 1. Lung—
abnormalities—atlases.   2. Lung—radiography—
atlases.   3. Lung Diseases—in infancy and childhood—
atlases. WF 17 S617r]

RJ433.5.R25S56 1988   618.92′240757   87–28383

ISBN 0–7216–2062–0

Editor: W. B. Saunders Staff
Designer: W. B. Saunders Staff
Production Manager: Carolyn Naylor
Manuscript Editor: Louise Robinson
Illustration Coordinator: Lisa Lambert
Indexer: Helene Taylor

Radiologic Atlas of Pulmonary Abnormalities in Children   ISBN 0–7216–2062–0

Last digit is the print number: 9   8   7   6   5   4   3   2   1

Preface to the Second Edition

Since the first edition of *Radiologic Atlas of Pulmonary Abnormalities in Children* was published in 1971, there have been many requests for updating this Atlas, and for enlarging it to encompass various conditions that were not originally included. Although the comments made in the preface to the first edition are still appropriate, the radiographic features of a number of conditions, particularly in the newborn, have been altered by the development of more sophisticated life-support systems and the increased intensive care given these infants. Similar alterations in the radiographic patterns of a number of the viral and bacterial pneumonias have occurred for similar reasons. In addition, neoplastic diseases of the lungs have shown an alteration in their natural progression because of the newer forms of chemotherapy that are now employed.

Computerized tomography is now an established and essentially indispensable method of evaluating mediastinal lesions and pulmonary neoplastic diseases. Digital subtraction studies of intrathoracic vessels is another major technologic development that was not available when the first edition was prepared. With the exception of echocardiography, diagnostic ultrasound has limited use in the evaluation of pulmonary lesions but may be helpful in imaging some areas of the chest wall, pleural space, and lungs.

Magnetic resonance imaging of the pediatric chest is currently less satisfactory than computerized tomography but continues to show promise in a number of conditions as the technology improves.

Consequently, although the format of this second edition remains essentially the same, there have been major changes in regard to the inclusion of newer conditions not recognized in the first edition, a discussion of the alterations of radiographic patterns associated with newer forms of treatment, and the application of new diagnostic modalities. It is hoped that these additions will provide an updated view of the varieties of abnormalities of the pediatric chest.

We wish to acknowledge the patient efforts of our secretary, Eloise Simons, in the typing and multiple retypings of this manuscript. Equally appreciated is the assistance provided by the Photographic Services Department of St. Luke's Episcopal Hospital, Texas Children's Hospital, and the Texas Heart Institute. We also thank the W. B. Saunders Company and Mr. Dean J. Manke, Mr. Dana Dreibelbis, Ms. Carolyn Naylor, and Ms. Lisa Lambert for their cooperation. As in the first edition, we hope that this atlas will be helpful to radiologists, pediatricians, and all those who care for children of all ages.

Edward B. Singleton
Milton L. Wagner
Robert V. Dutton

Introduction

Except for bronchial carcinoma and industrial pulmonary diseases, the variety of intrathoracic abnormalities found in the pediatric patient is as great as that encountered in the adult. In addition, because of the numerous congenital defects as well as the many specific and frequently esoteric neonatal pulmonary abnormalities, pediatric chest diseases and their accompanying radiologic features are the most important subjects in pediatrics and pediatric radiology.

Although the history and physical examination are of the utmost diagnostic importance, chest roentgenography is the single most important procedure in determining the diagnosis. This is especially true in the examination of the neonate, in whom physical findings are frequently less revealing than in the older patient and in whom significant historical details are unavailable.

An appreciation of the different conditions affecting the intrathoracic structures of this age group and a knowledge of the pulmonary physiology of the neonate are necessary for an adequate appreciation of the radiographic features of many pediatric conditions. The details of the pathogenesis and the clinical and physical findings of these conditions are described in textbooks of pediatrics. This text emphasizes the radiographic features but, because of the necessity for accurate correlation of clinical findings with the x-ray picture, it also includes a brief discussion of the pertinent clinical features.

The variations of normal structures in the growing infant and child require an appreciation of normalcy before the abnormal can be recognized. Consequently, the first portion of this monograph will include a description of the normal neonatal chest as well as changes in the radiographic appearance during growth. Because certain pulmonary diseases are more commonly found at specific ages, the description of most of the conditions presented herein will be divided into the neonatal period, older infants, and children.

A consideration of the numerous pulmonary abnormalities occurring in the young infant is of particular interest because of both the common and the unusual abnormalities. Many of these conditions are found only in the neonate, and, unless there is an awareness on the part of the obstetrician, pediatrician, or radiologist, they will go unsuspected even though the radiographic features may at times be characteristic.

In this age group the most common symptom requiring radiographic evaluation is respiratory distress, which may be in the form of tachypnea alone or may be associated with cyanosis. An x-ray study of the chest in these infants is the single most important examination in determining the cause of the respiratory distress. A disturbance in respiration may be the result of central nervous system abnormality, intestinal obstruction, diaphragmatic hernia, congenital heart disease, or alteration in the serum electrolyte level as well as of disease inherent in the lung. The absence of demonstrable radiographic pathology in the lungs excludes them as the cause for the infant's distress and should alert the clinician to check the other areas previously mentioned. Radiographic findings of congenital heart disease or intestinal tract abnormality may also be readily appreciated by film examination.

The discussion of pulmonary abnormalities will proceed according to the outline in the Table of Contents. It is hoped that the atlas format will be of greater diagnostic value to both the pediatrician and the radiologist than a textbook format.

Contents

1 TECHNIQUE

The most important consideration in obtaining high-quality radiographs of the pediatric chest is exposure time. A generator capacity of at least 300 mA and an exposure time of at least 1/60 sec are necessary for quality radiographs.

Although teleoroentgenograms are necessary in older children and in adult patients, they are not a major consideration in infants because of the relatively thin anteroposterior dimension of the infant chest, which eliminates the problem of distortion. Although a distance of 72 inches is preferred, 40- or even 36-inch tube film distances may be used. The important consideration is that the same distance is employed consistently (Fig. 1–1).

There are many commercial devices used to obtain upright chest films in infants. However, a practical and satisfactory approach is to radiograph all infants in a supine position and avoid the difficulties of positioning uncooperative patients in an upright position. The help of a parent, nurse, or aide protected with a lead apron will expedite the examination (Fig. 1–2). It is important to remember that, when supine films are made, the infant's elbows should be held against the ears to keep the head straight. Unless this is done, a distorted picture of the chest will be obtained. If the x-ray technologist does not have additional help, immobilization may be accomplished by use of a stockinette to hold the infant's arms above the head with a generous amount of masking tape (Fig. 1–3A). If upright radiographs are necessary, the Pigg-o-stat is the most practical (Fig. 1–3B). In unusually fat infants a supine position is preferable to obtain a better inspiratory film because, when the infant is in a sitting position, the thighs press against a protuberant abdomen; this in turn restricts the respiratory movements of the diaphragm (Fig. 1–4).

Although inspiratory films are preferable, it should be understood that an expiratory film is often a reflection of a normal chest, and incomplete aeration of the lungs in such cases should not be interpreted as abnormal (Fig. 1–5). The routine custom of making two x-ray exposures in an effort to obtain a deep inspiratory radiograph is still employed in many x-ray departments. This is unnecessary, exposes the infant to additional radiation, and reflects the radiologist's lack of knowledge in evaluating the pediatric chest. In most infants with upper or lower respiratory infections or with respiratory distress from other causes, a film will show the diaphragm in a low position because of tachypnea, air hunger, or air trapping. In such infants it is difficult to obtain an expiratory film. If the infant is crying it is easier to make an inspiratory film, but if the infant is happy and placid the film will usually be taken during expiration. Consequently, no attempt is made to quiet the crying infant when preparations are being made for a chest radiograph. On the contrary, steps are frequently made to encourage crying at this stage of the examination.

Struggling infants frequently arch their backs, producing a lordotic view of the chest. Similar distortion results from centering the central x-ray beam over the abdomen. In both situations the ribs appear to be horizontal, with upward deflection of the anterior portions. In addition, there is apparent bulging of the

Text continued on page 6

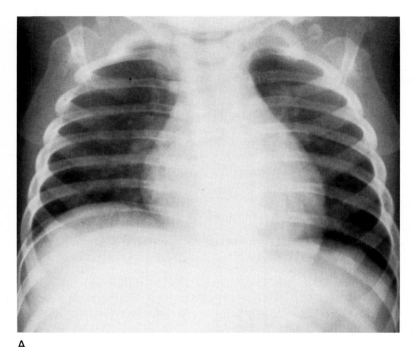

A

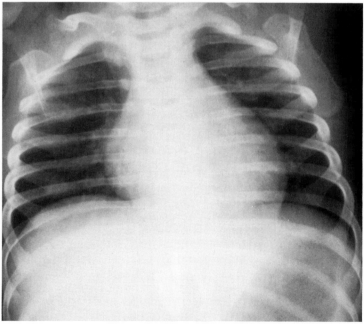

B

Figure 1–1. Chest radiographs made of an infant at 72 inches and 36 inches. A, 72-inch tube-film distance. B, 36-inch tube-film distance, with no apparent distortion.

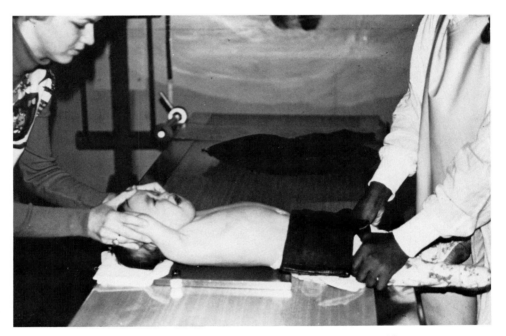

Figure 1–2. *Immobilization with assistance of parent and aide.*

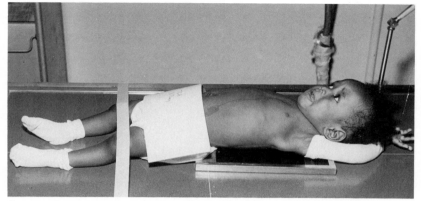

A

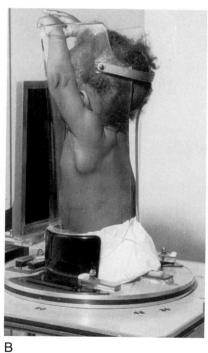

B

Figure 1–3. A, *Supine chest technique using elastic stockinette to hold the infant's arms.* B, *Pigg-o-stat using a plastic holding device.*

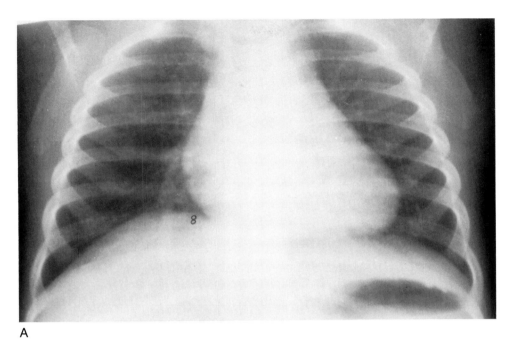

A

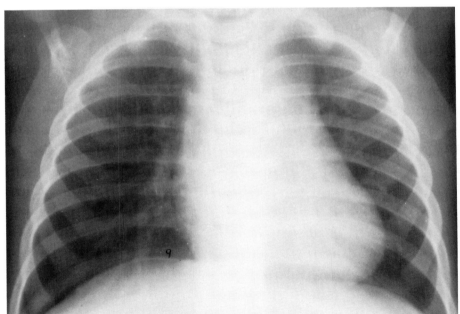

B

Figure 1–4. *Obese infant. A, Upright radiograph shows high position of the diaphragm. B, Supine film allows better inspiratory radiography.*

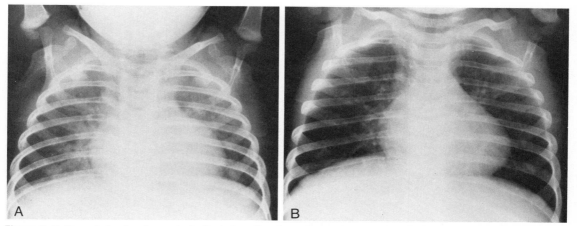

Figure 1–5. Normal chest radiograph. A, *Expiratory film shows incomplete aeration of lungs, simulating pneumonia.* B, *Inspiratory film of same infant.*

lungs in the intercostal spaces, which should not be misinterpreted as overinflation (Fig. 1–6).

It should be understood that, in all situations, lead-equivalent protectors are utilized to cover the gonadal portions of the body.

The intensive efforts currently employed to save the lives of low-birth-weight and premature infants require frequent portable radiographs of the chest and abdomen, not only for initial evaluation of the heart and lungs but also for localization of specialized equipment such as endotracheal tubes, umbilical artery and venous catheters, central venous lines, and nasogastric tubes. In addition, follow-up studies for the complications of prematurity—that is, interstitial air in the lungs, pneumothorax, and bronchopulmonary dysplasia—require frequent radiographs over a period of many weeks or months. These examinations must be made with the infant in the life support environment, and with as little handling

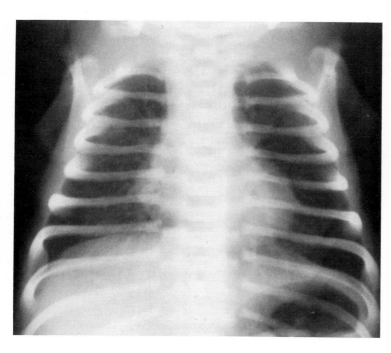

Figure 1–6. Chest radiograph of normal infant with x-ray tube centered over upper abdomen. The apparent bulging of the intercostal spaces and the horizontal position of the ribs are normal findings.

as possible. Capacity discharge portable units provide very rapid exposure times and are preferable for this type of examination.

Although magnification techniques may be used to advantage, particularly in newborn infants suspected of having hyaline membrane disease, they are usually impractical because of the risk involved in moving these critically ill infants to the x-ray department. Consequently, there is now less enthusiasm in employing magnification radiography in the evaluation of infantile respiratory distress. The development of newer portable x-ray units with smaller focal spots, however, and the use of incubators that can be altered to provide the necessary distance between the infant and cassette, may provide practical methods for magnification without disturbing the infant.

Since the first edition of this book newer modalities of chest imaging have become available, greatly enhancing and broadening the diagnostic armamentarium. These techniques include ultrasound, computerized tomography (CT), digital subtraction angiography and, more recently, magnetic resonance imaging (MRI). In most instances these procedures are required to answer specific questions suggested by results obtained from the initial radiograph of the chest, which remains the centerpiece for imaging the chest.

The initial use of ultrasound was very limited because of mechanical problems of static scanning, as well as the inherent complexity of the chest that is compounded by the breathing child. With the advent of gray scale and real-time scanners these problems have diminished, although the physical complexity of soft tissue, bone, and air will always limit the utility of chest ultrasonography to some extent. Nevertheless, much useful information can now be derived by the use of real-time scanners and water bath equipment (Octoson). For sector scans, a simple explanation to the older child, warm gel, and gentle hands are all that is needed. Intercostal, subxyphoid, subcostal, suprasternal, and parasternal examinations can be performed in various positions, depending on the information needed. Unlike CT and MRI, the examination is operator-dependent but also very versatile. Lesions of the chest wall, pleural space, diaphragm, and lung bases can be demonstrated, and some mediastinal and pulmonary parenchymal lesions may also be seen. A wide selection of transducers are available from 2.5 to 10 mHz; the choice depends on the age of the patient and on the nature of the suspected lesion. Portable real-time scanners are readily available, allowing bedside scanning. Sector scanners are also very helpful in defining pleural fluid or masses, which may also be biopsied under ultrasound guidance.

In contrast to ultrasound, CT of the chest is uniquely suited to differentiate soft tissue, bone, and air, with excellent spatial detail. It has become invaluable in its ability to detect and characterize disease processes that may only be suggested or completely unrevealed by conventional radiography. Like ultrasound, it has undergone evolutionary stages related to improved equipment. Older scanners requiring 18 sec/scan have now been largely replaced by third- and fourth-generation scanners capable of 1-sec scans at reduced radiation dosages. Cine CT scanners provide multiple images per second without the necessity of sedation. In spite of these refinements, respiratory motion and the paucity of fat remain significant problems in pediatric CT imaging. Each patient must be monitored individually to obtain diagnostic studies. Because of the cool temperature required in most CT suites, some effort must be made to keep small infants and children warm by using thermal blankets or heaters. A properly shielded parent may be left in the room to reassure the apprehensive child, and sedation may be unnecessary. As a rule, an infant under 6 to 10 months of age does not require sedation if warm and properly wrapped. Children from 1 to 4 years of age usually require sedation and various schedules are available. For children up to 2 years of age we usually use oral chloral hydrate in a dose of 50 to 70 mg/kg. This is safe and is usually quite satisfactory. For older children a combination of meperidine (2 mg/kg), promethazine (0.5 mg/kg), and chlorpromazine (0.5 mg/kg)

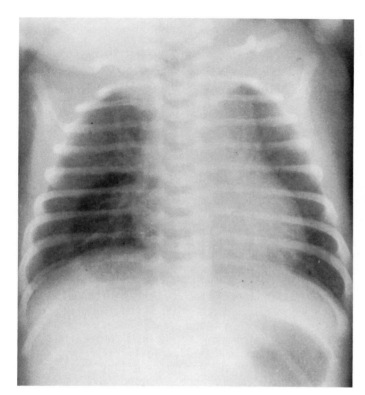

Figure 1–7. *Radiolucent defect in right hem-ithorax of newborn. This is an artifact pro-duced by an opening in the top of the isolette.*

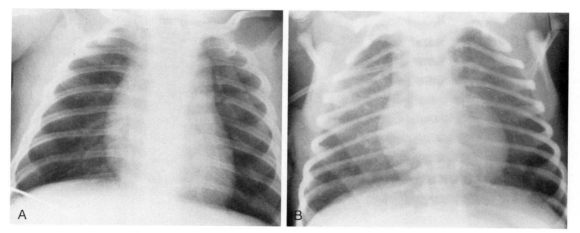

Figure 1–8. A, *Skin fold simulating pneumothorax.* B, *Multiple skin folds, right lower hemithorax.*

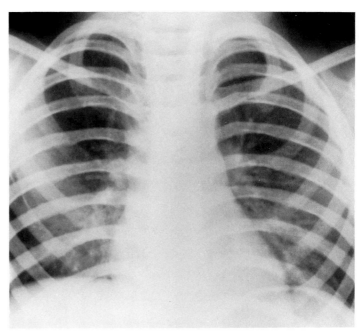

Figure 1–9. A, *Pectoral muscles, simulating pneumonia.* B, *Chest radiograph of same patient made moments later.*

A

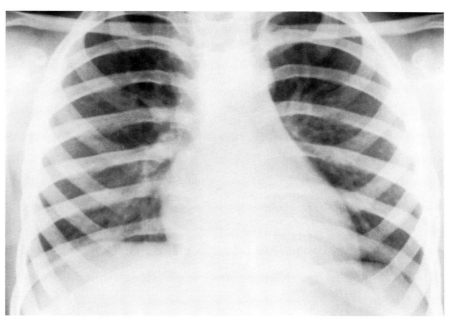

B

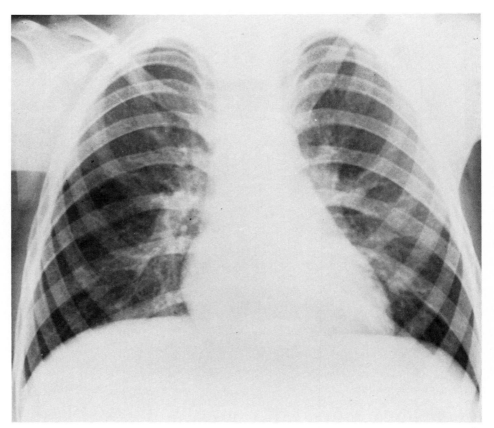

Figure 1–10. *Poland's syndrome in a 5-year-old boy showing absence of the right pectoral muscle, resulting in increased radiolucency of the right hemithorax.*

can be given (DPT, cardiac cocktail). The total dose of meperidine should not exceed 50 mg, and no more than 15 mg of promethazine or meperidine should be given. For proper identification of vascular structures and masses, pre- and postcontrast scans are necessary. Only contrast studies may be necessary for follow-up, reducing the number of scans. Intravenous iodinated contrast (60%) in doses of 2 ml/kg (not over 100 ml) may be given by bolus injection for dynamic scans, or a combination of bolus and drip infusion may be given for routine examinations.

Digital subtraction angiography in infants and children provides satisfactory visualization of the pulmonary arteries and other intrathoracic vessels, and is accomplished by pressure injection through a No. 18 or 20 Cathlon in a peripheral vein. In infants, because of their shorter circulation time and lower blood volume, hand injection of a small amount of contrast material may suffice. DPT sedation as recommended for CT is necessary for those in this age group, including the young infant. If the recommended amount of medication does not maintain the necessary sedation, or if the patient awakens during the examination, ketamine hydrochloride may be used as a supplement, either intramuscularly (2 mg/kg) or intravenously (0.5–1.0 mg/kg). However, this dose is only administered to children 10 years of age or younger because of its ability to produce vivid dreams or hallucinations in older children. Ketamine may also produce a transient increase in blood pressure, and should not be used in patients with hypertension or increased intracranial pressure. If ketamine is used, a one-time injection of 0.1 mg/55 kg of atropine is administered intramuscularly to counteract the excessive bronchial secretions produced by ketamine. Additional titration with intravenous pentobarbitol (1–2 mg/kg) is given if needed. Thorazine is contraindicated in patients with a history of seizures and, if deleted, the dose of promethazine is doubled to 1 mg/kg.

Although the basic concepts of magnetic resonance imaging were reported independently by Bloch and Purcell in 1946, it was not until the early 1970s that the first images in humans were obtained by Damadian, Lauterbur, Mansfield, and others. Since then, there has been great interest and exceptional growth of this modality. Experience in MRI of the chest in children is currently limited, but will obviously play a significant role for selected problematic cases. The apparent safety of presently available scanners and the nonionizing nature of MRI are major advantages. Soft tissue contrast is very good. Cardiac chambers and vascular structures are clearly defined without injection of contrast. The disadvantages are expense and the long duration of the scan, during which the patient must remain perfectly still. For children older than 4 or 5 years, an explanation of what is to be done and reassurance that there will be no pain or injury are usually enough. Infants under 1 year of age generally fall asleep when comfortably wrapped and warm. Children between 1 and 4 years of age must be individualized and some will require sedation, usually chloral hydrate. Parents are encouraged to stay in the room with the child while visual and voice contact are maintained by the scan operator. Ferromagnetic objects, monitors, and currently available resuscitation equipment cannot be brought into the scan room. Patients with pacemakers and vascular clips should not be scanned.

It is important to recognize the artifacts that are commonly seen in chest radiographs of infants and children. Radiographs of newborn infants taken through plastic isolettes may show the small circular opening on the top of the isolette as a radiolucent defect in the lung (Fig. 1–7). Skin folds are commonly seen in chest radiographs of young infants, especially newborns, and should not be mistaken for pneumothorax or atelectasis (Fig. 1–8). Contraction of pectoral muscles at the time of exposure may produce density, simulating pneumonia (Fig. 1–9). This should not be mistaken for Poland's syndrome, in which the pectoral muscle is absent (Fig 1–10).

SUGGESTED READINGS

Ablow RC, Greenspan RH, and Gluck L: The advantages of direct magnification technic in a newborn chest. Radiology, 92:745, 1969.

Bloch F, Hansen WW, and Packard ME: Nuclear induction. Phys Rev 69:127, 1946.

Brasch RC et al.: Magnetic resonance imaging of the thorax in children. Work in progress. Radiology, 150:463, 1984.

Cohen MD: Pediatric Magnetic Resonance Imaging. Philadelphia, W.B. Saunders, 1986.

Darling DB: Radiography of Infants and Children. Springfield, IL, Charles C Thomas, 1962.

Davis LA: Standard roentgen examination in newborns, infants and children: Technic, "portable" films, immobilization devices and fluoroscopy. Prog Pediatr Radiol, 1:3, 1967.

Gasie G, Dominguez R, and Young LW: Comparison of A-P supine vs P-A upright methods of chest roentgenography in infants and young children. J Natl Med Assoc, 76:171, 1984.

Haller JO et al.: Sonographic evaluation of the chest in infants and children. Am J Roentgenol, 134:1019, 1980.

Kirks DR: Practical techniques for pediatric chest computed tomography. J Comput Assist Tomogr, 7:31, 1983.

Poznanski AK: Practical Approaches to Pediatric Radiology. Chicago, Year Book Medical Publishers, 1976.

Poznanski AK, Borer RC, and Roloff DW: Adaptation of infant warmer for magnification radiography. Radiology, 112:219, 1974.

Purcell EM, Torrey HC, and Pound RV: Resonance absorption by nuclear magnetic moment in a solid. Phys Rev, 69:37, 1946.

Shurtleff RT: Children's Radiographic Technique, 2nd ed. Philadelphia, Lea & Febiger, 1962.

Wagner ML, Singleton EB, and Egan ME: The use of digital subtraction angiography in evaluating pulmonary abnormalities in children. Pediatr Radiol, 12:73, 1985.

White JD and Wisniewski HM: An improved method of radiographing premature infants in the nursery. Radiology, 100:696, 1971.

2 NORMAL CHEST

Because respiratory movements are known to occur during fetal life, and because it has been demonstrated that amniotic fluid enters the tracheobronchial tree during this period, it seemed reasonable to believe that inflation of the lungs in the newborn occurs gradually, depending on the vigor of the respiratory effort, the amount of fluid present, and the adhesiveness of the alveoli. However, cinefluorographic studies of pulmonary inflation in the newborn have demonstrated that the normal healthy neonate, who cries spontaneously after birth, inflates the lungs completely, by radiologic standards, during the first few breaths (Fig. 2–1). Serial measurements of functional pulmonary capacity have also emphasized the rapidity with which normal aeration and respiratory exchange occur. The pressures required have been carefully evaluated and, apparently, the effort required for the first breath is essentially the same as that for a cry in an infant several days old. Consequently, descriptive radiographic terms, such as persistent fetal atelectasis, neonatal atelectasis, and incomplete expansion of the neonatal lung, which at one time were considered normal variations in the pulmonary aeration of the neonate, have no place in the roentgenographic interpretation of the normal newborn chest. In addition, several important cardiovascular changes occur during the first postnatal day. These include a decrease in pulmonary vascular resistance and constriction of the ductus arteriosus: clamping the umbilical cord decreases the blood flow to the right atrium, with an increase in left atrial pressure, thereby establishing the normal circulatory pathway.

Radiographs of the normal newborn show symmetric radiolucency of the lungs. The diaphragm is usually at an inspiratory level of the eighth to ninth ribs posteriorly, or the anterior portion of the sixth ribs, and the anteroposterior

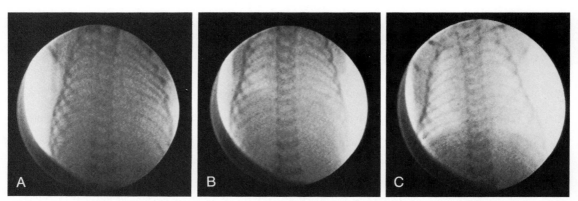

Figure 2–1. Cineradiography demonstrating pulmonary aeration during the first few breaths. A, First inspiratory effort shows partial pulmonary aeration. B, Second inspiratory effort shows more complete pulmonary aeration. C, Third inspiratory effort shows complete aeration of the lungs.

dimension of the chest is approximately the same as the transverse dimension (Fig. 2–2). Frequently, the lungs appear to be slightly overaerated and overly radiolucent. This is probably due to the physiologic acidosis that is commonly present at this age. The ribs may appear horizontal, and convexity of the aerated lung at the intercostal space levels can frequently be identified. This is usually the

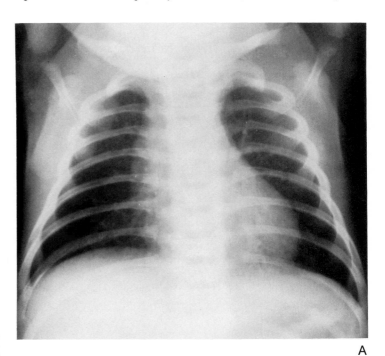

Figure 2–2. Normal neonatal chest. A, Frontal projection shows complete aeration of the lungs, with the diaphragm at the level of the eighth intercostal space posteriorly. B, Lateral view shows the anteroposterior diameter to be approximately the same as the transverse diameter.

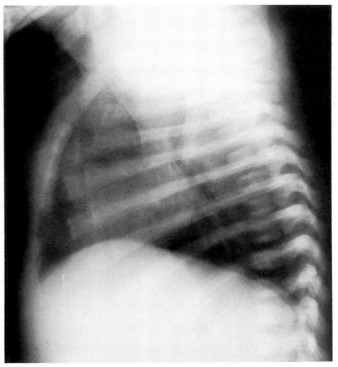

A

B

result of positioning the central beam of the x-ray tube over the upper abdomen, thus giving the chest a lordotic appearance (see Fig. 1–6).

The transverse diameter of the heart may be from 50 to 70% of the transverse diameter of the chest and, consequently, evaluation of the cardiothoracic ratio is meaningless because it is impossible to obtain a standard degree of inspiration at this age. The width of the superior mediastinum varies but is usually full because of the abundant thymic tissue. Occasionally the thymus may be large in the newborn, particularly if the baby is postmature, and lateral chest radiographs will show obliteration of the anterior mediastinum by the thymus. If the exposure is

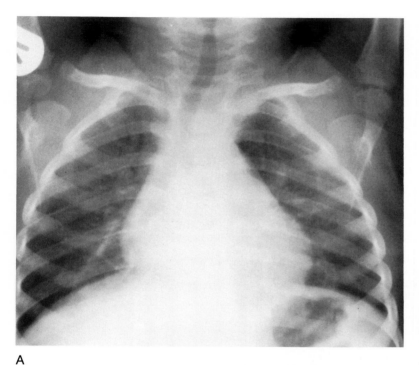

A

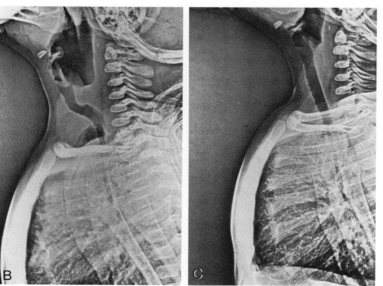

B   C

Figure 2–3. Changes in the trachea during expiration. A, Frontal projection shows the trachea deviated to the right, with the diaphragm at the level of the posterior portion of the seventh rib. B, Lateral view shows anterior buckling of the trachea below the hypopharynx. C, Lateral view with inspiration shows the trachea to be straight.

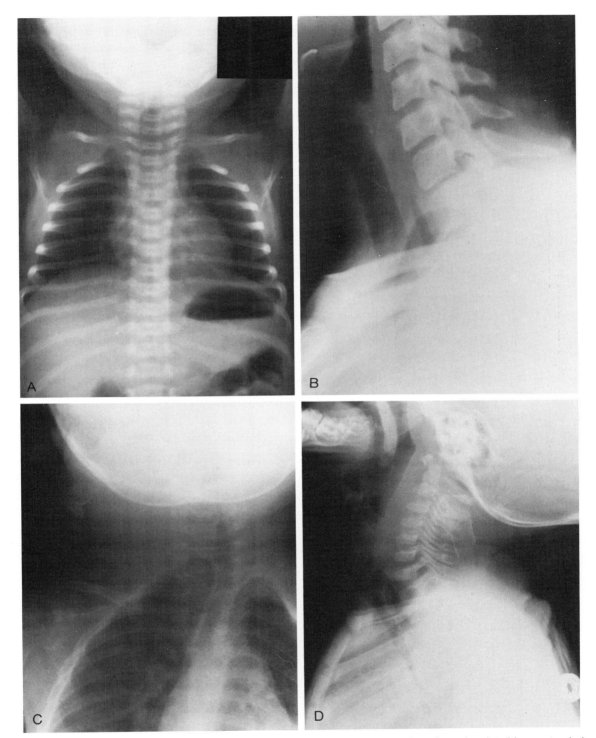

Figure 2–4. *Herniation of the pulmonary apices in an infant. A, Anteroposterior view shows herniated lung extended above the lines of the first ribs bilaterally. B, Lateral view. C, A unilateral herniation of the apex of the right lung in a young infant, using high-kilovoltage filtered technique. D, Lateral view showing the herniated apical portion of the right lung. (A, B, Courtesy of Dr. L. Swischuk.)*

made during expiration there will generally be buckling of the trachea to the right and anteriorly (Fig. 2–3). This should be recognized as normal, and should not be mistaken for a retrotracheal or retropharyngeal mass. Also, an expiratory film in a term newborn should not be cause for alarm. Frequently this represents indirect evidence that there is no problem of respiratory distress, because it is extremely unusual to see a high-positioned diaphragm in an infant who is experiencing labored respirations. Aeration of the apical segments of the lungs above the level of the clavicles is not uncommon in the infant and young child, and should not be interpreted as abnormal (Fig. 2–4). A slightly overpenetrated film will usually demonstrate the pleuroazygoesophageal line (Fig. 2–5). Obliteration of this line may occur in hilar or subcarinal adenopathy.

Normal changes in the appearance of the thymus occur during infancy. There is usually an increase in size during the first few weeks and months of life, with the prominence of the thymus apparently reflecting the health of the infant. Frequently, the edges of the thymus will have a wavy configuration, the thymic "wave sign." This may be especially prominent in infants with bronchiolitis (Fig. 2–6). The angular corner of the thymus, usually the right side, has been described as the "sail sign" (Fig. 2–7). A large or unusually shaped thymus, even accompanied by breathing and cardiac difficulties, should not be considered a threat to the life of the infant (Fig. 2–8). A mass in the anterior-superior portion of the mediastinum in a healthy infant should be regarded as a normal thymus unless there is obvious growth in a short period of time. After a period of illness or stress, or after surgical correction of congenital heart disease or some other chronic defect, regeneration of the thymus frequently occurs (see Fig. 3–9). Occasionally the thymus may extend posteriorly between the innominate artery and superior vena cava, displacing the superior vena cava laterally, simulating mediastinal mass (Fig. 2–9A–F). Magnetic resonance imaging in such cases shows the thymus to have a smooth configuration, whereas lymphomas usually show lumps or nodules. Magnetic resonance imaging has shown that approximately 15% of children will

Text continued on page 26

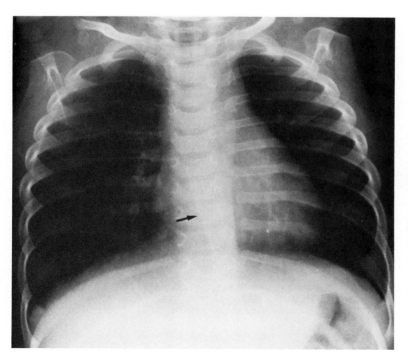

Figure 2–5. *Pleuroazygoesophageal line (arrow).*

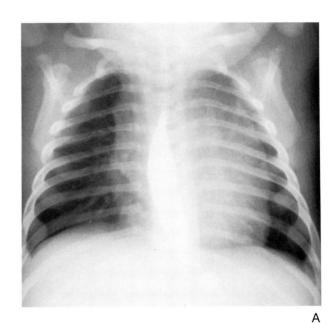

A

Figure 2–6. *Thymic wave sign. A, Compression of the thymus by the anterior portions of the costal cartilages produces a wavy configuration of the thymus. B, Exaggeration of the thymic wave sign in infant with bronchiolitis. Note the hyperaeration of the lungs.*

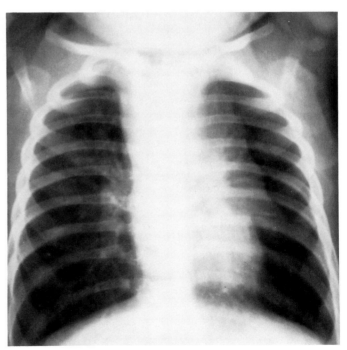

B

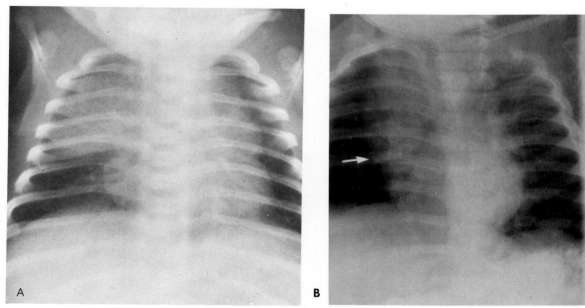

Figure 2–7. *Thymic sail sign. A, Frontal view of the chest shows prominence in the anterosuperior mediastinum. B, Oblique view shows angulation of the inferior lateral border of the thymus (arrow).*

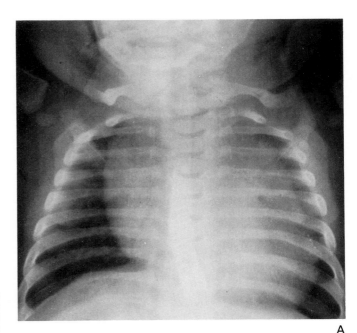

A

Figure 2–8. Variations in the size and the configuration of the thymus. A, Large thymus obscures cardiac silhouette, extending on the right from the apex inferiorly to the diaphragm and on the left from the apex to the lower left cardiac border. B, Large right lobe of the thymus produces apparent mass in the hilar area.

Illustration continued on following page

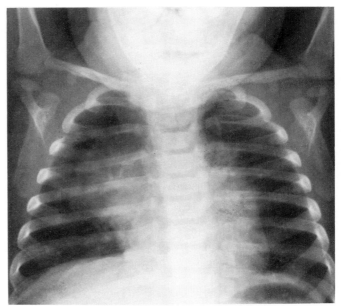

B

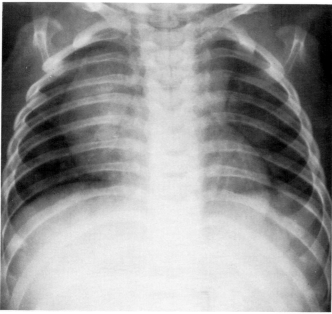

C

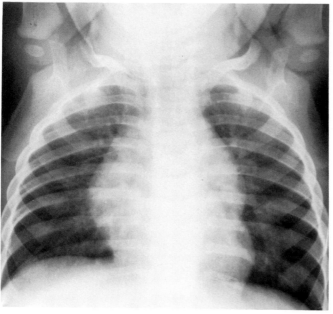

D

Figure 2–8. *C, Large right lobe of the thymus obscures the right cardiac border. D, Prominent thymus cloaks the superior mediastinal silhouette.*

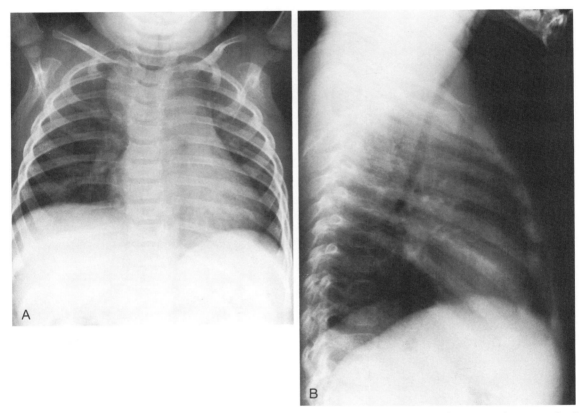

Figure 2–9. A, *Anteroposterior view shows mass in superior mediastinum.* B, *Lateral view shows mass in paratracheal location.*

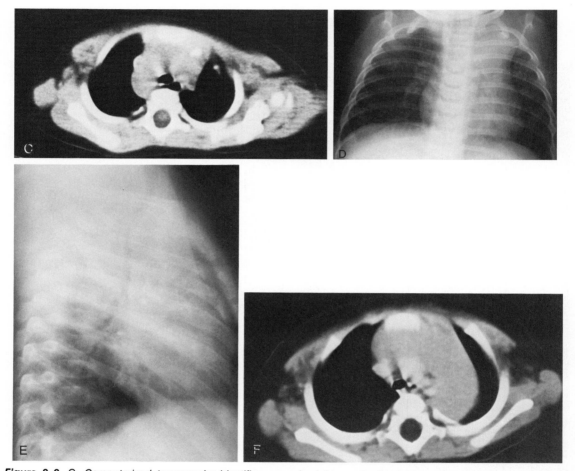

Figure 2–9. *C, Computerized tomography identifies mass in right paratracheal area extending into the posterior mediastinum. Normal thymus found at exploration. D, Thymus simulating left superior mediastinal mass in a 6-month-old infant. E, Lateral projection shows mass in anterior mediastinum. F, Computerized tomography demonstrates the extension of the thymus into the right posterior mediastinum.*

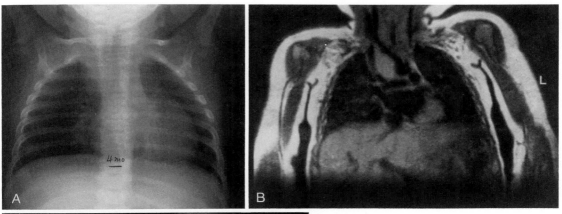

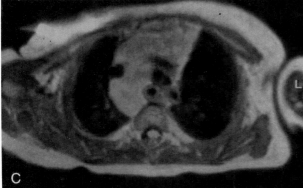

Figure 2–10. A, A 4-month-old boy with right superior mediastinal mass. A chest radiograph shows the mass in the right superior mediastinum. B, Gated T1 weighted magnetic image shows high-intensity signal of the thymus extending between the superior vena cava and the brachiocephalic artery. C, Cross-sectional T1 gated image shows the posterior extent of the high-intensity thymic signal extending into the posterior mediastium. (Courtesy of Dr. G. Currarino, Dallas, Texas.)

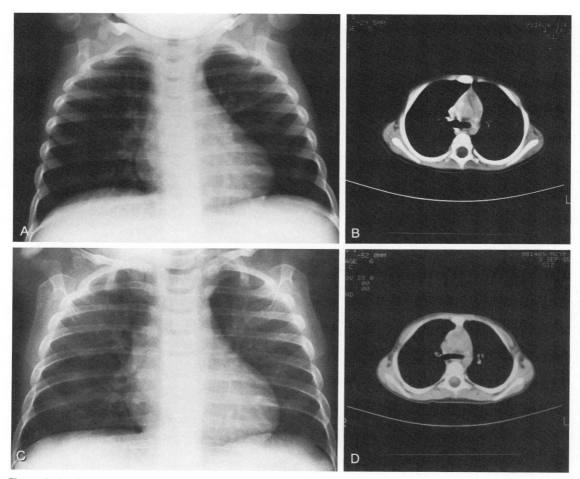

Figure 2–11. A, *Anteroposterior view of the chest in a normal 1-year-old infant. B, Computerized tomography of the mediastinum at the level of the carina demonstrates the thymus adjacent to the heart. C, Anteroposterior chest view of a normal 2-year-old child. D, Computerized tomography of the mediastinum shows the thymus anterior to the aortic arch.*

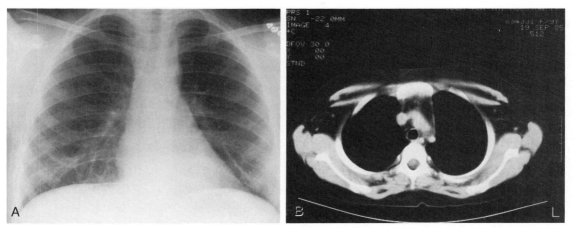

Figure 2–12. A, *Chest radiograph of a 14-year-old child. B, Computerized tomography shows replacement of the thymus by fat.*

Figure 2–13. *Premature infant. Chest radiographs show incomplete expansion of the lungs, with vague areas of increased density occupying both lungs.*

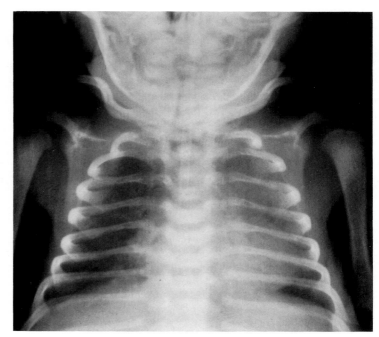

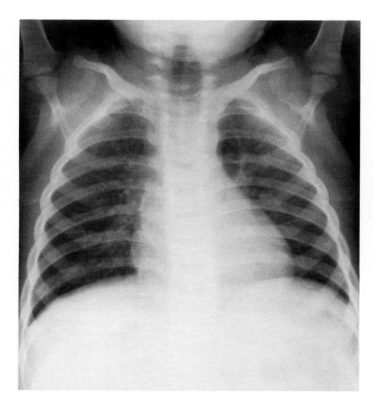

Figure 2–14. *Normal chest radiograph of a 3-year-old child. There has been normal growth of the chest and mediastinum, obliterating the thymus and resulting in the overall configuration of the mediastinal structure seen in the older child and adult.*

have a portion of their thymus extending posterior to the superior vena cava (Fig. 2–10).

Computerized tomography of the chest also demonstrates the variety of sizes and shapes of the thymus; if not appreciated, these may be mistaken for an abnormal mediastinal mass. In the axial projection the thymus usually appears bilobed, with the left lobe slightly higher and larger than the right lobe (Fig. 2–11). The normal thymus may also have a triangular configuration. Although the maximum thickness of either lobe prior to 20 years of age is stated to be 1.8 cm, this is subject to considerable variation in the infant. In the pediatric patient the density of the thymus is similar to that of the muscles of the chest wall. After puberty there is a gradual replacement of the thymus by fat, with resulting lowering of the attenuation coefficient (Fig. 2–12).

Although complete aeration occurs in the vigorous infant in the first few breaths of life, the premature or weak baby, or the infant who is born of an overly sedated mother, may show abnormal areas of pulmonary aeration (Fig. 2–13). In addition, specific forms of neonatal pulmonary disease have characteristic roentgenographic patterns. (Each of the pulmonary diseases in this age group will be discussed in detail in Chapter 3.)

By the end of infancy (the third year), the configurations of the chest, mediastinum, and heart are usually similar to those seen in the older child and adult (Fig. 2–14). Although conventionally it has been taught that during late infancy and childhood the thymus undergoes a normal involution process, direct coronal and sagittal measurements of the thymus utilizing magnetic resonance imaging have shown that the thymus probably does not change significantly in size from approximately 6 months to puberty.

SUGGESTED READINGS

Avery ME, Fletcher BD, and Williams R: Lung And Its Disorders In The Newborn Infant, 4th ed. Philadelphia, W.B. Saunders, 1981.

Baron RL et al.: Computed tomography of the normal thymus. Radiology, 142:121, 1982.

Chang LWN, Lee FA, and Gwinn JL: Normal lateral deviation of the trachea in infants and children. Am J Roentgenol, 109:247, 1970.

Cohen MD et al.: The diagnostic dilemma of the posterior mediastinal thymus: CT manifestations. Radiology, 146:691, 1983.

Davis ME, and Potter EL: Intrauterine respiration of the human fetus. JAMA, 131:1194, 1946.

Fawcett J, Lind J, and Wegelius C: The first breath. Acta Paediatr Scand (Suppl 123), 49:5, 1960.

Heiberg E et al.: Normal thymus: CT characteristics in subjects under 20. Am J Roentgenol, 138:491, 1982.

Karlberg P et al.: Respiratory studies in newborn infants. II. Pulmonary ventilation and mechanics of breathing in the first minutes of life, including the onset of respiration. Acta Paediatr Scand, 51:121, 1962.

Klaus M et al.: Lung volume in the newborn infant. Pediatrics, 30:111, 1962.

Kuhn JP, and Seidel FG: Magnetic resonance imaging of the thymus in infancy and childhood. Presented before the International Pediatric Radiology Society, June 1987.

Lee JKT, Sagel SS, and Stanley SS: Computed Body Tomography. Raven Press, New York, 1983.

Nadelhaft J, and Ellis K: Roentgen appearance of the lungs in 1000 apparently normal full-term newborn infants. Am J Roentgenol, 78:440, 1957.

Singleton EB: Respiratory distress syndrome. Prog Pediatr Radiol, 1:109, 1967.

Wilds PL: Observations of intrauterine fetal breathing movements. A review. Am J Obstet Gynecol, 131:315, 1978.

3 NONINFECTIOUS PRIMARY PULMONARY DISEASES IN THE NEWBORN AND YOUNG INFANT

TRANSIENT TACHYPNEA OF THE
  NEWBORN
RESPIRATORY DISTRESS
  SYNDROME
AIR BLOCK COMPLICATIONS
BRONCHOPULMONARY DYSPLASIA
CHRONIC PULMONARY
  INSUFFICIENCY OF THE
  PREMATURE INFANT

MECONIUM ASPIRATION
PERSISTENT FETAL CIRCULATION
PULMONARY HEMORRHAGE
ASPIRATION PNEUMONITIS
WILSON-MIKITY SYNDROME

Respiratory distress in the newborn may be secondary to central nervous system abnormalities, neuromuscular disorders, intestinal obstruction, ascites, congenital heart disease, or a pulmonary abnormality, either primary parenchymal disease or mechanical interference with pulmonary aeration. It is beyond the scope of this text to consider causes other than those directly related to pulmonary aeration. However, it should be recognized that a normal chest radiograph in an infant with respiratory distress should suggest that the cause is due to other abnormalities, as already mentioned, and is unrelated to lung disease.

TRANSIENT TACHYPNEA OF THE NEWBORN (WET LUNG SYNDROME)

Transient tachypnea of the newborn is a clinical description of a type of respiratory distress occurring most often in full-term infants who are usually normal at birth but who, during the first few hours of life, show a gradual onset of tachypnea frequently accompanied by retraction, grunting, and, occasionally, mild cyanosis. The respiratory rates usually range from 80 to 140/min, but become normal after 2 to 5 days. The clinical symptomatology may simulate that of hyaline membrane disease (HMD) but this is minimal, with no alteration of blood gases or pH values. In contradistinction to HMD there is a prompt response to oxygen therapy and a visible "pink" color.

Although the radiographic features are not diagnostic, they are consistent with the clinical phenomenon of transient respiratory distress. The overall appearance is suggestive of congestive heart failure: the heart is frequently slightly enlarged, the pulmonary vascular markings are more prominent than normal, and small pleural effusions are often present. Consequently, the diagnosis of congenital heart disease is often suspected, but no cardiovascular abnormalities may be found. Cardiac failure in the first week of life is usually a result of a hypoplastic left ventricle or severe coarctation with ventricular septal defect, patent ductus arteriosus, or both. These can be excluded by their distinctive clinical and echocardiographic features.

Several mechanisms have been postulated as the cause of transient tachypnea; the most widely accepted hypothesis is that there is a delay or interference in clearing of the fetal lung fluid. One function of the fetal lung, beginning at 25 to 28 weeks of intrauterine life, is the manufacture of fluid that passes up the tracheobronchial tree and becomes part of the amniotic fluid. If an excessive amount of fluid is formed, or if it is not removed during the compression of the thorax during birth, wet lung syndrome results. The prominent vascular markings are secondary to delayed absorption of fluid by lymphatic and capillary drainage, with resulting engorgement of the vascular tissues.

The newborn with respiratory distress, whose chest x-ray shows prominent linear vascular markings radiating from the hilar areas and whose heart is borderline or slightly enlarged, may have transient tachypnea rather than congenital heart disease. Normal blood gases and prompt improvement with oxygen therapy is presumptive evidence that transient tachypnea of the newborn is present, and follow-up radiographs in several days will show a decrease in heart size and in the prominence of the pulmonary vascular channels (Figs. 3–1 and 3–2). Some cases of transient tachypnea may demonstrate prominent Kerley's B lines, and radiographic differentiation from obstructive pulmonary venous return is difficult (Fig. 3–3).

RESPIRATORY DISTRESS SYNDROME

Through common usage, the terms "idiopathic respiratory distress syndrome of the newborn" and "hyaline membrane disease" have become synonomous. It is the most common serious pulmonary abnormality in the newborn. The infant with hyaline membrane disease is usually premature. Larger infants with hyaline membrane disease are commonly cesarean, with maternal diabetes frequently playing a predisposing role. Term infants rarely suffer from hyaline membrane disease.

Although disturbance in respiration is usually evident at birth, it may not be observed until the first few hours of life. Onset of symptoms after a 6- to 8-hour period of normal breathing is practically unknown in this condition. The onset is accompanied by a progressive increase in respiratory rate with retraction of the lower sternum during inspiration, accompanied by a fullness or increased convexity of the upper portion of the thorax. Cyanosis may become severe as the disease progresses. Since the first edition of this text there has been a remarkable decrease in the mortality of infants with hyaline membrane disease, largely due to assisted ventilation and oxygenation techniques that have been developed over the past 20 to 25 years. Unfortunately this has been accompanied by an increase in morbidity, especially air block complications, bronchopulmonary dysplasia, intracranial hemorrhage, and ischemic bowel disease.

Etiologic Considerations. Our purpose here is not to discuss the controversial aspects of the pathogenesis of hyaline membrane disease, but a brief description of fetal lung development is helpful in appreciating the pulmonary complications of prematurity (Table 3–1). The underlying abnormality is the immaturity of the lung and the inability of type II pneumocytes of the alveoli to synthesize and secrete surfactant in sufficient quantities to achieve alveolar elasticity and stability. Many other contributing factors have been incriminated, including aspiration, anoxia, hypovolemia, cardiac failure, hypotension, fibrinolytic enzyme defects, acidosis, hypoproteinemia, a deficient alveolar lining layer, oxygen toxicity, and neurohormonal deficits. A combination of prenatal anoxia and other unexplained events apparently results in pulmonary arteriolar constriction, which in turn leads to necrosis and fibrinous hyaline membranes of the bronchiolar and alveolar duct epithelium.

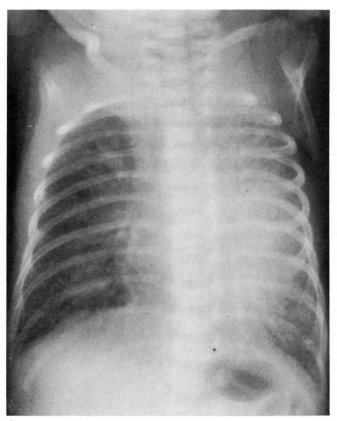

A

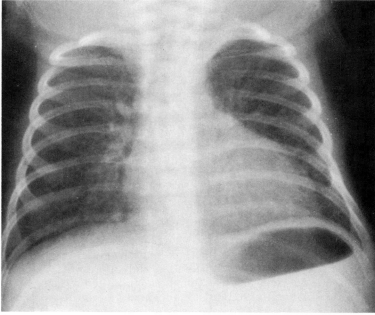

B

Figure 3–1. Transient tachypnea of the newborn. A, Chest radiograph made during the first day of life shows linear areas of density extending from the hilus into each lung, with associated cardiac enlargement. B, Repeat chest radiograph 1 week later shows no abnormality.

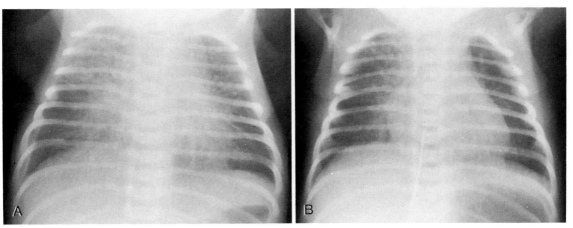

Figure 3–2. *Transient tachypnea of the newborn. A, The heart is enlarged, the pulmonary veins are dilated, and there is right pleural effusion. B, Repeat chest radiograph 3 days later shows regression of the vascular congestion, decrease in heart size, and resolution of the pleural effusion.*

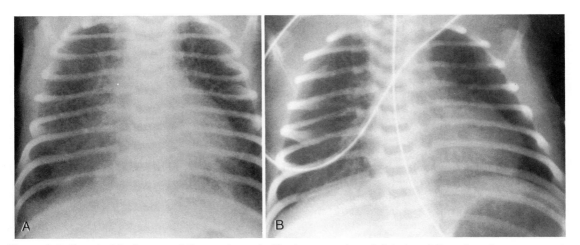

Figure 3–3. *Transient tachypnea of the newborn. A, The lungs are hyperinflated and there is pulmonary vascular congestion, with Kerley's B lines identified above each costophrenic sulcus. B, Repeat chest radiograph 1 day later shows a normal chest.*

Table 3–1. *Chronology of Fetal Lung Development*

Gestation Age (weeks)	Feature(s)
Less than 20	Closed air spaces; lack of alveoli; decreased capillary development in interstitium
25–28	Development of alveoli; proliferation of pulmonary capillary network; formation of lung fluid; development of surfactant
27–31	Increase in weight to 1–1.5 kg
34–36	Increase in weight to 2–2.5 kg

Radiographic Findings. There is a lack of complete agreement as to the specificity of the radiographic findings. By the time the infant has developed clinical evidence of respiratory distress, positive radiographic findings should be present. It is obvious that a normal chest roentgenogram in a newborn infant with respiratory distress after the first 5 to 6 hours of life excludes hyaline membrane disease and suggests abnormality of the central nervous system or of other extrathoracic systems.

Although there are exceptions, the usual roentgenographic findings consist of uniform reticulogranular densities distributed evenly throughout both lungs (Figs. 3–4 and 3–5). These minute areas of opacity represent atelectatic alveoli. Magnification techniques may be used to enhance the granular pattern, but these are usually impractical because of the critical condition of the infant and the hazard of moving the patient to the x-ray department. Some have had success with adaptations allowing magnification by the use of portable radiographic units. The heart is normal or slightly enlarged and bronchial air spaces (air bronchograms) are prominent, especially in the lower lobes. In the nonintubated infant the lungs do not appear overly inflated but, if aspiration of meconium or associated infectious pneumonitis is present, segmental areas of air trapping will be seen. Even though acidosis commonly leads to overinflation of the lungs in most young infants, this does not occur in the respiratory distress syndrome because of the loss of lung volume due to the alveolar atelectasis. Lateral projections made during inspiration show an increased convexity of the upper thorax with retraction of the lower sternum. Occasionally, a better view of the granular densities and the air bronchogram is obtained in this position than in the frontal view. The smaller the infant the more difficult it is to detect the granular opacities, but the air bronchogram is usually obvious (Fig. 3–6). As the disease progresses the reticulogranular pattern becomes more prominent and coalescence of many of the small atelectatic areas occurs, resulting in more opaque lung fields (Fig. 3–7). In mild uncomplicated cases gradual clearing of the lungs usually occurs and, at the end of a week, the roentgenographic appearance is normal (Fig. 3–8).

The radiographic findings have now been considerably altered in modern intensive care units, in which tracheal intubation and positive pressure ventilation are quickly employed at the first sign of respiratory distress. The lungs of these infants usually show hyperinflation and a low position of the diaphragm, and the granular appearance and peripheral air bronchograms may be more distinct. Residual pulmonary opacifications are frequent and often prolonged in infants requiring assisted ventilation.

It is important for radiologists and x-ray technologists to recognize the precarious condition of these infants. Unnecessary handling during the x-ray examination should be avoided. Portable roentgenographic examinations are recommended, and the infant should remain in the isolette or incubator during the x-ray exposure.

The severity of the radiographic findings is usually proportional to the severity of the clinical picture. Mild cases show poorly defined granular densities, and recovery is usually rapid. More severe forms show more characteristic roentgenographic features. The thymus of an infant with hyaline membrane disease is usually very small. This may be due to the infant's prematurity or to antenatal steroids, which may have been given to the mother in an effort to enhance lung maturation and surfactant production. However, regeneration of the thymus is a common finding in those infants who thrive after recovery (Fig. 3–9).

Preliminary studies are in progress in regard to the direct instillation of surfactant to the lungs. Results are not yet conclusive, but some alteration of radiographic manifestations may be anticipated.

The problem of a hemodynamically significant ductus arteriosus is suggested in the low-birth-weight infant who is recovering from hyaline membrane disease and develops apnea, increasing oxygen requirements, bounding pulses, and a

Text continued on page 37

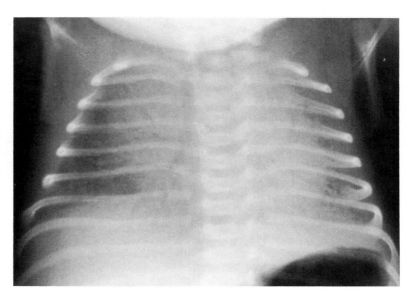

Figure 3–4. Hyaline membrane disease. Both lungs show diffuse granularity, with air bronchograms extending into the lung periphery. The diaphragm is at a relatively high level.

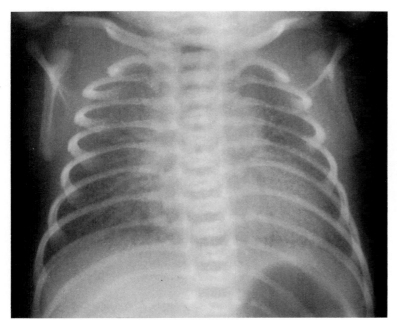

Figure 3–5. Respiratory distress syndrome. Chest radiographs show small punctate densities scattered throughout both lungs and slight cardiac enlargement. A faint air bronchogram is identified and seen to best advantage in the left lower lobe. The diaphragm is at a normal level.

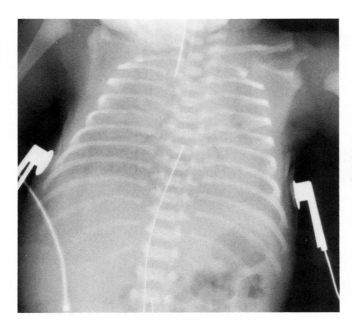

Figure 3–6. Hyaline membrane disease. The diffuse alveolar atelectasis is prominent, but the air bronchograms are clearly identified.

Figure 3–7. Hyaline membrane disease. More advanced alveolar atelectasis has resulted in nearly complete opacification of the lungs.

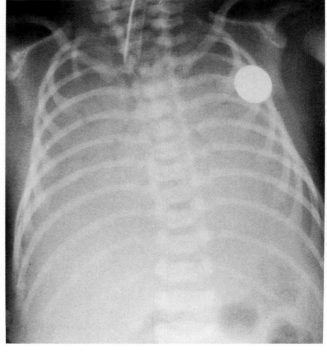

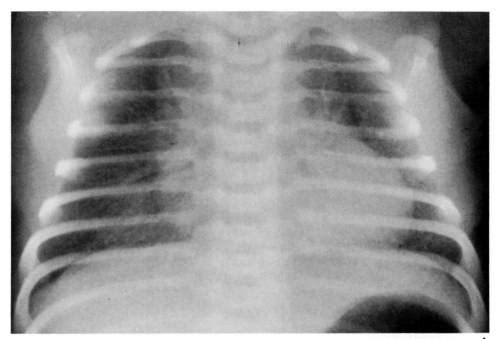

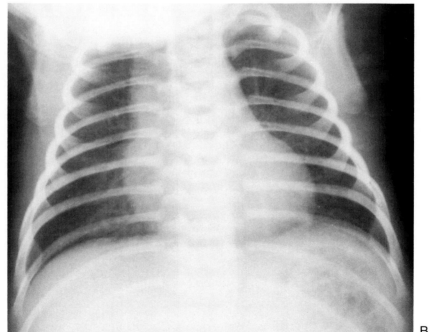

Figure 3–8. *Respiratory distress syndrome.* A, *Characteristic granular pattern of hyaline membrane disease.* B, *Repeat radiograph at the end of 1 week shows no abnormality.*

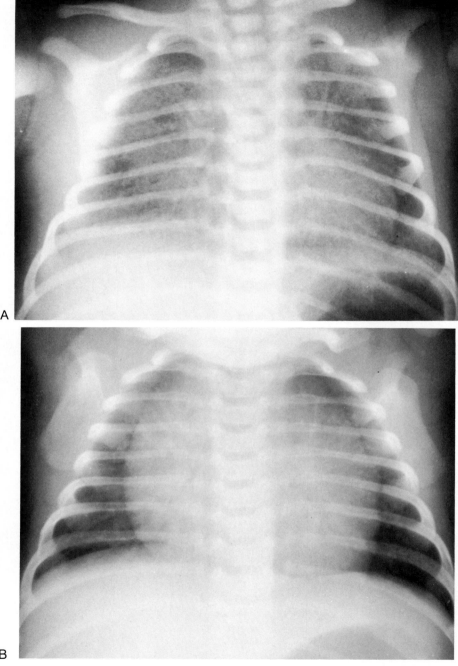

Figure 3–9. Respiratory distress syndrome with recovery and thymic regeneration. A, Characteristic radiographic changes of hyaline membrane disease at 1 day of age. B, Repeat chest radiograph 2 months later shows normal chest with large thymus.

characteristic murmur. The radiographic findings may be subtle, but often very suggestive, showing an increase in heart size and pulmonary edema not previously evident or otherwise explained (Fig. 3–10). Echocardiography is often diagnostic, showing left atrial and ventricular enlargement and direct visualization of an enlarged ductus by Doppler studies.

Variations in the roentgenographic appearance may occasionally be encountered, consisting of more unilateral distribution of the granular densities (Fig. 3–11). In such cases differentiating between hyaline membrane disease and pulmonary hemorrhage may be impossible. In cases in which the histologic appearance is that of hyaline membrane disease, but the radiographic appearance is not, one must not necessarily be critical of either method of diagnosis. The histologic examination of a small segment of lung taken at autopsy does not necessarily reflect the overall pathologic picture.

AIR BLOCK COMPLICATIONS

Air block complications secondary to positive pressure ventilators and oxygen therapy may occur in any of the newborn lung diseases but are more frequently

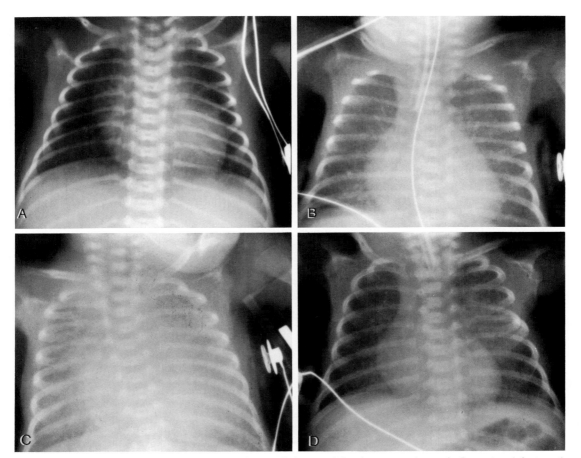

Figure 3–10. Left ventricular failure secondary to failure of closure of the ductus arteriosus. A, Premature infant on the first day of life shows a normal chest. B, At 5 days of age there are changes of hyaline membrane disease, in addition to slight increase in heart size and in the prominence of the pulmonary vascular markings. C, At 13 days of age there is increase in heart size with evidence of bilateral pulmonary edema. D, Postoperative regression of heart size and clearing of the lungs following closure of the ductus arteriosus.

seen in infants with hyaline membrane disease and bronchopulmonary dysplasia, and consequently will be considered in this chapter.

The most common initial complication is interstitial pulmonary emphysema. In this condition, air apparently escapes from the alveoli into the surrounding interstitial tissues. The change may initially produce a radiograph that enhances the granular densities of hyaline membrane disease. Progression usually occurs to a radiolucent reticular pattern, readily identified as air in the interstitial structures of the lung (Figs. 3–12 and 3–13). Invariably the lungs are hyperinflated, and one lung may be more affected than the other (Fig. 3–14). Severe localized pulmonary interstitial emphysema with mediastinal displacement may be treated with selective bronchial intubation and obstruction of the air-trapped segment.

Dissection along the perivascular sheaths results in pneumomediastinum. In its mildest form, this is identified as air beneath the thymus and surrounding the pericardium (Fig. 3–15). Progression of the dissection may occur upward into the neck or downward, separating the muscular portion of the diaphragm from the visceral pleura (Fig. 3–16). This complication may easily be confused with pneumoperitoneum, but decubitus or other radiographs using different positions do not show the air to move as it would in the peritoneal cavity.

Dissection of air into the inferior pulmonary ligament, either unilaterally or bilaterally, is another form of pneumomediastinum (Fig. 3–17). These collections of air are located in a parasagittal position above the diaphragm and posterior to the heart. Midline collection of air in approximately the same location is in the infra-azygous compartment of the mediastinum. The midline radiolucency between the air in the inferior pulmonary ligaments seen in Figure 3–17C is probably in this compartment.

Dissection of air into the pleural space results in pneumothorax, which is usually an emergency situation requiring the insertion of a chest tube. Pneumothorax will frequently develop on one side, only to be followed by a bilateral pneumothorax (Figs. 3–18 and 3–19). Pneumothorax may simulate pneumomediastinum (medial pneumothorax) because of the location of the air beneath the anterior chest wall (Fig. 3–20). Cystic pulmonary emphysema may develop (Fig. 3–21) and perforate into the pleural space, with resulting pneumothorax (Fig. 3–22).

Dissection of air into the pericardial sac is a less frequent complication, but can occur and produce cardiac tamponade that requires aspiration of the air or insertion of a tube into the pericadial sac (Fig. 3–23). Pneumoperitoneum may result from air in the pleural space extending through the pleuroperitoneal foramina into the peritoneum, or through the inferior pulmonary ligaments or infra-azygous region into the peritoneal space (Fig. 3–24). Differentiation between pneumoperitoneum as a complication of pulmonary air block and pneumoperitoneum secondary to perforated bowel may be difficult, but usually in the latter situation air and fluid levels will be present in the peritoneal space. Air within the heart and thoracic vessels is usually a fatal complication (Figs. 3–25 and 3–26). Presumably in such cases there is rupture of air from the alveoli into the pulmonary capillary bed.

BRONCHOPULMONARY DYSPLASIA

Bronchopulmonary dysplasia (BPD), first described in 1967 by Northway, is a common complication of treatment of infants with hyaline membrane disease. The etiology is apparently secondary to the necessary oxygen administered to these patients, and the mechanical factor of positive pressure ventilation may play a secondary role. During the past 10 years there has been an alteration in the radiographic pattern of BPD. Originally, one expected to see stages (as described by Northway) of hyaline membrane disease, progressing from an acute state to a

Text continued on page 47

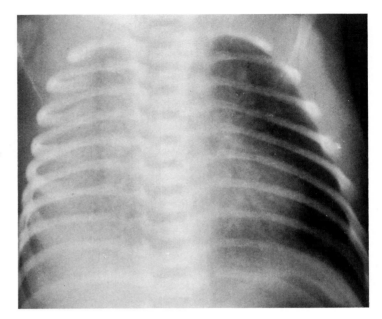

Figure 3–11. Respiratory distress syndrome. Abnormality of the right lung has radiographic features very suggestive of hyaline membrane disease, whereas the left lung shows only minimal changes (confirmed at autopsy).

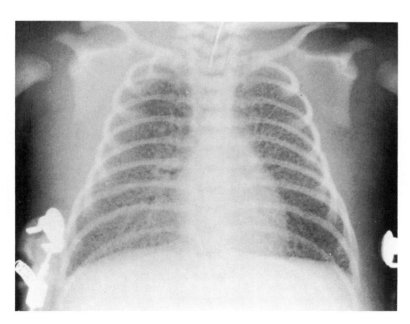

Figure 3–12. Hyaline membrane disease with pulmonary interstitial air. Multiple minute linear and round areas of radiolucency are identified within the lung parenchyma.

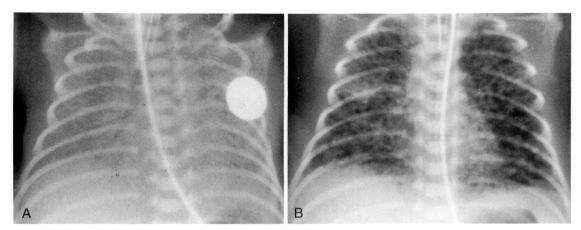

Figure 3–13. *Hyaline membrane disease with development of bilateral interstitial emphysema. A, Characteristic findings of hyaline membrane disease are present. B, Interstitial air is identified as linear and round areas of radiolucency within the hyperinflated lungs.*

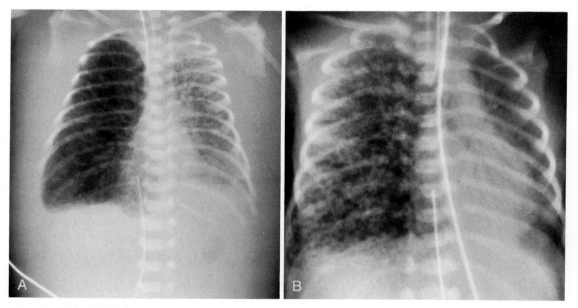

Figure 3–14. *A, Air block with pulmonary interstitial air involving predominantly the right lung. Increase in soft tissues of the chest wall and abdomen is secondary to Pavulon therapy. B, Unilateral pulmonary interstitial air block with resulting pulmonary emphysema. The left lung is essentially clear, except for air bronchogram associated with the patient's hyaline membrane disease.*

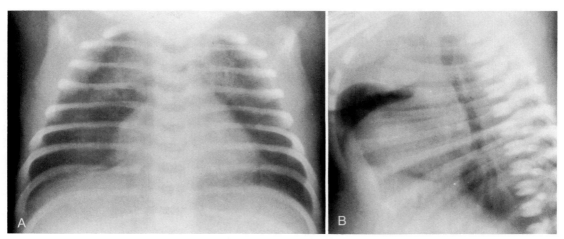

Figure 3–15. *Pneumomediastinum.* A, *Chest radiograph shows air elevating the thymus and adjacent to the pericardium.* B, *Lateral view shows air beneath the thymus to better advantage.*

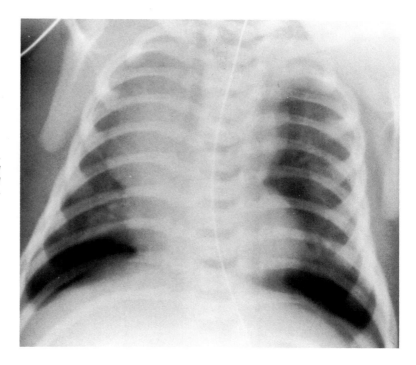

Figure 3–16. *Dissection of air. Supine chest view shows subpleural air between the parietal pleural and muscular portions of the diaphragm, bilaterally.*

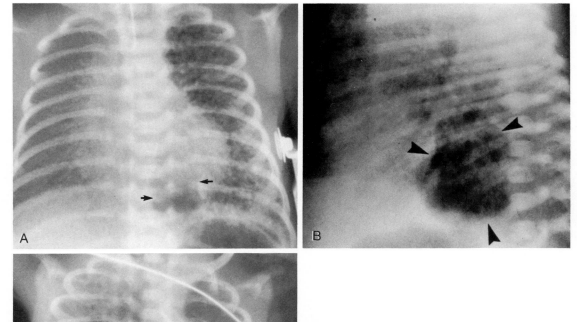

Figure 3–17. Pneumomediastinum with air in the inferior pulmonary ligament. A, There is interstitial emphysema of the left lung as well as collection of air within the inferior pulmonary ligament on the left (arrows). B, Lateral view shows air in the inferior pulmonary ligament in the retrocardiac area (arrowheads). C, Air is present within both right and left inferior pulmonary ligaments. Chest tubes were inserted because of complicating pneumothorax.

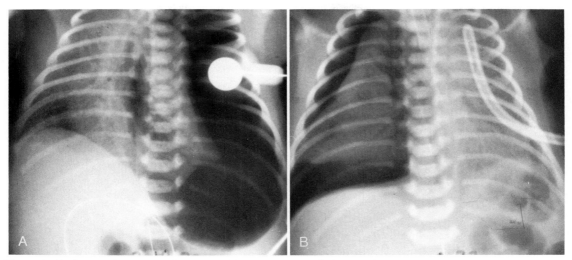

Figure 3–18. Pneumothorax complicating positive pressure ventilation in infant with hyaline membrane disease. A, Tension pneumothorax has developed on the left, with resulting shift of mediastinal structures to the right. B, Pneumothorax on the left has been successfully corrected by insertion of a thoracic tube. Several hours later tension pneumothorax developed on the right.

Figure 3–19. Bilateral pneumothoraces in infant with severe pulmonary interstitial emphysema, which has prevented complete collapse.

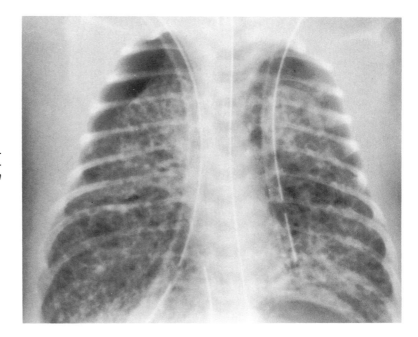

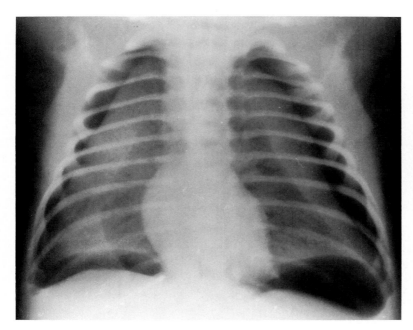

Figure 3–20. Medial pneumothorax. Although bilateral pneumothoraces are present, the radiolucency surrounding the mediastinum is air beneath the anterior chest wall rather than air within the mediastinum.

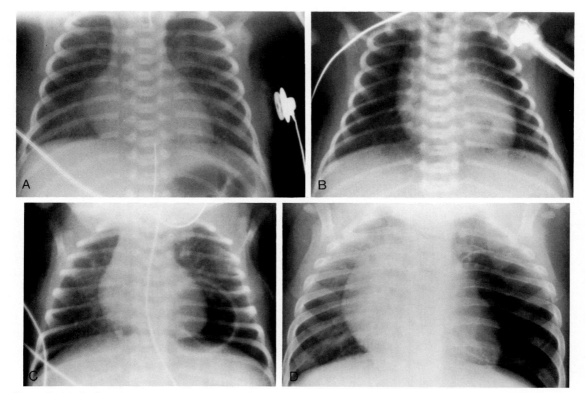

Figure 3–21. A, Cystic pulmonary emphysema. Premature infant with an essentially normal chest on the first day of life. B, At 2 days of age there is a local cystic collection of air in the left lower lobe. C, At 2 weeks of age the cyst has increased in size. D, Further increase in the cyst is present at 6 months of age. The infant was asymptomatic.

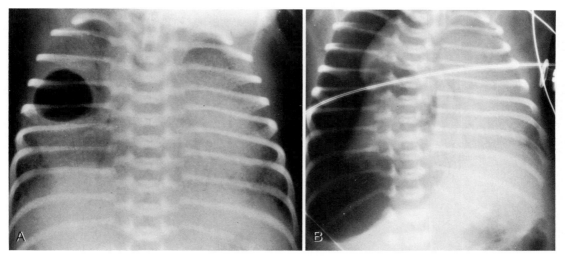

Figure 3–22. A, *Localized subpleural interstitial emphysema in a patient with hyaline membrane disease on positive pressure ventilation. B, Repeat radiograph made the same day shows rupture of the cystic pulmonary emphysema into the pleural space, with resulting tension pneumothorax.*

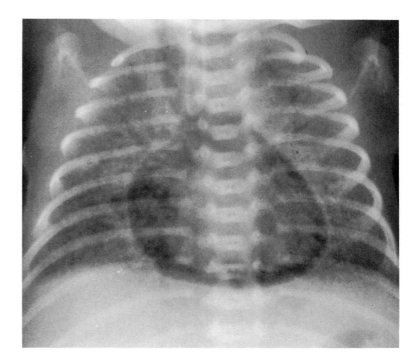

Figure 3–23. *Pneumopericardium.*

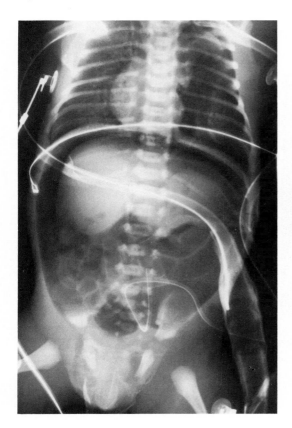

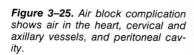

Figure 3–24. *Pneumoperitoneum secondary to air block. A small pneumothorax is seen on the left, and extensive pneumoperitoneum is present with extension of air into the tunica vaginalis bilaterally. Note the absence of air-fluid levels in the peritoneal cavity.*

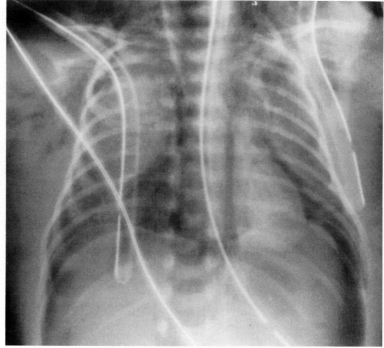

Figure 3–25. *Air block complication shows air in the heart, cervical and axillary vessels, and peritoneal cavity.*

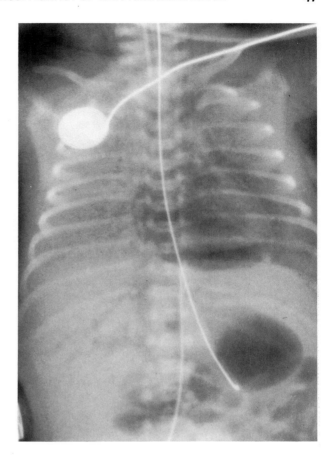

Figure 3–26. *Air block complication showing air within the mediastinum, pericardial sac, heart, and vessels within the neck axillae and portal circulation.*

regenerative stage, and then on to a transitional and chronic stage with marked alteration of lung architecture. This alteration consisted of multiple vacuoles of variable sizes, hyperinflation of the lungs, and a spectrum of linear densities interspersed throughout the vacuoles (Fig. 3–27). For those infants who are oxygen- and respirator-dependent, there is progression of the disease with extensive alteration of lung architecture (Fig. 3–28). Large solitary blebs or bullae may also develop (Fig. 3–29). Pneumothorax may be a complication at any time. During more recent years, presumably because of a decrease in the amount of oxygen administered to patients and possibly also because of a decrease in ventilatory pressure, the radiographic findings are frequently less severe (Fig. 3–30). Consequently, although vacuoles may develop occasionally, the major radiographic alteration is that of bilateral pulmonary hyperinflation (Fig. 3–31). Infants who survive BPD will show gradual improvement in the appearance of the lungs, often with restoration of normal roentgenographic appearance after 2 to 3 years. However, recurrent infection during this period is common.

CHRONIC PULMONARY INSUFFICIENCY OF THE PREMATURE INFANT

Chronic pulmonary insufficiency of prematurity (CPIP; immature lung syndrome) is clinically and radiographically different from hyaline membrane disease. Although both conditions occur in the premature infant, CPIP is usually found in

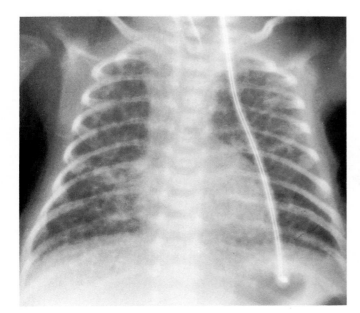

Figure 3–27. Bronchopulmonary dysplasia. Multiple vacuoles within a spectrum of linear densities and associated hyperinflation of the lungs are seen.

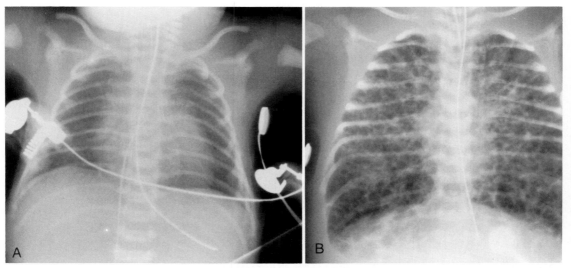

Figure 3–28. Advanced bronchopulmonary dysplasia. A, Extensive vacuolation and hyperaeration of both lungs is present. B, Five weeks later there has been progressive air trapping, with herniation of a segment of the lung beyond the confines of the rib cage on the left.

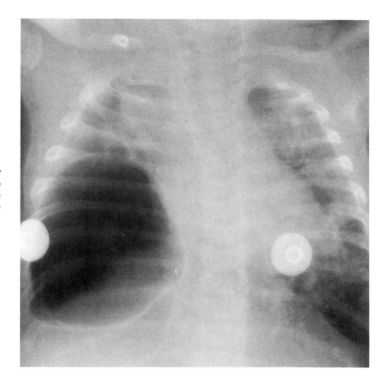

Figure 3–29. Residual bronchopulmonary dysplasia in a 6-month-old. The large bleb occupies the right lower lobe and chronic interstitial lung disease is present in the left lung and right upper lobe.

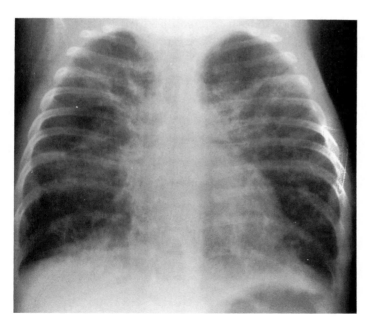

Figure 3–30. Bronchopulmonary dysplasia in a 3-month-old. There is bilateral air trapping with interstitial lung disease, but absence of severe honeycombing.

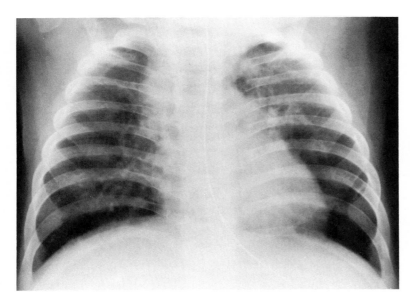

Figure 3–31. *Bronchopulmonary dysplasia in a 6-month-old, showing bilateral hyperinflation.*

lower birth weight prematures (under 1500 g), and the respiratory distress does not begin until 4 to 7 days of life. The reason for the clinical and radiographic differences has not been satisfactorily explained. The absence of surfactant in infants with hyaline membrane disease has been clearly established. However, analysis of tracheal or gastric aspirates in the more premature infant with CPIP demonstrates surfactant, possibly because of intrauterine stress that results in accelerated and premature manufacture of surfactant.

The radiographic findings consist of ill-defined densities having a "smudged" appearance, located primarily in the perihilar areas (Fig. 3–32). Air bronchograms are usually absent or are much less prominent than in hyaline membrane disease. These findings usually remain unchanged for 1 to 2 months, with gradual recovery. Although the complication of intracranial hemorrhage may develop, in our experience the development of air trapping complications and bronchopulmonary

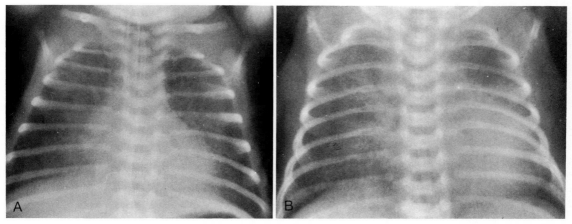

Figure 3–32. *Chronic pulmonary insufficiency of the premature (immature lung syndrome). A, One-week-old infant showing ill-defined, homogeneous density in the medial portions of each lung. B, Another infant, 2 weeks of age, showing similar radiographic changes.*

dysplasia, which are so common in hyaline membrane disease, occur infrequently in CPIP. In fact, the major clinical findings are those related to apnea of prematurity.

MECONIUM ASPIRATION

There is general agreement that fetal respiratory movements normally occur in utero because a certain amount of amniotic fluid extends into the respiratory pathways. The exact amount of aspirated fluid that the newborn infant can tolerate without significantly interfering with inflation of the lungs is unknown. It is reasonable to assume that a certain amount of particulate matter in the form of squamous cells and lanugo hairs may also be aspirated and may not cause respiratory distress. Particulate material of this type has been found in the respiratory tract at autopsy of infants whose deaths were not pulmonary in origin. However, the aspiration of amniotic fluid in which there is meconium is associated with a severe form of fetal distress. These infants are usually postmature, and a history of meconium in the amniotic fluid at birth is of value in the diagnosis. In most cases, fetal hypoxia or anoxia is probably responsible for vagal stimulation, which in turn leads both to intrauterine respirations and intestinal peristalsis. Meconium is expelled into the amniotic fluid, in which it becomes dispersed and aspirated during intrauterine respiratory efforts.

Clinical examination of these infants frequently shows them to be meconium-stained, and to have labored respiration. Inspiratory retractions may be present, but are usually not as obvious as those in the infant with hyaline membrane disease. Tachypnea is common, and rales may or may not be present. The radiographic findings are similar to those seen in older infants with severe bronchopneumonia. Coarse linear peribronchial infiltrations are present, extending to both lungs from the hilar areas. Segmental or larger areas of atelectasis are commonly present, as are areas of obstructive emphysema (Fig. 3–33). The diaphragm is at a low level and frequently shows reverse curvature because of the air trapping. The anteroposterior diameter of the chest is increased, with increased convexity of the anterior chest wall similar to that seen in infants with other forms of severe obstructive emphysema (Fig. 3–34). Milder forms of meconium aspiration may show only hyperinflation of the lungs, presumably caused by air block limited to the trachea. Pulmonary interstitial air, pneumomediastinum, pneumothorax, and other forms of air block may be complications of the aspiration syndrome (Fig. 3–35). Lateral supine films of the chest are frequently helpful in demonstrating small amounts of mediastinal air. As in other neonatal pulmonary diseases, careful follow-up radiographic studies are important. Identical radiographic findings may accompany infectious pneumonitis of the newborn.

Treatment is mainly supportive and consists of oxygen therapy in whatever concentration is necessary, with an appropriate humidity and temperature environment. Mechanical ventilation is often necessary, with a resultant increase in the complications of air leak. A decrease in the severity of the meconium aspiration can be accomplished by meticulous suctioning of the trachea prior to the first inspiratory efforts. Every infant who is meconium-stained and who has a disturbance of respiration should have gastric aspiration to remove swallowed meconium and prevent further aspiration.

Postmortem studies frequently show the presence of associated hyaline membranes, but the more gross changes of aspiration dominate the roentgenographic picture. Clinical improvement precedes radiographic clearing and, in those infants who recover, gradual regression of atelectasis and infiltration, as well as disappearance of the areas of air trapping, occur over a period of several days to several weeks.

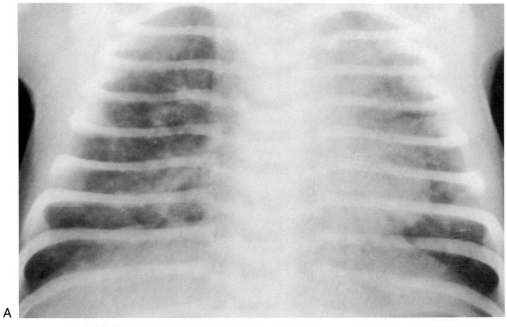

A

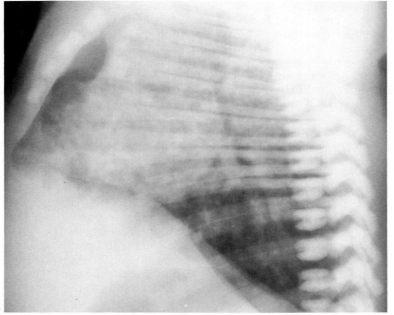

B

Figure 3–33. *Meconium aspiration. A, Frontal projection shows hyperaeration of the lungs, with cɔarse linear peribronchial infiltrations radiating from the hilar areas into the lungs. B, Lateral view shows increased anteroposterior diameter of the chest, and emphasizes the air trapping associated with this condition.*

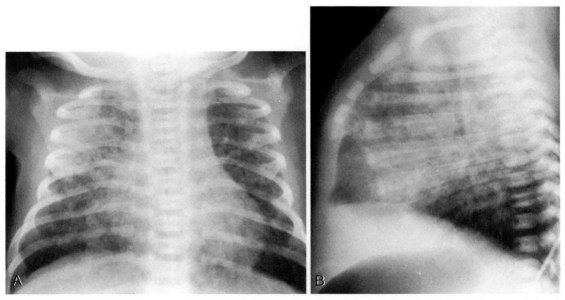

Figure 3–34. *Meconium aspiration in the newborn infant. A, The lungs are hyperinflated and there is increased density throughout both lung fields. B, Lateral radiograph shows increase in anteroposterior dimension of the chest and flattening of the diaphragm.*

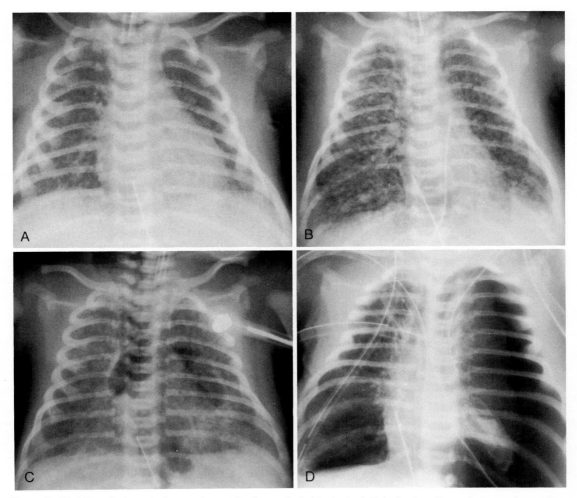

Figure 3–35. *Meconium aspiration and complications of air block. A, Initial chest radiograph in newborn shows hyperinflation of the lungs, with pulmonary changes consistent with meconium aspiration. B, Repeat radiograph 2 days later shows pulmonary interstitial air within the meconium aspiration pneumonitis. C, Pneumomediastinum has developed 2 days later. Note the air within the soft tissues of the neck and also within the inferior pulmonary ligament on the left. D, One week later bilateral pneumothoraces have developed. The right lung has expanded following insertion of chest tubes and the left lung has collapsed.*

PERSISTENT FETAL CIRCULATION

In some infants the pulmonary vascular resistance is unusually high, for unknown reasons. This results in pulmonary hypertension with right-to-left shunting across the ductus arteriosus and persistent fetal circulation (PFC) at birth. These infants have primary pulmonary hypertension of unknown cause. PFC may also be secondary to obvious anoxic conditions such as hyaline membrane disease, meconium aspiration, diaphragmatic hernia, or other ischemic conditions. Both primary and secondary pulmonary hypertension result in respiratory distress and cyanosis.

The radiographic changes are not specific in the idiopathic primary variety. Pulmonary vascular markings are diminished, and mild cardiomegaly is frequently present (Fig. 3–36). If there is left ventricular overload with resulting left ventricular decompensation, changes of congestive heart failure can be identified, but evaluation of blood gases and clinical and electrocardiographic findings are more specific. Treatment includes appropriate oxygen therapy with positive pressure ventilation, pulmonary arterial vasodilators, and pulmonary hyperventilation. Prompt response to treatment may occur in 24 to 48 hours. However, the mortality is high in those infants requiring prolonged ventilation.

PULMONARY HEMORRHAGE

Pulmonary hemorrhage in the newborn is another neonatal respiratory problem that is secondary to anoxia or stress. Theoretically, in this situation, the capillary permeability may be so affected that there is gross hemorrhage into the alveolar bed. The clinical picture of respiratory distress associated with gross blood being suctioned from the trachea or endotracheal tube suggests this complication. Differentiation between fetal blood and swallowed maternal blood may be determined by appropriate laboratory tests (e.g., Apt test). The radiographic diagnosis is generally determined by excluding other more typical pictures of pulmonary respiratory distress. The chest radiographs of an infant with pulmonary hemorrhage usually show ill-defined areas of density in one or more pulmonary segments (Fig. 3–37), or even diffuse bilateral "white out" of the lungs (Fig. 3–38). These findings and the absence of other more typical radiographic evidence, characteristic of hyaline membrane disease or of the aspiration syn-

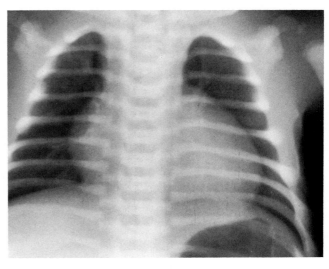

Figure 3–36. Persistent fetal circulation. The pulmonary vascular markings are diminished and the heart is enlarged.

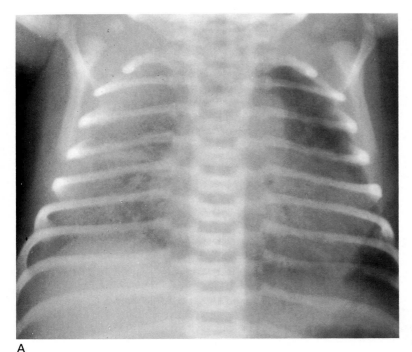

A

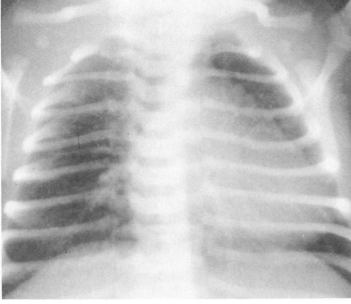

B

Figure 3–37. Pulmonary hemorrhage. A, Abnormal density occupies most of the right lung. Clinically the infant was thought to have pulmonary hemorrhage. B, Repeat radiograph 3 days later shows complete resolution of the hemorrhage.

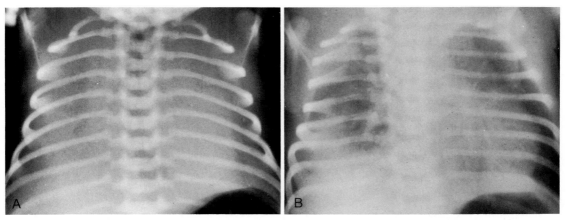

Figure 3–38. *Pulmonary hemorrhage in two premature infants. Radiographic findings mimic those of severe hyaline membrane disease.*

drome, should alert the radiologist or pediatrician to the possibility of pulmonary hemorrhage. It should be recognized, though, that bilateral lung opacification of severe hyaline membrane disease may be identical to that of pulmonary hemorrhage and, in each situation, careful correlation of the radiographic findings with the clinical impression is, of course, important. After 2 or 3 days resolution occurs in those infants who survive, and the chest has a normal appearance. Frequently, however, any underlying cerebral anoxic or stress phenomenon that is severe enough to produce pulmonary hemorrhage is fatal to the infant.

ASPIRATION PNEUMONITIS

Aspiration pneumonitis in the neonate may be secondary to a number of conditions, including esophageal atresia, tracheoesophageal fistula, pharyngeal incoordination, gastroesophageal reflux, congenital intestinal obstruction, and intracranial abnormality. Any situation resulting in vomiting or in the inability of the infant to swallow properly may result in aspiration pneumonia. Although infants with this type of aspiration have respiratory distress, the severity of the symptoms is usually less than that seen in hyaline membrane disease and in the meconium aspiration syndrome.

The pulmonary abnormality in infants with aspiration pneumonitis is usually located in the right upper lobe and in the perihilar areas; these are the most dependent areas of the lungs (Fig. 3–39). A combination of atelectasis and pneumonia in the right upper lobe of a young infant strongly suggests aspiration due to esophageal atresia, tracheoesophageal fistula, or gastroesophageal reflux (Fig. 3–40). If the aspiration is secondary to intestinal obstruction the obstruction is usually high, and abdominal scout films will show distention of the stomach and small bowel proximal to the obstruction. Esophageal atresia is readily diagnosed by passing a catheter under fluoroscopic control until the obstruction is met. A minute amount of contrast medium may then be introduced to outline the upper esophageal pouch and to determine if there is fistulous communication between the upper pouch and the tracheobronchial tree. Careful fluoroscopic examinations, including videotape recordings of deglutition, are extremely helpful in the evaluation of pharyngeal incoordination. This physiologic abnormality, in which swallowed material is aspirated into the trachea, is particularly common in weak premature infants, in brain-damaged babies, and in infants suffering from generalized muscular deficiencies, cerebral palsy, or congenital dysautonomia.

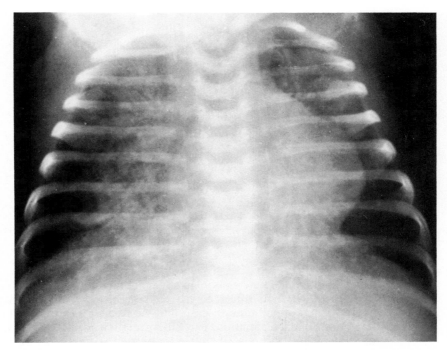

Figure 3–39. Aspiration pneumonitis. Chest radiograph made after episode of vomiting and strangling shows parenchymal abnormality involving the right upper and lower lobes.

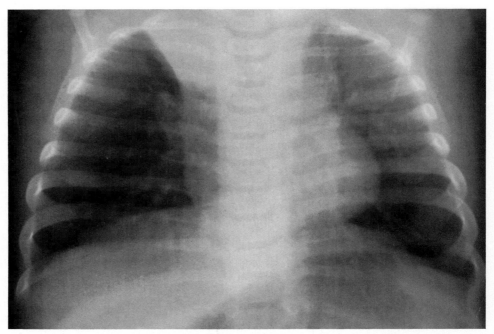

Figure 3–40. Aspiration pneumonitis. Chest radiograph shows atelectasis of the right upper lobe secondary to aspiration following vomiting in an infant with duodenal obstruction. Pneumonia or atelectasis in this area is characteristic of aspiration pneumonia.

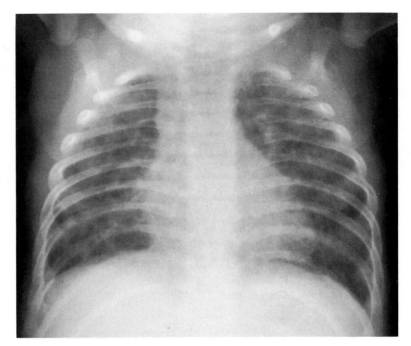

Figure 3–41. Wilson-Mikity syndrome. Reticular densities are scattered throughout both lungs and contain multiple focal radiolucent areas of hyperaeration characteristic of this condition.

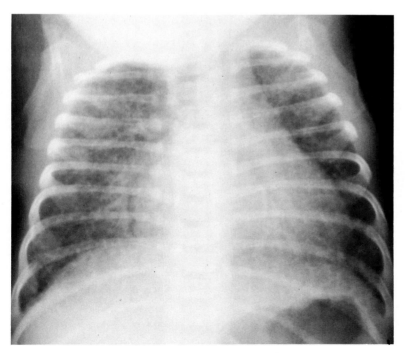

Figure 3–42. Another infant with Wilson-Mikity syndrome showing focal areas of hyperaeration and reticular parenchymal densities.

WILSON-MIKITY SYNDROME

This rare condition was first reported by Wilson and Mikity and later described as pulmonary dysmaturity. Although the clinicial manifestations may not become evident until several weeks after birth, the infant is more commonly premature and shows evidence of respiratory disturbance after the first few days of life. The respiratory distress is initially not as severe as that seen in hyaline membrane disease but eventually becomes very severe, with a high mortality rate. This diagnosis seems to be made less frequently now, probably because of the frequency of ventilator and oxygen use early in the course of the condition. In those infants who survive there is gradual improvement in the chest roentgenograms and in the clinical appearance over a period of 6 to 12 months.

The radiographic features consist of diffuse linear and reticular areas of density, within which are multiple small cystlike areas of hyperaeration (Figs. 3–41 and 3–42). Both lungs are usually symmetrically involved. Although the course is unknown, the radiographic features frequently resemble those seen in bronchopulmonary dysplasia. The histologic features are considered diagnostic, and, consequently, reports of this condition in biopsy or postmortem specimens suggest that the radiographic features may not always be typical.

SUGGESTED READINGS

TRANSIENT TACHYPNEA OF THE NEWBORN

Avery ME: The Lungs And Its Disorders In The Newborn Infant, 4th ed. Philadelphia, WB Saunders, 1981.

Avery ME, Gatewood OD, and Brumley G: Transient tachypnea of the newborn: Possible delayed resorption of fluid at birth. Am J Dis Child, 111:380, 1966.

Kuhn JP, Fletcher BD, and DeLomos RA: Roentgen findings in transient tachypnea of the newborn. Radiology, 92:751, 1969.

Steele RW, and Copeland GA: Delayed resorption of pulmonary alveolar fluid in the neonate. Radiology, 103:637, 1972.

Swischuk LE: Transient respiratory distress of the newborn (TRDN): A temporary disturbance of a normal phenomenon. Am J Roentgenol, 108:557, 1970.

Wesenberg RL, Graven SN, and McCabe EB: Radiological findings in wet-lung disease. Radiology, 98:69, 1971.

RESPIRATORY DISTRESS SYNDROME

Ablow RC: Respiratory distress syndrome (hyaline membrane disease). CRC Crit Rev Diagn Imag, 14:321, 1981.

Avery ME: The Lung and Its Disorders In the Newborn Infant, 4th ed. Philadelphia, WB Saunders, 1981.

Burney B et al.: Chest film diagnosis of patent ductus arteriosus in infants with hyaline membrane disease. Am J Roentgenol, 130:1149, 1978.

Capitanio MA, and Kirkpatrick J: Roentgen examination in the evaluation of the newborn infant with respiratory distress. J Pediatr, 75:896, 1969.

Felman AH: The Pediatric Chest—Radiological, Clinical and Pathological and Observations, pp 92–101. Springfield, IL, Charles C Thomas, 1983.

Fujiwara T et al.: Artificial surfactant therapy in hyaline membrane disease. Lancet, 1:55, 1980.

Gewolh IH, Lebowitz RL, and Taeusch HW Jr.: Thymus size and its relationship to respiratory distress syndrome. J Pediatr 95:108, 1979.

Higgins MA et al.: Patent ductus arteriosus in preterm infant with idiopathic respiratory distress syndrome. Radiographic and echocardiographic evolution. Radiology, 124:189, 1977.

Madansky DL et al.: Pneumothorax and other forms of pulmonary air leak in newborns. Am Rev Respir Dis, 120:729, October 1979.

Papagerogiou AN et al.: The antenatal use of betamethasone in the prevention of respiratory distress syndrome: A controlled double-blind study. Pediatrics, 63:73, 1979.

Reilly BJ: Regional distribution of atelectasis and fluid in the neonate with respiratory distress. Radiol Clin North Am, 13:225, 1975.

Rudhe U, Margolin FR, and Robertson B: Atypical roentgen appearance of the lung and hyaline membrane disease of the newborn. Acta Radiol, 10:57, 1970.

Singleton EB: Special treatment article. Progr Pediatr Radiol, 1:109, 1967.

Tchou CS et al.: Asymmetric distribution of roentgen pattern in hyaline membrane disease. J Can Assoc Radiol, 23:85, 1972.

Usher R, McLean F, and Maughan GB: Respiratory distress syndrome in infants delivered by cesarean section. Am J Obstet Gynecol, 88:806, 1964.

Wesenberg RL, Wax RE, and Zachman RD: Varying roentgenographic patterns of patent ductus arteriosus in the newborn. Am J Roentgenol, 114:340, 1972.

AIR BLOCK COMPLICATIONS

Aranda JV, Stern V, and Dunbar JS: Pneumothorax with pneumoperitoneum in a newborn infant. Am J Dis Child, 123:163, 1972.

Bowen A, and Quattromani FL: Infra-azygous pneumomediastinum in the newborn. Am J Roentgenol, 135:1017, 1980.

Chopra DR et al.: Arteriovenous air embolism: A complication of mechanical ventilation in respiratory distress syndrome. Clin Pediatr, 15:178, 1976.

Clark TA, and Edwards DK: Pulmonary pseudocysts in newborn infants with respiratory distress syndrome. Am J Roentgenol, 133:417, 1979.

Donahoe PK et al.: Pneumoperitoneum secondary to pulmonary air leak. J Pediatr, 81:797, 1972.

Grossfield JL, Boger D, and Clatworthy HW: Hemodynamic and manometric observations in experimental air block syndrome. J Pediatr Surg, 6:339, 1971.

Heitzman ER: The Mediastinum: Radiologic Correlation with Anatomy and Pathology, p 237. St Louis, C.V. Mosby, 1977.

Kirkpatrick BV, Felman AH, and Eitzman DV: Complications of ventilator therapy in respiratory distress syndrome. Am J Dis Child, 128:496, 1974.

Kogutt MS: Systemic air embolism secondary to respiratory therapy in the neonate: Six cases including one survivor. Am J Roentgenol, 131:425, 1978.

Leonidas JC, Hall RT, and Rhodes PG: Conservative management of unilateral pulmonary interstitial emphysema under tension. J Pediatr, 87:776, 1975.

Macklin MT, and Macklin CC: Malignant interstitial emphysema of the lungs and mediastinum as an important occult complication in many respiratory diseases and other conditions: An interpretation of the clinical literature in the light of laboratory experiments. Medicine, 23:281, 1944.

Magilner AD et al.: Persistent localized intrapulmonary interstitial emphysema: An observation in three infants. Radiology, 111:379, 1974.

Moskowitz PS, and Griscom NT: The medial pneumothorax. Radiology, 120:143, 1976.

Sagel SS, Wimbush P, and Goldenberg DB: Tension pneumopericardium following assisted ventilation in hyaline membrane disease. Radiology, 106:175, 1973.

Siegle RL et al.: Air embolus following pulmonary interstitial emphysema in hyaline membrane disease. Clin Radiol, 27:77, 1976.

Steele RW et al.: Pneumothorax and pneumomediastinum in the newborn. Radiology, 98:629, 1971.

Stocker JT, and Madewell JE: Persistent interstitial pulmonary emphysema: Another complication of respiratory distress syndrome. Pediatrics, 59:847, 1977.

Thibeault DW et al.: Pulmonary interstitial emphysema, pneumomediastinum and pneumothorax. Am J Dis Child, 126:611, 1973.

Vahey TN, Pratt GB, and Baum RS: Treatment of localized pulmonary interstitial emphysema with selective bronchial intubation. Am J Roentgenol, 140:1107, 1983.

Vinstein AL et al.: Pulmonary venous air embolism in hyaline membrane disease. Radiology, 105:627, 1972.

Volberg, FN, Everett CJ, and Brill PW: Radiological features of inferior pulomary ligament air collections in neonates with respiratory distress. Radiology, 130:357, 1979.

Wescott JL, and Cole SR: Interstitial pulmonary emphysema in children and adults: Roentgenographic features. Radiology, 111:367, 1974.

Wood BP, Anderson VM, Mauk JE and Merritt TA: Pulmonary lymphatic air: Locating "Pulmonary Interstitial Emphysema" of premature infant. Am J Roent; 138:809–814, May 1982.

BRONCHOPULMONARY DYSPLASIA

Edwards DK: Radiographic aspects of bronchopulmonary dysplasia. J Pediatr, 95:823, 1979.

Edwards DK, Colby TV, and Northway WH Jr: Radiographic pathologic correlation in bronchopulmonary dysplasia. J Pediatr, 95:834, 1979.

Northway WH Jr, Rosen RC, and Porter DY: Pulmonary disease following respirator therapy of hyaline membrane disease: Bronchopulmonary dysplasia. N Engl J Med, 276:357, 1967.

Siassi B et al.: Patent ductus arteriosus complicating prolonged assisted ventilation in respiratory distress syndrome. J Pediatr, 74:11, 1969.

Tsai SH et al.: Bronchopulmonary dysplasia associated with oxygen therapy in infants with respiratory distress. Radiology, 105:107, 1972.

CHRONIC PULMONARY INSUFFICIENCY OF THE PREMATURE INFANT

Edwards DK, Jacob J, and Gluck L: The immature lung: Radiographic appearances, course, and complications. Am J Roentgenol, 135:659, 1980.

Kraus AN, Klain DB, and Auld PAM: Chronic pulmonary insufficiency of prematurity (CPIP). Pediatrics, 55:55, 1975.

Parker BR et al.: Immature lung syndrome (abstr). Clin Res, 24:194A, 1976.

MECONIUM ASPIRATION

Ahvenainen EK: On changes in dilation and signs of aspiration in foetal and neonatal lungs. Acta Paediatr Scand [Suppl 3], 35:1, 1948.

Desmond MM et al.: Meconium staining of the amniotic fluid. A marker of fetal hypoxia. Obstet Gynecol, 9:91, 1957.

Gooding CA, Gregory GA: Roentgenographic analysis of meconium aspiration of the newborn. Radiology, 100:131, 1971.

Hoffman RR, Campbell RE, and Dicker JP: Fetal aspiration syndrome, clinical roentgenographic, and pathologic features. Am J Roentgenol, 122:90, 1974.

PERSISTENT FETAL CIRCULATION

Drummond WH: Persistent pulmonary hypertension of the neonate. Adv Pediatr, 30:61, 1983.

Fox WW, and Duare S: Persistent fetal circulation in the neonate: Diagnosis and management. J Pediatr, 103:505, 1983.

Haworth SG, and Reid L: Persistent fetal circulation: Newly recognized structural features. J Pediatr, 88:614, 1976.

Merten DF, Goetzman BW, and Wennberg RP: Persistent fetal circulation: An evolving clinical and radiographic concept of pulmonary hypertension in the newborn. Pediatr Radiol, 6:74, 1977.

Riemenschneider TA et al.: Disturbances of the transitional circulation: Spectrum of pulmonary hypertension and myocardial dysfunction. J Pediatr, 89:622, 1976.

PULMONARY HEMORRHAGE

Easterly JR, and Oppenheimer EH: Massive pulmonary hemorrhage in the newborn. I. Pathologic considerations. J Pediatr, 69:3, 1966.

Rowe S, and Avery ME: Massive pulmonary hemorrhage in the newborn. II. Clinical considerations. J Pediatr, 69:12, 1966.

Wesenberg RL: The Newborn Chest, pp 71–83. Hagerstown, MD, Harper & Rowe, 1973.

ASPIRATION PNEUMONITIS

Frank MM, and Gatewood OMB: Transient pharyngeal incoordination in the newborn. Am J Dis Child, 111:178, 1966.

Matsaniotis N, Karpouzas J, and Gregoriou M: Difficulty in swallowing with aspiration pneumonia in infancy. Arch Dis Child, 42:308, 1967.

McCauley RGK et al.: Gastroesophageal reflux in infants and children: A useful classification and reliable radiologic technique for its demonstration. Am J Roentgenol, 130:47, 1978.

WILSON-MIKITY SYNDROME

Baghdassarian OM, Avery ME, and Neuhauser EBD: Form of pulmonary insufficiency in premature infants: Pulmonary dysmaturity? Am J Roentgenol, 89:1020, 1963.

Edwards DK, Jacob J, and Gluck L: The immature lung: Radiographic appearance, course and complications. Am J Roentgenol, 135:659, 1980.

Grossman H et al.: Neonatal focal hyperaeration of the lungs (Wilson-Mikity syndrome). Radiology, 85:409, 1965.

Hodgman JE et al.: Chronic respiratory distress in the premature infant. Wilson-Mikity syndrome. Pediatrics, 44:179, 1969.

Thibeault DW et al.: Radiologic findings in the lungs of premature infants. J Pediatr, 74:1, 1969.

Wilson MG, and Mikity VG: New form of respiratory disease in premature infants. Am J Dis Child, 99:489, 1960.

4 SURGICAL OR MECHANICAL ABNORMALITIES IN THE NEWBORN INFANT AND CHILDREN

There are many abnormalities of the respiratory tract that may produce respiratory distress in the newborn and young infant. Many of these conditions are in the form of mechanical obstructions, and some are amendable by surgery. Early recognition, particularly of the surgical cases, is necessary if the infant is to survive. Although severe disturbance in respiration may be caused by many extrathoracic problems, such as intracranial abnormalities, intestinal obstruction, intra-abdominal masses or fluid, and many forms of congenital heart disease, only those extracardiac intrathoracic abnormalities that are radiologically demonstrable will be considered here.

The initial assessment of the child with respiratory distress is by anteroposterior and lateral radiographs. When upper airway obstruction is suggested, a high-kV filtration anteroposterior radiograph may be very helpful for further evaluation. Also, xerography may be used for special circumstances. Recently, examination by computerized tomography (CT) has been utilized to define normal and abnormal tracheal dimensions. Fluoroscopic examination of the chest is extremely important in the evaluation of obstructive lesions and of many surgically correctable abnormalities. Fluoroscopic observations of pulmonary aeration, mediastinal position, and diaphragmatic motion, and of the hypopharynx and tracheobronchial tree during inspiration and expiration, should be part of the radiographic study if the infant's condition permits this additional effort. It should be recognized, however, that the health of an infant with respiratory distress is precarious, and the additional handling necessary for fluoroscopic examination in the x-ray department may not be tolerable. A portable image intensifier and television monitoring should be used, because these permit fluoroscopic evaluation with less disturbance of the infant.

OBSTRUCTION OF UPPER AIR PASSAGES

The use of fluoroscopy in evaluating retropharyngeal soft tissues in the normal dynamics of the upper air passages during inspiration and expiration has been greatly aided by radiologic videotape techniques. The thickness of the retropharyngeal structures varies considerably in different age groups and with normal respirations. The normal anterior buckling of the infant's trachea during expirations, with the resulting increased thickness of the retropharyngeal soft tissues, should not be mistaken for a retropharyngeal mass (Fig. 4–1). With deep inspiration and with the neck in extension, the distance between the anterior portion of the cervical spine and the posterior edge of the trachea is approximately the same as the anteroposterior dimension of a cervical vertebra. Although adenoid tissue normally produces a recognizable mass in the nasopharynx of older infants and young children, there is insufficient lymphoid tissue in the nasopharynx during the first few months of life to produce such a density. Consequently, the age factor is also a consideration in the evaluation of the upper air passages.

Choanal atresia, as well as malformations of the tongue and mandible, may produce severe respiratory embarrassment in the newborn infant. Unless the nares are patent, the young infant has a great deal of difficulty breathing, especially while nursing. Not only is respiration affected, but attempts at mouth breathing during feeding are commonly accompanied by strangling and aspiration of milk into the tracheobronchial tree. Instillation of contrast medium into the nasal cavities confirms the diagnosis. Aspiration of mucus from the nasal cavities and instillation of topical decongestants prior to injection frequently delineates the site of obstruction more accurately (Fig. 4–2). Dionosil or one of the nonionic contrast agents are less irritating than some water-soluble compounds. Fluoroscopic examinations show paradoxic dilatation of the hypopharynx during expiration. The use of CT scanning has been shown to be very helpful in the evaluation of choanal atresia (Fig. 4–2C).

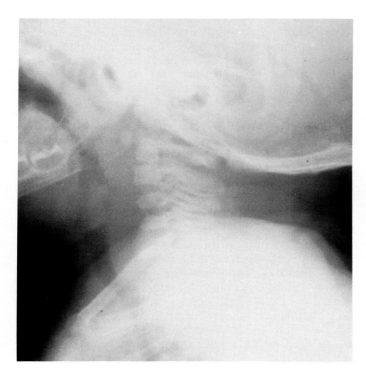

Figure 4–1. *Lateral view of the pharynx during expiration shows anterior buckling of the trachea, simulating retrotracheal mass.*

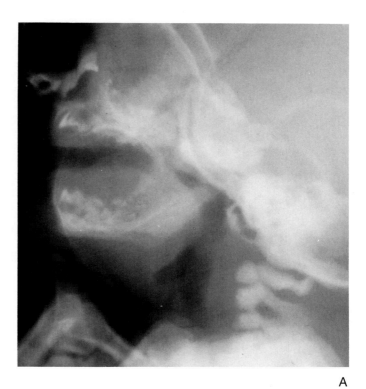

A

Figure 4–2. Choanal atresia. A, *Initial instillation of contrast medium into the nasal cavity.* B, *Instillation of contrast medium into the nasal cavity after aspiration of mucus shows the site of obstruction more accurately. Paradoxic distension of the hypopharynx during expiration is prominent in B, as compared to absence of distension in inspiration in A.*

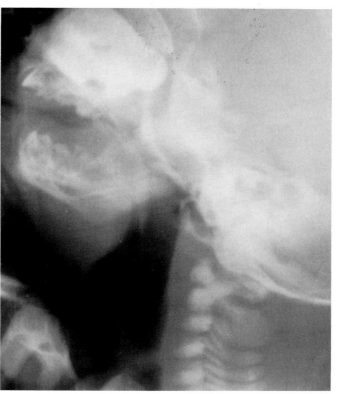

B

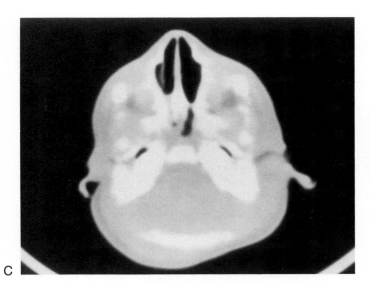

Figure 4–2. C, *Computerized tomography demonstrates enlargement of the vomer (posterior portion of the nasal septum), medial bowing and thickening of the lateral wall of the nasal cavity, and the posterior obstruction that may be the bony or soft tissue atresia.*

C

Marked enlargement of the adenoids or tonsils may interfere with respirations (Fig. 4–3), and severe cases may produce chronic hypoxia and congestive heart failure. Neoplasms of the nasopharynx (e.g., angiofibroma, Burkitt's lymphoma) may also produce respiratory difficulties (Fig. 4–4).

Malformations of the mandible, particularly those conditions in which there is mandibular hypoplasia, such as the Pierre Robin, Treacher Collins, Hallermann-Streiff, and trisomy E syndromes, are responsible for respiratory obstruction (Fig. 4–5). In these cases, as in conditions associated with macroglossia—cretinism, Beckwith-Wiedemann syndrome (Fig. 4–6), lymphangioma (Fig. 4–7), hemangioma, or lingual cyst (Fig. 4–8)—the posterior portion of the tongue encroaches on the pharynx and produces respiratory obstruction. Lateral views of the pharynx are frequently helpful in demonstrating the malformations. Lingual thyroid (Fig. 4–9), submaxillary gland cysts (ranula, Fig. 4–10), and nasopharyngeal encephaloceles (Fig. 4–11); are rare causes of airway obstruction.

Congenital Laryngeal Stridor

Congenital laryngeal stridor is occasionally present in the neonatal period, but is more often recognized by the parents after the infant has reached several weeks of age. Clinically the stridor is most pronounced during inspiration while the infant is asleep. Expiratory stridor may also be present if there is associated tracheal obstruction. Fluoroscopic observation of the larynx in the lateral view shows distention of the hypopharynx during inspiration, associated with downward and forward displacement and bowing of the aryepiglottic folds (Fig. 4–12). Characteristic inspiratory vibrations may occasionally be seen. The stridor diminishes as the infant grows, and usually disappears by the second year.

Congenital Tracheal Stridor

Congenital tracheal stridor, or tracheomalacia, is another cause of stridulous breathing in the young infant, and may occur with or without laryngeal stridor. Infants with this condition produce expiratory sounds rather than the inspiratory stridor heard in congenital laryngeal stridor. Normally, the tracheal lumen diminishes in size during expiration and increases in size during inspiration. In

Text continued on page 74

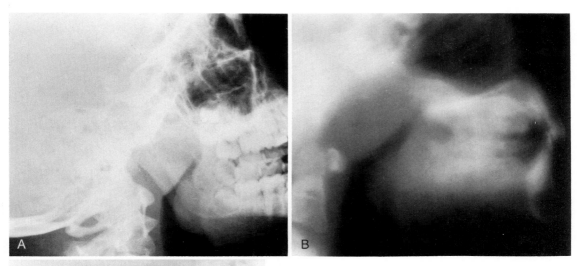

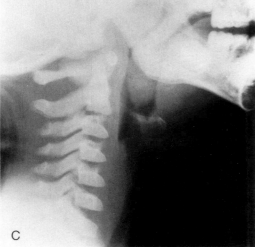

Figure 4–3. Large adenoids simulating nasopharyngeal neoplasm in a 10-year-old boy. A, Lateral view shows soft tissue mass in the nasopharynx displacing the nasopharyngeal air column anteriorly. B, Tomography emphasizes the large size of the mass, which at biopsy was found to be normal adenoid tissue. C, Large tonsils extending into the hypopharynx of a 4-year-old child. Note also the enlargement of the adenoids.

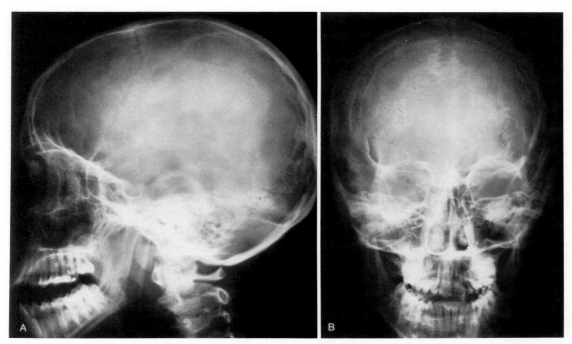

Figure 4–4. Nasopharyngeal mass in a 14-year-old boy with epistaxis. A, Lateral radiograph of the skull shows obliteration of the nasopharyngeal air column. B, Frontal projection shows increased density obliterating the right nasal cavity and ethmoid cells.

Illustration continued on opposite page

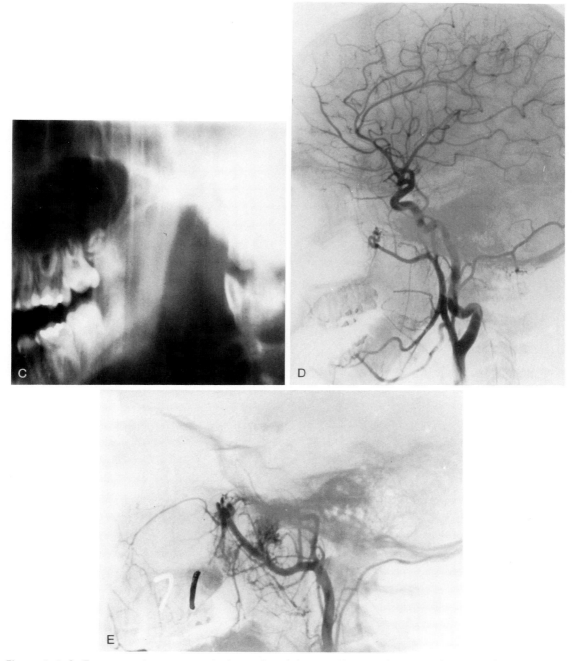

Figure 4–4. *C, Tomogram demonstrates the large size of the nasopharyngeal mass and erosion of pterygoids. D, Arteriogram shows absence of the hypervascularity expected with an angiofibroma. The histologic diagnosis was Burkitt's lymphoma. E, Arteriogram in another patient with angiofibroma showing the hypervascularity associated with this tumor.*

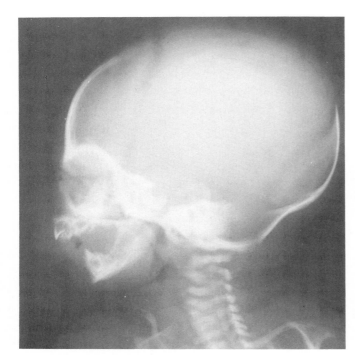

Figure 4–5. Mandibular hypoplasia associated with trisomy E syndrome. The hypoplastic mandible is associated with narrowing of the nasopharyngeal air passages.

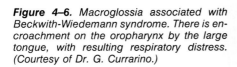

Figure 4–6. Macroglossia associated with Beckwith-Wiedemann syndrome. There is encroachment on the oropharynx by the large tongue, with resulting respiratory distress. (Courtesy of Dr. G. Currarino.)

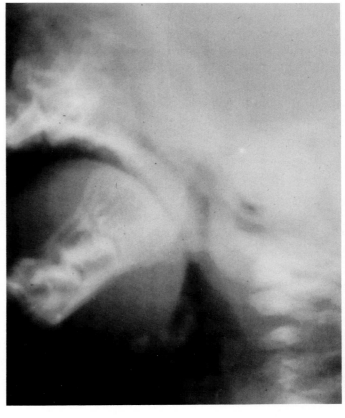

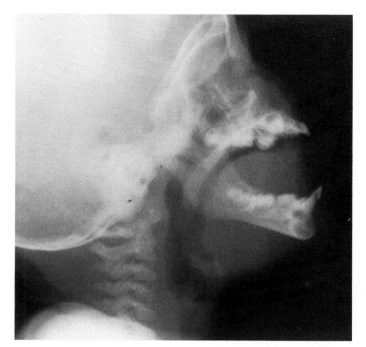

Figure 4–7. *Infant with large lymphangioma of the tongue, which displaces an air column in the oropharynx upward and posteriorly.*

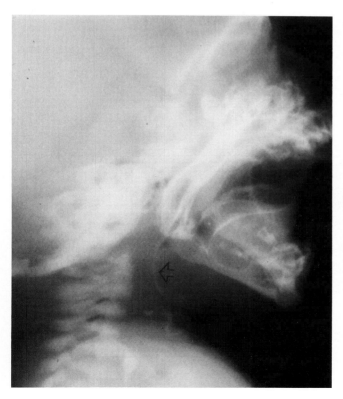

Figure 4–8. *Lingual cyst* (arrow) *in a 1-week-old infant.*

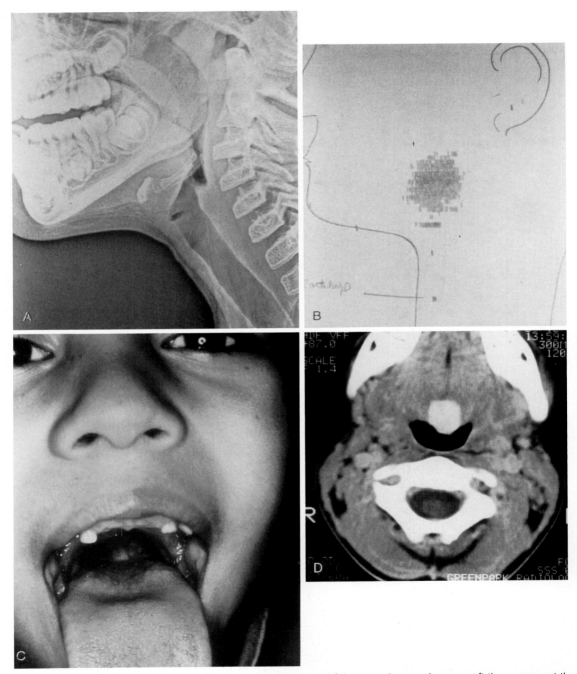

Figure 4–9. A, *Large lingual thyroid in a 5-year-old girl. Xerogram of the nasopharynx shows a soft tissue mass at the base of the tongue. B, ^{131}I uptake shows concentration of the isotope at the base of the tongue without evidence of thyroid tissue in the neck. C, Large lingual thyroid is identified at the base of the patient's tongue. D, Lingual thyroid in a 7-year-old child. Enhanced computerized tomography scan shows the marked vascularity of the ectopic thyroid tissue.*

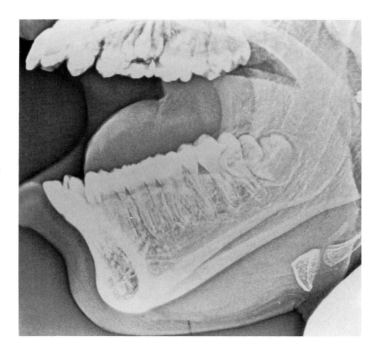

Figure 4–10. Xerogram of a child with a large submaxillary gland cyst (ranula).

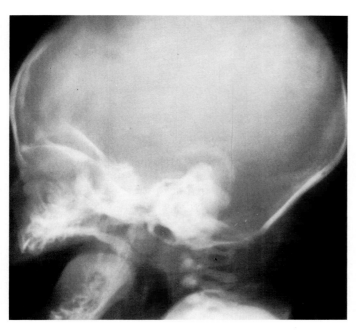

Figure 4–11. Infant with a soft tissue mass extending into the nasopharynx from the base of the skull. The mass was proven to be an encephalocele. (Courtesy of Dr. G. Blank.)

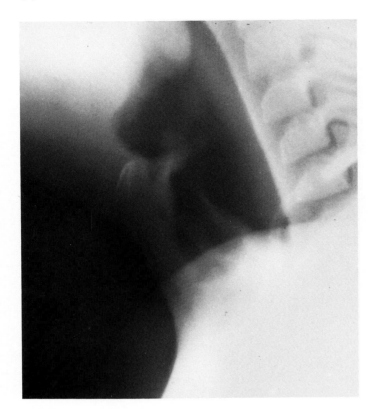

Figure 4–12. Congenital laryngeal stridor.

congenital tracheal stridor the trachea, during expiration, collapses much more than normally (Fig. 4–13), apparently because of inadequacy of the cartilaginous structures. Tracheomalacia is also common in infants with tracheoesophageal fistula. By the time infancy has passed, the growth of the tracheobronchial tree will have alleviated the stridor, but during this time croup or tracheobronchitis may become a serious complication.

Croup

Croup is a common form of upper airway obstruction in infants and children, and is the result of inflammatory edema of the subglottic area (conus elasticus). Various types of viruses (usually parainfluenza virus) cause the infection. The radiographic findings are best appreciated in the frontal projection and show the subglottic airway to be constricted, producing a "pencil" configuration (Fig. 4–14). A high-kV filter technique is helpful in demonstrating the laryngeal and tracheal air columns. The lateral view is less helpful, with the subglottic area being ill-defined. Fluoroscopy is unnecessary but will show inspiratory dilatation of the hypopharynx and expiratory dilatation of the cervical trachea. Radiographic studies are usually requested to exclude epiglottitis. Unless there is associated bronchopneumonia, there is no evidence of air trapping in the lungs.

Membranous croup (membranous laryngotracheobronchitis) is a diffuse inflammatory disease of the larynx, trachea, and bronchi that produces adherent membranes, which may be radiographically demonstrated on lateral views of the neck. Edema of the conus elasticus and trachea causes narrowing of these structures (Fig. 4–15). Various bacterial, viral, and fungal infections, separately or in combination, may produce these membranes, which may have to be removed endoscopically.

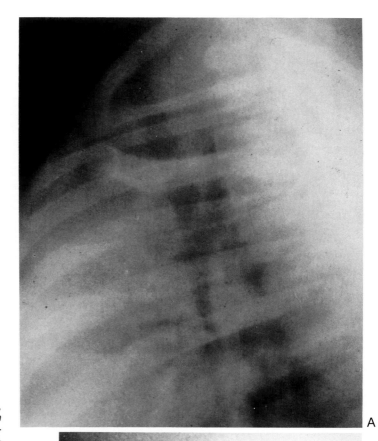

Figure 4–13. Congenital tracheal stridor. A, Lateral radiograph made during inspiration shows normal tracheal lumen. B, Radiograph made during expiration shows collapse of the tracheal air column.

A

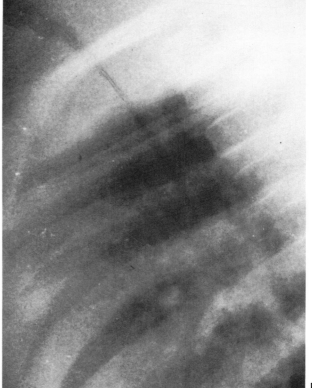

B

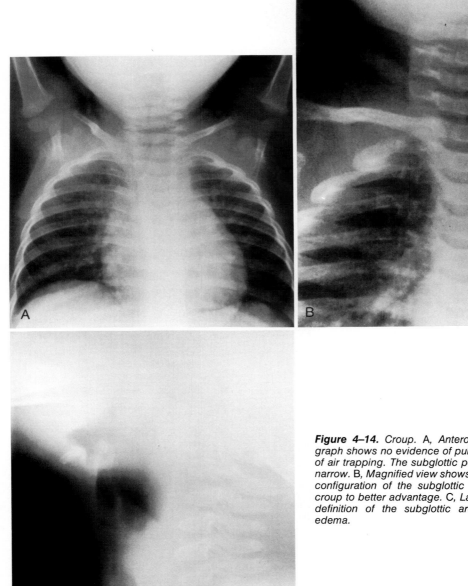

Figure 4–14. Croup. A, Anteroposterior chest radiograph shows no evidence of pulmonary abnormality or of air trapping. The subglottic portion of the trachea is narrow. B, Magnified view shows the tapered subglottic configuration of the subglottic area characteristic of croup to better advantage. C, Lateral view shows poor definition of the subglottic area secondary to the edema.

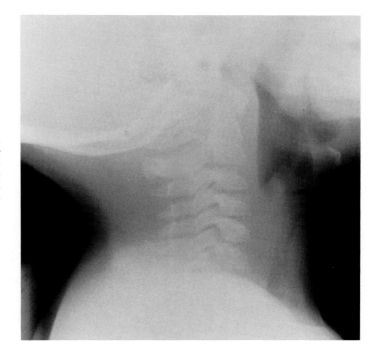

Figure 4–15. Membranous laryngotracheo-bronchitis in a young child. There is slight distension of the hypopharynx. The sub-glottic area is narrowed and, there is opaque material within the lumen, representing inflammatory membranes associated with this condition.

Epiglottitis

Epiglottitis is a serious infection occurring in infants and children usually over 18 to 24 months of age, and requires immediate diagnosis and treatment. Clinically, the infants have an expression of panic, hold their heads forward, breathe through their mouths, and drool because of the difficulty in swallowing. The upper airway may be rapidly obstructed with resulting asphyxia—hence, the urgency in the diagnosis. Direct inspection of the epiglottis is contraindicated. Lateral radiographs of the neck result in less struggling and crying, and are less disturbing to the patient. Lateral radiographs of the neck show increased size of the epiglottis, particularly of its tip (Fig. 4–16). Associated thickening of the aryepiglottic folds adds to the obstruction. There is usually associated dilatation of the hypopharynx because of the inspiratory obstruction. The etiologic agent is usually Haemophilus influenzae. Other causes of epiglottic enlargement include angioneurotic edema, hemorrhage, trauma (Fig. 4–17), and neoplasms. Fluoroscopy should be avoided, not only because it is unnecessary but because it also prolongs treatment, which may be of an emergency nature.

Postintubation strictures, granulomas, and other complications (Fig. 4–18) may develop, particularly in the newborn, and require respiratory support. The ingestion of caustic substances may produce cicatrical changes of the hypopharynx and larynx, and rare conditions such as epidermolysis bullosa may produce similar changes (Fig. 4–19). Sublaryngeal hemangioma and laryngeal papillomas may occur in older children, and may reach a size that interferes with respiration (Fig. 4–20). Seeding of the papillomas into the distal bronchi frequently results in advanced bronchiectasis (Fig. 4–21).

Peritracheal cysts, which are probably a variety of retention cysts, may encroach on the subglottic or tracheal area, producing respiratory compromise (Fig. 4–22). Calcification of tracheal cartilages may occur in chondrodystrophia calcificans congenita (Conradi's disease), and interfere with respiration (Fig. 4–23).

Text continued on page 84

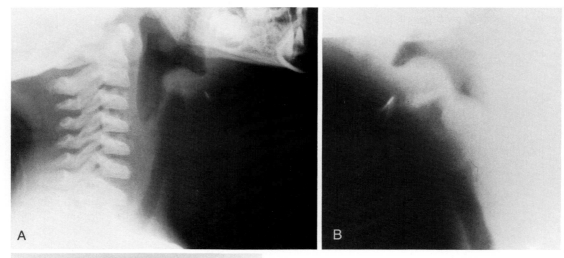

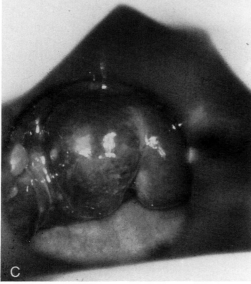

Figure 4–16. *Epiglottitis in a 2-year-old child. A, Lateral view of the nasopharynx shows the enlarged epiglottis extending into the hypopharynx. B, Enlargement shows the enlarged round tip of the epiglottis and prominent aryepiglottic folds to better advantage, producing partial obstruction of the hypopharynx. C, Epiglottitis.*

Figure 4–17. Thermal injury of the epiglottis. This 2½-year old boy was perfectly well until choking on "hot dressing." He was seen in the emergency room, at which time he had mild stridor and some difficulty in swallowing. The lateral view shows the characteristic swelling usually associated with acute epiglottitis. The patient had no fever or signs of sepsis, and made an uneventful recovery.

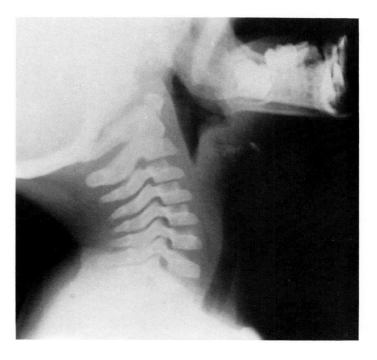

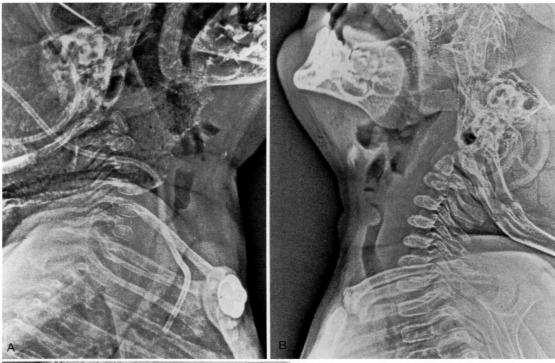

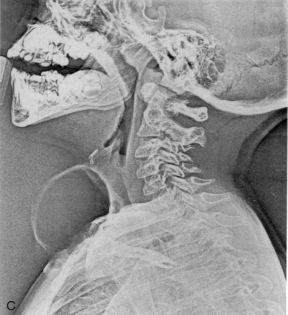

Figure 4–18. A, *Tracheal stricture secondary to long-standing endotracheal intubation. B, Granuloma in the subglottic area of the trachea following long-standing endotracheal intubation. C, Cervical pneumatocele in a 5-year-old girl who had a tracheostomy at 5 weeks of age because of seizures and hypocalcemia secondary to thyroid agenesis, resulting from* [131]*I therapy of the mother for thyroid carcinoma. The tracheostomy remained for 3 years. Following closure of the tracheostomy fistula, the patient developed a cervical pneumatocele.*

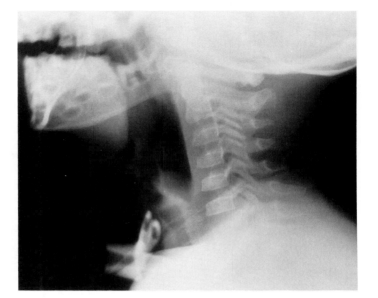

Figure 4–19. Epidermolysis bullosa dystrophica. Lateral view of the infant's neck shows distension of the hypopharynx secondary to partial obstruction of the glottis and subglottic area due to the cicatricial changes produced by this condition.

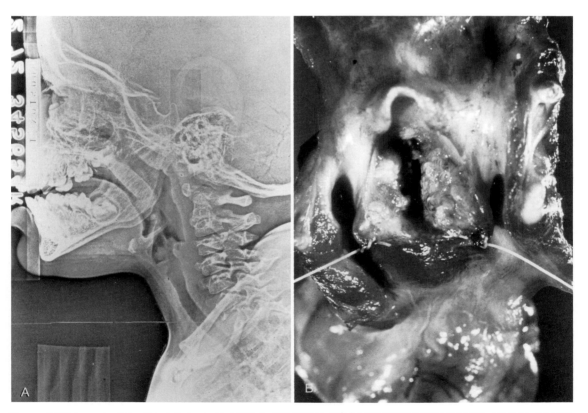

Figure 4–20. Laryngeal papilloma in a young child. A, Papillomas can be identified adjacent to the vocal cord and in the subglottic area. B, Autopsy specimen of a patient with laryngeal papillomatosis, which covered the vocal cords.

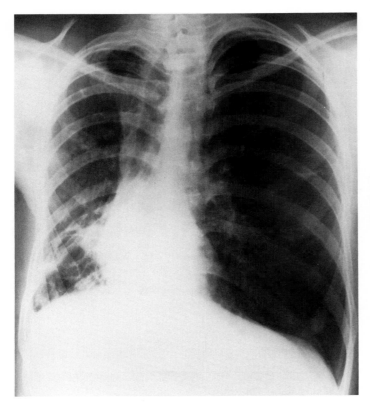

Figure 4–21. Advanced bronchiectasis and loss of lung volume in an older patient with papillomatosis and seeding of the distal bronchi. Compensatory emphysema of the left lung is present. (Courtesy of Dr. J. Kirpatrick.)

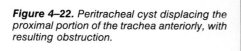

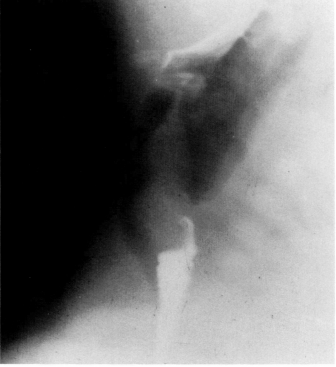

Figure 4–22. Peritracheal cyst displacing the proximal portion of the trachea anteriorly, with resulting obstruction.

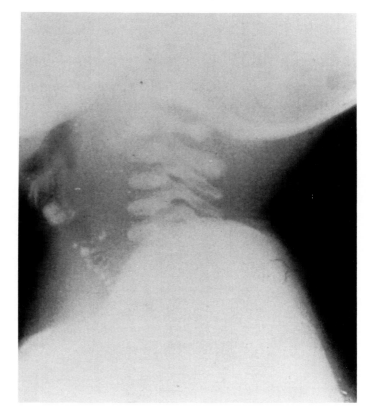

Figure 4–23. Chondrodystrophia calcificans congenita (Conradi's disease). This young infant had extensive calcifications in the laryngeal and tracheal cartilages.

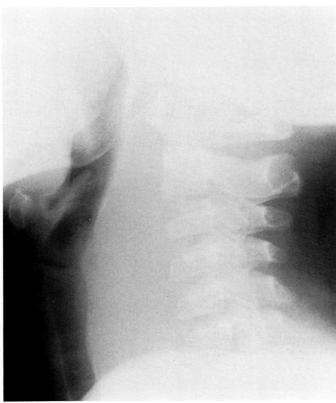

Figure 4–24. Twelve-year-old boy with hemophilia. The retropharyngeal and retroesophageal spaces are occupied by a large hematoma resulting from trauma to the neck.

Retropharyngeal masses secondary either to hemorrhage (Fig. 4–24), abscess, or cellulitis may also interfere with respiration (Figs. 4–25, 4–26, and 4–27). Goiter in the newborn is a rare cause of respiratory distress (Fig. 4–28). Masses lateral and posterior to the trachea such as cystic hygroma duplication and neurenteric cysts may also displace or compress the trachea (Figs. 4–29 and 4–30). Cervical pneumatocele may be a complication of tracheostomy closure, and produce tracheal compression (see Fig. 4–18C).

ASPIRATION OF FOREIGN BODIES

The aspiration of a foreign object into the trachea or bronchi is secondary in frequency to croup in producing respiratory difficulty in the older infant and young child. Most of these objects are usually food products (particularly peanuts), with resulting rapid onset of coughing and wheezing. Routine chest radiographs may be strikingly normal if the chest radiograph is made at the time of deep inspiration. Consequently, fluoroscopy is invaluable in the evaluation of pulmonary aeration. During fluoroscopic examination no attempt should be made to keep the infant from crying to evaluate the dynamics of respiration more accurately. In addition, every effort should be made to position the child in a direct frontal position. This is most easily accomplished by performing the examination with the infant supine and the elbows held against the ears, thereby maintaining a straight position of the head. Any deviation of the head to the right or left may produce slight rotation of the chest, and could interfere with accurate fluoroscopic observations. During

Text continued on page 93

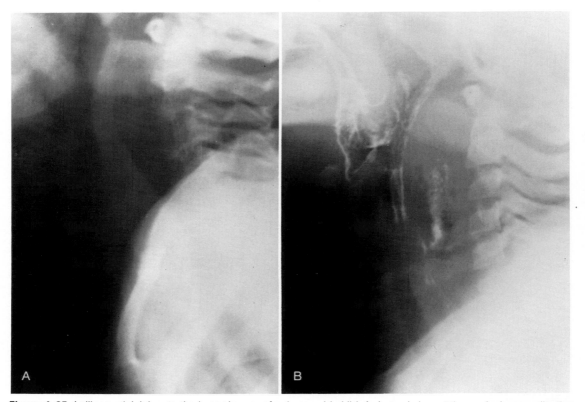

Figure 4–25. *Lollipop stick injury to the hypopharynx of a 4-year-old child. A, Lateral view of the neck shows collection of gas in retropharyngeal space. B, Following ingestion of contrast medium, there is extension of the material into the precervical area at the site of perforation.*

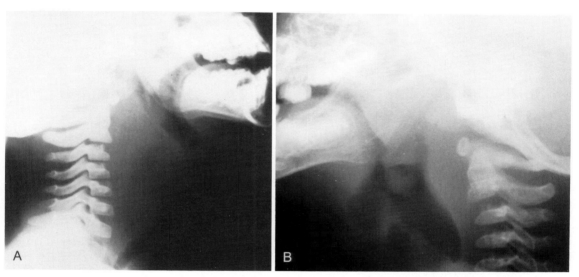

Figure 4–26. A, *Retropharyngeal abscess secondary to acute tonsillitis.* B, *Cellulitis.*

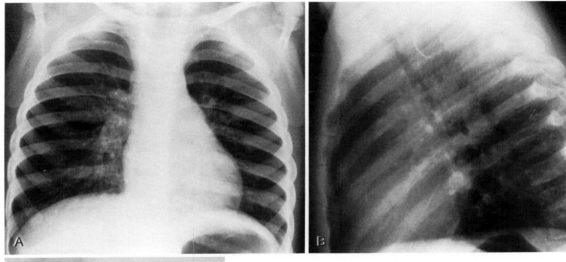

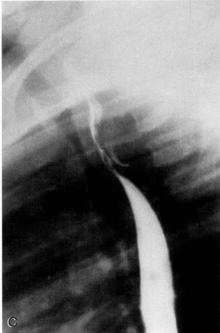

Figure 4–27. Three-year-old child with history of fever and cough. A, Frontal chest radiograph shows no abnormality. B, Lateral chest radiograph shows area of metallic density posterior to the narrowed tracheal air column. C, Following swallow of contrast medium the aluminum pull-tab is seen posterior to the esophagus. Note also the constriction of the trachea secondary to the inflammatory process.

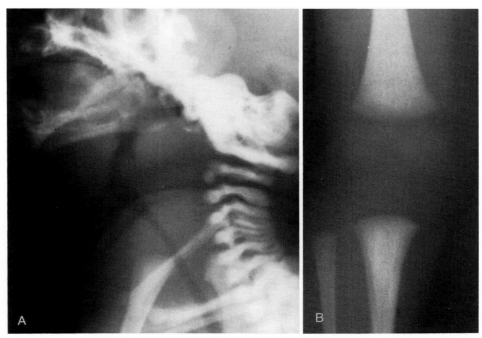

Figure 4–28. Goiter in a newborn. A, Lateral view of the neck shows displacement of the pharynx and tracheal air column anteriorly by a large mass, located anteriorly and posteriorly to these structures. B, Radiograph of the knee shows absence of term gestational ossification centers. Although the gestation period was normal, the mother had been on therapeutic doses of potassium iodide expectorant during most of her pregnancy, which resulted in congenital hypothyroidism.

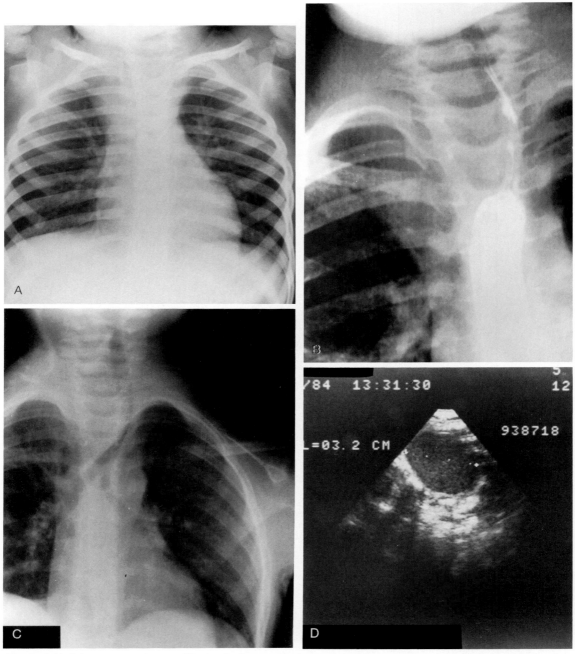

Figure 4–29. *Infant with respiratory difficulty. A, Chest radiograph shows fullness in the right superior mediastinum. B, Barium swallow shows displacement of the trachea and proximal esophagus to the left. C, Filtered high-kV technique of the trachea emphasizes the tracheal displacement. D, Ultrasound studies show a hypoechoic mass. Surgical exploration demonstrated a neurenteric cyst (esophageal duplication). The preoperative diagnosis was cystic hygroma.*

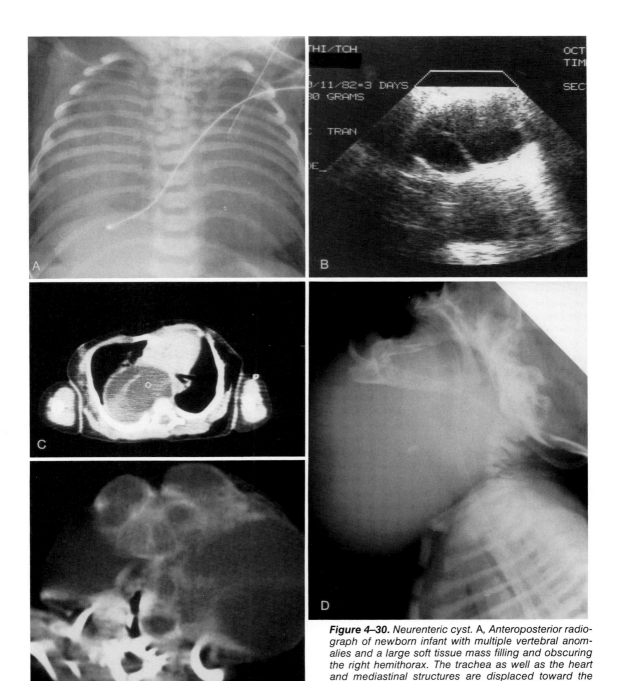

Figure 4–30. Neurenteric cyst. A, Anteroposterior radiograph of newborn infant with multiple vertebral anomalies and a large soft tissue mass filling and obscuring the right hemithorax. The trachea as well as the heart and mediastinal structures are displaced toward the left side. A left chest tube is in place because of previous pneumothorax. B, Longitudinal ultrasound of the chest shows a large septated cystic mass filling the right hemithorax. C, Computerized tomography demonstrates the smooth wall posterior mediastinal mass, with the septum within it. Note lower attenuation center. D, Large cystic hygroma in the neck of the newborn infant. Lateral radiograph shows the large mass occupying the interior portion of the neck. Note the dysplastic changes of the mandible. E, Computerized tomography shows the large mass to be of low density, with associated compression of the larynx and proximal trachea.

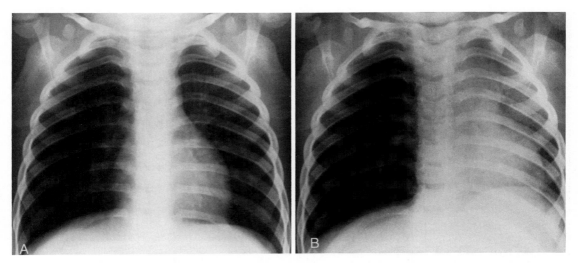

Figure 4–31. *Alteration of pulmonary aeration and mediastinal position caused by nonopaque foreign body in the right main stem bronchus, producing air trapping in the right lung. A, Inspiratory film shows a mediastinum in a normal position, and the lungs are equally aerated. B, Expiratory radiograph shows shift of mediastinal structures to the normal side, with air trapping of the right lung.*

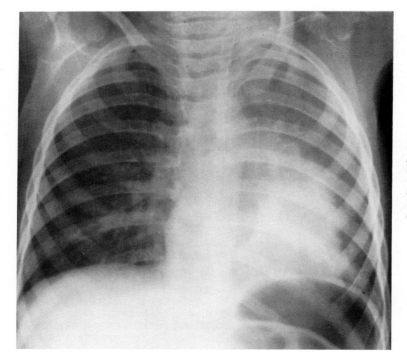

Figure 4–32. *Atelectasis of upper lobe in 2-year-old infant following aspiration of popcorn. Frontal chest radiograph shows shift of mediastinal structures to the left, with increased density of the left lung.*

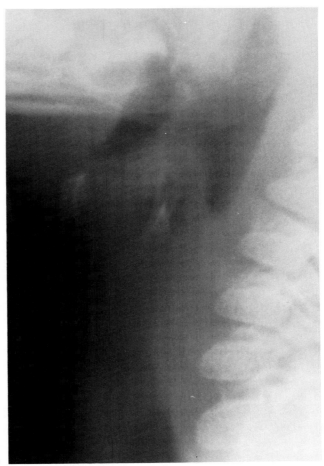

Figure 4–33. A, Aspirated chicken bone in the hypopharynx. B, Metallic straight pin in left main stem bronchus.

A

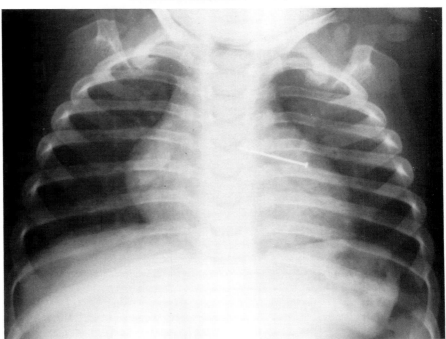

B

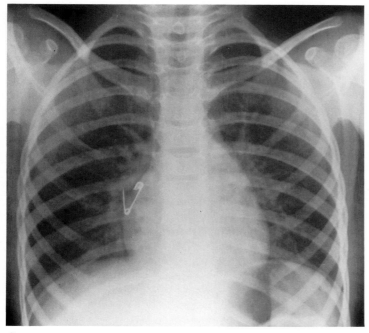

C

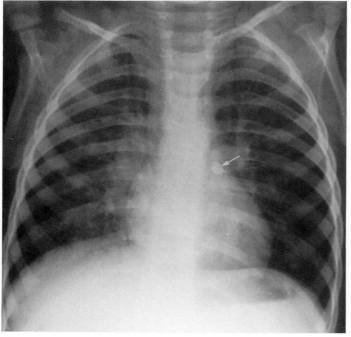

D

Figure 4–33. *C, Open safety pin in right main stem bronchus. D, Tooth in left main stem bronchus (*arrow*).*

inspiration mediastinal structures are in a normal midline position and the diaphragm is low, with equal aeration of the lungs. However, during expiration, the unobstructed lung evacuates its air contents normally, with resulting movement of the mediastinal structures to the normal side because of the air block of the opposite lung (Fig. 4–31). The diaphragm of the obstructed lung remains in a low position. With inspiration the mediastinum shifts back to its normal position, and the lungs appear to be aerated equally. This to-and-fro motion of the mediastinum with expiration and inspiration is indicative of air block, and is readily explained by the normal increase in luminal size of the bronchi during inspiration and the normal decrease in size during expiration. Consequently, during expiration, the lumen closes on the foreign body, which prohibits exit of the air from the obstructed lung.

Occasionally, the foreign body may shift from one lung to the other. If there is complete bronchial obstruction prohibiting air from entering the lung, resorption of air distal to the obstruction occurs with atelectasis (Fig. 4–32). This is usually a late finding and is easily recognized on routine chest radiographs, in which the mediastinum is displaced to the atelectatic side. Fluoroscopy in these cases demonstrates mediastinal displacement to the obstructed side during inspiration, with partial return of mediastinal structures to the midline during expiration. Opaque foreign objects in the bronchus are usually recognized readily, and fluoroscopy is unnecessary (Fig. 4–33). Tracheal or midline foreign bodies will result in paradoxic changes in the size of the heart with inspiration.

The lodgement of a foreign body in the esophagus is another common recurrence in this age group. Unless they pass into the stomach, they usually lodge in the thoracic inlet or at the lower esophageal segment. Coins in the lower esophageal segment will generally pass to the stomach if the infant is given a carbonated beverage or something to eat. However, objects at the thoracic inlet usually must be removed, either by endoscopy or by catheter technique. Catheter technique is preferred by many referring physicians and radiologists. The procedure consists of passing a symmetrically distensible Foley catheter past the object, inflating it under fluoroscopic observation with opaque contrast medium and, with the patient in a prone or semiprone Trendelenburg position, withdrawing the catheter and, hopefully, the object. If undue resistance is encountered, the procedure should be abandoned because of possible damage to the esophagus. It is mandatory to have someone in the fluoroscopic room who is trained in laryngoscopy in case the coin is aspirated into the larynx on its removal into the pharynx.

Coins that are aspirated into the upper trachea are seen on edge in the anteroposterior view because of the normal anatomic position of the vocal cords and the configuration of the tracheal cartilages. These objects obviously require laryngoscopy before removal.

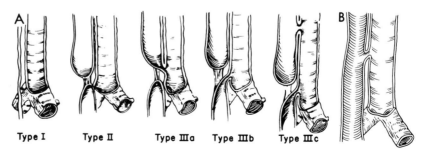

Type I   Type II   Type IIIa   Type IIIb   Type IIIc

Figure 4–34. *Types of esophageal atresia and tracheoesophageal fistulas. A, Atresia without fistula (types I and II) and atresia with fistula (type III). B, H-type tracheoesophageal fistula. (From Singleton, E. B., Wagner, M. L., and Dutton, R. V.: Radiology of the Alimentary Tract in Infants and Children. Philadelphia, W. B. Saunders, 1977.)*

ESOPHAGEAL ATRESIA AND TRACHEOESOPHAGEAL FISTULA

Esophageal atresia may take many forms (Fig. 4–34), but, in 85 to 90% of cases, it is associated with tracheal communication between the lower esophageal segment and the tracheobronchial tree. The condition is suspected clinically by the presence of an excessive amount of mucus and saliva in the infant's mouth. Frontal and lateral radiographs of the chest and abdomen frequently show distention of the upper esophageal pouch (Fig. 4–35) and, because of the fistulous communication between the lower esophageal segment and the tracheobronchial tree, there is usually air in excessive amounts in the stomach and small bowel. The upper esophageal pouch is frequently distended, and may cause respiratory distress by pressure on the trachea.

The diagnosis may be confirmed by passage of a small nasogastric tube through the nose into the obstructed esophageal pouch. Fluoroscopic visualization of this procedure is advisable because the catheter, if passed blindly, may coil up on itself and give the erroneous impression that it is passing into the stomach. After the catheter has been positioned in the upper esophageal segment, the infant should be placed in a semiprone or prone position and a small amount, approximately 1 ml, of contrast material (e.g., thin barium, Dionosil, or iohexol) should be injected (Fig. 4–36) under fluoroscopic control.

This procedure not only actively outlines the location of the upper esophageal pouch, but is also useful in determining if there is fistulous communication between the upper pouch and the trachea. Atelectasis and pneumonia, or a combination of these conditions, are commonly present in the right upper lobe, because this is the most dependent portion of the pulmonary bed and consequently the most common site for aspiration pneumonia. Right upper lobe pneumonia in the neonate suggests esophageal atresia, tracheoesophageal fistula, or pharyngeal incoordination, and radiologic investigation is indicated.

The absence of gas in the gastrointestinal tract in an infant with esophageal atresia is presumptive evidence that a fistulous connection between the lower esophageal segment and the tracheobronchial tree does not exist (and that only esophageal atresia is present). However, the judicious use of a small amount of contrast medium to outline the upper pouch is helpful in eliminating the possibility of an upper segment tracheoesophageal fistula.

An H-type fistula is best demonstrated with the infant in a prone position and with the lower portion of the infant elevated. This position facilitates filling the communication because of the cephalic direction of the fistula from the esophagus to the trachea. A catheter should be positioned in the upper esophagus, usually just above the thoracic inlet. Under fluoroscopic visualization the esophagus should be forcefully distended by a bolus of contrast medium (either thin barium, Dionosil, or nonionic contrast medium), resulting in the opacification of the fistula and the trachea. Several attempts may be necessary before the fistula is identified. Careful fluoroscopic observation and videotape recordings are extremely important in demonstrating the lesion accurately (Fig. 4–37). Suction equipment should always be available if needed. Radiographs of the chest and abdomen usually show excessive accumulation of air in the stomach. Localized tracheomalacia or abnormal cartilaginous rings may result in tracheal narrowing associated with esophageal atresia and tracheoesophageal fistula (Figs. 4–38 and 4–39).

FOREGUT MALFORMATIONS

Rare foregut malformations, such as congenital absence of the trachea (Fig. 4–40), are naturally incompatible with life. An unusual tracheobronchial anomaly

Text continued on page 100

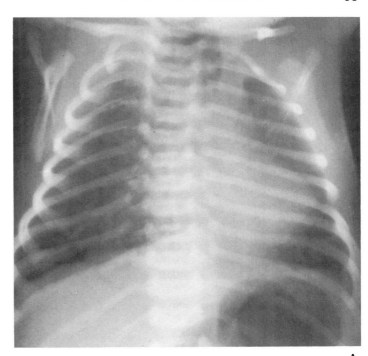

A

Figure 4–35. Esophageal atresia. A, Frontal radiograph shows distension of the upper esophageal pouch. Gas in the intestinal tract indicates communication of the lower esophageal segment and the tracheobronchial tree. B, Lateral view shows the dilated esophageal pouch displacing the trachea anteriorly.

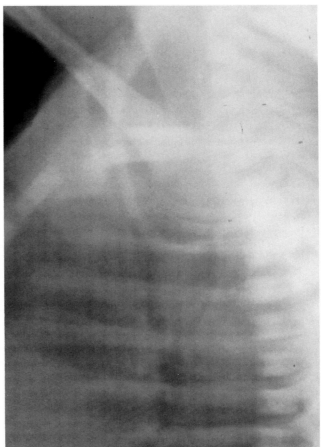

B

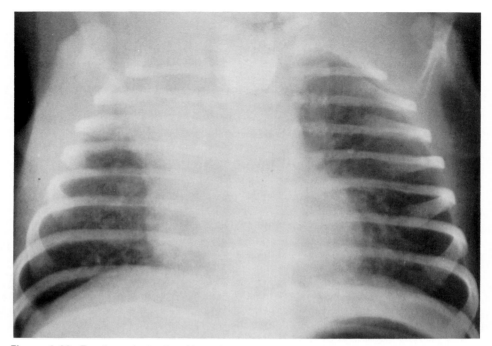

Figure 4–36. Esophageal atresia with aspiration pneumonia involving right upper lobe. A small amount of contrast medium has been injected into the esophageal pouch outlining the atresia. There is aspiration pneumonia involving the right upper lobe.

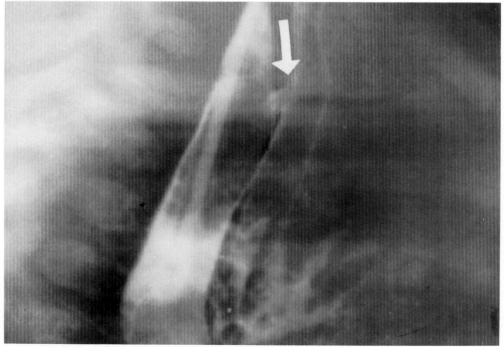

Figure 4–37. Tracheoesophageal fistula. Lateral view following injection of contrast medium into the upper esophagus demonstrates the tracheoesophageal fistula (arrow).

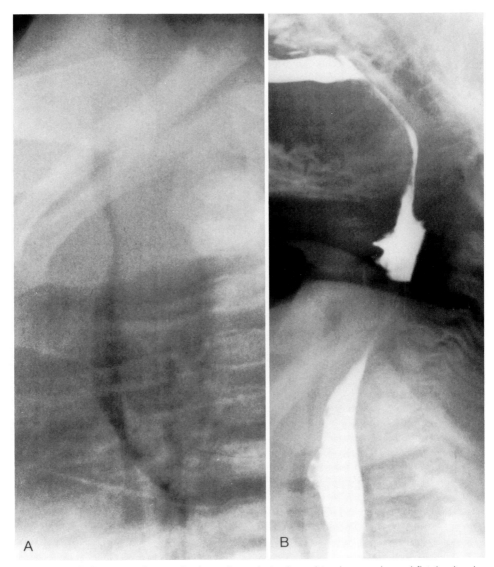

Figure 4–38. A, Postoperative repair of esophageal atresia and tracheoesophageal fistula showing a persistent narrowing of the trachea just beneath the thoracic inlet. B, Esophagram shows a narrowed tracheal lumen unrelated to any type of postoperative distension of the proximal esophageal segment.

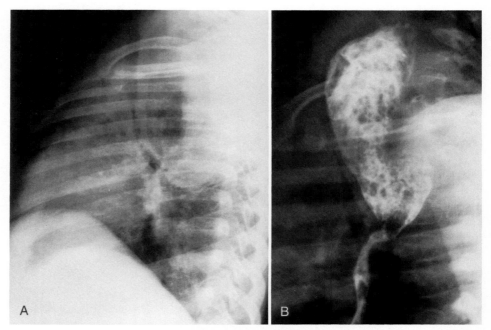

Figure 4–39. A, *Postoperative esophageal atresia and tracheoesophageal fistula. The trachea is narrowed, and there is air within the distended proximal esophageal segment.* B, *The distended portion of the esophagus above the anastamosis has produced slight anterior displacement of the trachea, but inherent tracheal narrowing is also present.*

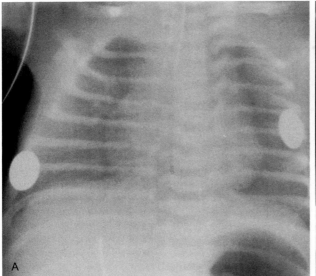

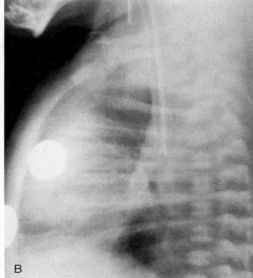

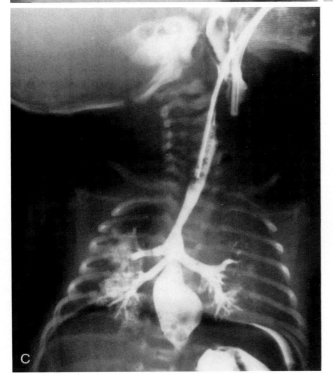

Figure 4–40. Tracheal agenesis in a premature infant with severe respiratory distress. Intubation was not possible. A, Anteroposterior radiograph suggests that the endotracheal tube is in a normal position; however, it is actually in the esophagus, through which the lungs were ventilated via esophageal bronchi for several days. B, Lateral radiograph shows the short anterior upper catheter blindly ending in the trachea and the posterior catheter positioned in the midesophagus. C, Postmortem injection of barium demonstrates a laryngoesophageal cleft, tracheal agenesis, and distal esophageal fistula. There is also a pneumoperitoneum from perforation of the stomach and a small amount of positive contrast medium outlining the left hemidiaphragm.

is an aberrant right upper lobe bronchus (pig bronchus), which arises from the trachea above the carina. Wheezing rather than respiratory distress is the usual symptom (Fig. 4–41). Additional foregut and bronchopulmonary-foregut malformations are described in Chapter 6 (sequestrations and esophageal bronchus) and in Chapter 7 (neurenteric cysts).

PNEUMOMEDIASTINUM AND PNEUMOTHORAX

Most cases of pneumomediastinum and pneumothorax in the newborn are secondary to positive pressure therapy and air block complications (see Chap. 3). However, pneumomediastinum and pneumothorax may occur in normal infants who have not undergone resuscitative measures. It may be presumed that, in such cases, birth trauma or perhaps congenital alveolar or pleural defects are present. The pathogenesis usually consists of alveolar rupture into the perivascular spaces, with medial dissection of air to the mediastinum. Frontal projections commonly show elevation of the thymus (Fig. 4–42). Progression of the condition produces pleural rupture, with resulting pneumothorax. Lateral supine films of the chest are particularly helpful in the diagnosis of pneumomediastinum.

The radiographic identification of pneumothorax in this age group is usually not difficult in that the degree of collapse is frequently complete unless there is underlying hyaline membrane disease. Pneumothorax may also be a complication in newborn infants with renal agenesis. In this condition there is associated pulmonary hypoplasia. Presumably the introduction of positive intrapulmonary pressure either due to voluntary respiratory measures or to resuscitative efforts results in rupture of the noncompliant hypoplastic lungs (Fig. 4–43).

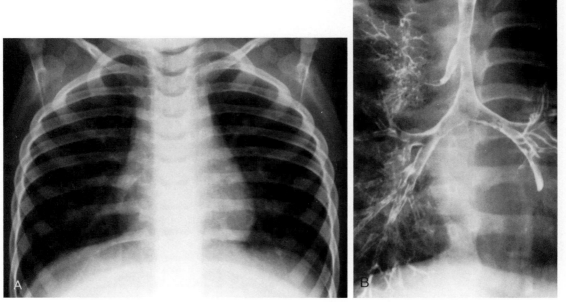

Figure 4–41. *Aberrant right upper lobe bronchus (pig bronchus) in a 2-year-old child with wheezing. A, Frontal chest radiograph shows no abnormality. B, Bronchogram shows aberrant right upper lobe bronchus arising from the trachea.*

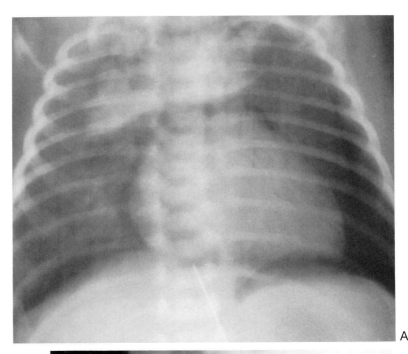

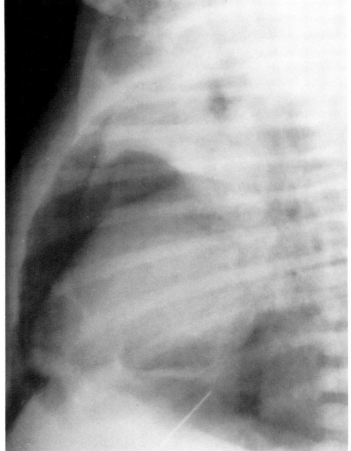

Figure 4–42. Pneumomediastinum and pneumothorax. A, Frontal projection shows elevation of the thymus by air in the mediastinum. There is associated pneumothorax, with collapse of the left lung. B, Lateral supine film shows air in the anterior mediastinum, with elevation of the thymus. Subcutaneous emphysema is also present.

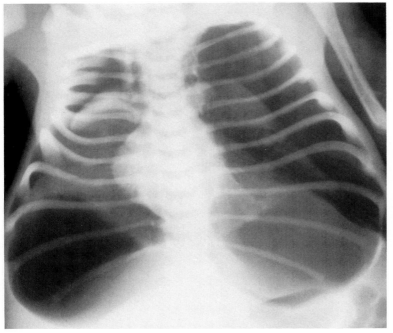

A

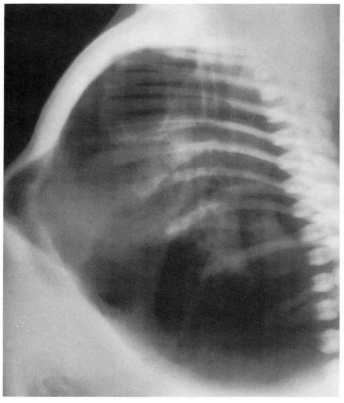

B

Figure 4–43. Extensive bilateral pneumothorax in newborn with renal agenesis and pulmonary hypoplasia after attempted resuscitation. A, Frontal projection shows tension pneumothorax, with collapse of both lungs. B, Lateral view shows marked downward displacement of diaphragm.

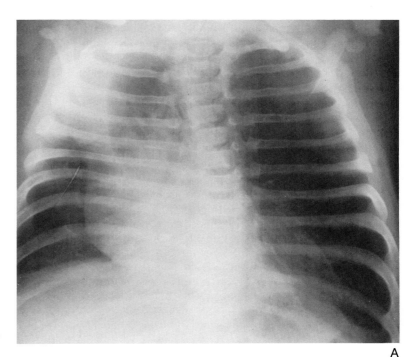

A

Figure 4–44. Congenital lobar emphysema. A, Frontal chest radiograph shows overinflation of the left upper lobe, with herniation across the anterior mediastinum into the right hemothorax. There is compression atelectasis of the left lower lobe, and mediastinal structures are displaced to the right. B, Lateral view shows the herniated hyperexpanded left upper lobe in the anterior mediastinum.

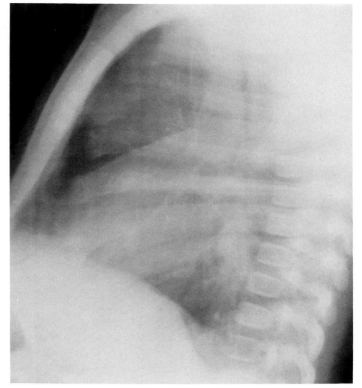

B

CONGENITAL LOBAR EMPHYSEMA

Congenital lobar emphysema may cause serious respiratory embarrassment in the young infant. Chest radiographs show hyperinflation of the lobe, usually the left upper lobe, with displacement of the mediastinum to the opposite side and compression atelectasis of the adjacent lobe (Fig. 4–44). The right middle lobe is the next most common location. Involvement of the lower lobes is rare (Fig. 4–45). Fluoroscopy is helpful in milder cases by demonstrating failure of deflation of the overexpanded segment during expiration. The mediastinum in such cases will move away from the obstructed side during expiration, and back to a more midline position during deep inspiration. In more severe cases the displacement of adjacent structures by the overinflated lobe prohibits changes in position during respiratory efforts (Fig. 4–46). The overly expanded lung, enlargement of the ipsilateral hemithorax, and relative smallness of the opposite hemithorax should not be mistaken for alveolar hypoplasia.

The theories regarding etiology include localized deficiency of cartilage and redundancy of the mucosa, with resulting air trapping of the affected bronchus. However, definite gross or histologic causes are rarely demonstrable. In severe cases surgical removal of the affected lobe is usually necessary, but milder cases may be closely watched and checked; improvement occasionally occurs in later infancy and early childhood. Bronchography is usually uninformative, and is contraindicated in severe cases.

In rare cases congenital lobar emphysema may be present in the first few days of life as an area of consolidation; after absorption of the fluid and replacement by air, it then assumes the more characteristic picture of lobar emphysema (Fig. 4–47). The fluid in the lobe is probably a combination of aspirated amniotic fluid and fluid derived from the fetus. Experimental evidence indicates that the fetal lung contains an ultrafiltrate of fetal serum, which accumulates in the lung and passes through the respiratory tract into the amniotic fluid. Consequently, congenital bronchial obstruction will result in fluid being trapped in the lung, and appears radiographically as a fluid-filled cyst (Fig. 4–48). Its appearance during this phase, or even after partial aeration has occurred, may be similar to the radiographic findings of cystic adenomatoid malformation of the lung.

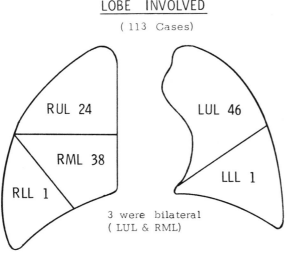

LOBE INVOLVED

(113 Cases)

RUL 24

RML 38

RLL 1

LUL 46

LLL 1

3 were bilateral
(LUL & RML)

Figure 4–45. *Sites of involvement in lobar emphysema in infants. (From Hendren WH, and McKee DM: Lobar emphysema of infancy. J Pediatr Surg, 1:24, 1966.)*

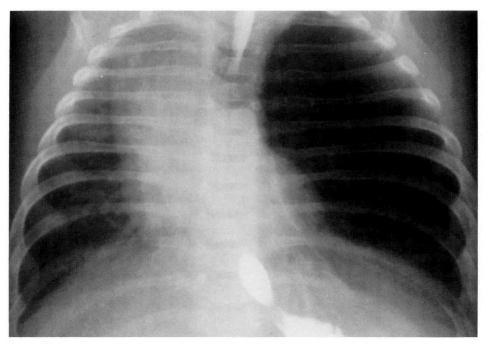

Figure 4–46. Congenital lobar emphysema. The left upper lobe is overinflated and displaces the mediastinum to the right. The left hemithorax is larger than the right but the absence of increased pulmonary vascular markings on the left, and the respiratory distress of the infant, indicate congenital lobar emphysema.

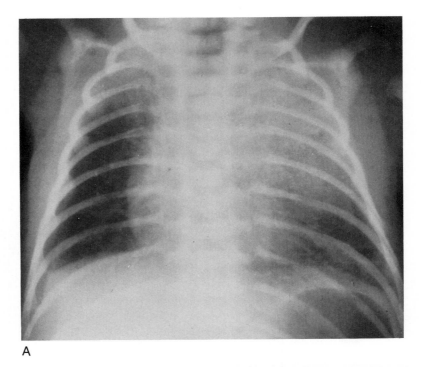

A

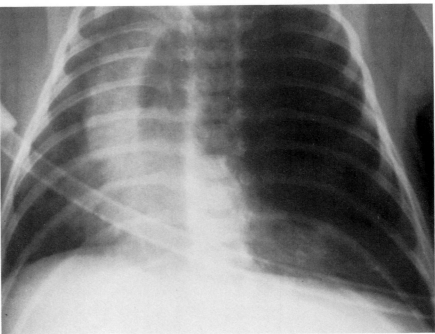

B

Figure 4–47. A, *Newborn infant with pulmonary density.* B, *This assumed the characteristics of lobar emphysema after a few days.* (Courtesy of Dr. M. Capitanio.)

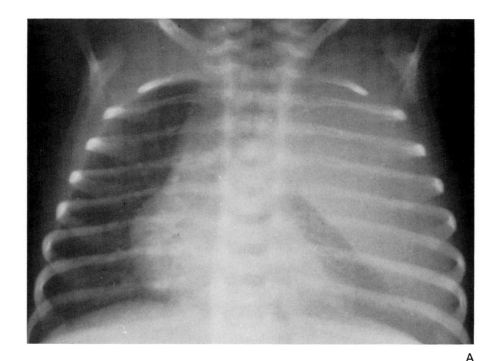

A

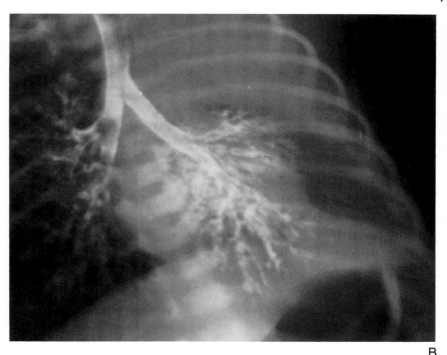

B

Figure 4–48. Bronchial atresia. A, Area of fluid density seen in left upper lobe. B, Bronchogram demonstrates normal bronchial segments. Surgical exploration disclosed anomalous atretic bronchus with fluid in lung distal to this. (From Griscom, N. T., et al.: Fluid-filled lung due to airway obstruction in the newborn. Pediatrics, 43:383, 1969.)

CONGENITAL CYSTIC ADENOMATOID MALFORMATION

Congenital cystic adenomatoid malformation of the lung represents one of the few truly congenital pulmonary cystic abnormalities consisting of multicystic pulmonary tissue associated with the proliferation of bronchial structures at the expense of alveolar development. Three types are recognized histologically. In type 1 there are single and multiple large cysts lined by ciliated pseudostratified columnar epithelium with smooth muscle in the cyst walls. Type 2 consists of multiple small cysts lined by cuboidal or columnar epithelium and without mucous cells. Type 3 is a large noncystic lesion containing bronchus-like structures lined by ciliated cuboidal epithelium. The prognoses of types 2 and 3 are less favorable than that of type 1 because of associated anomalies.

Although respiratory distress may not be present at birth it eventually occurs, and chest radiographs show an intrapulmonary mass within which radiolucent areas are scattered (Figs. 4–49 and 4–50). The areas of loculated air may simulate a diaphragmatic hernia. Occasionally, the lesion may appear as a large cyst (Fig. 4–51), or the mass may have a solid consistency without areas of radiolucency (Fig. 4–52). This is the expected finding if radiographs are made during the first few hours of life, before the trapped fetal lung fluid has been absorbed. Overlapping of cystic adenomatoid malformation with pulmonary sequestration may occur

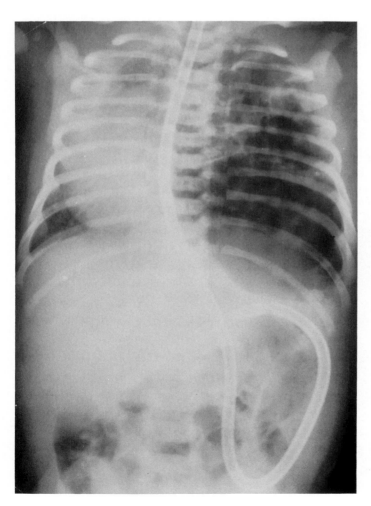

Figure 4–49. *Cystic adenomatoid malformation. Multiple areas of loculated air in the left hemithorax represent the congenital cystic disease simulating diaphragmatic hernia. However, the intestinal pattern is normal.*

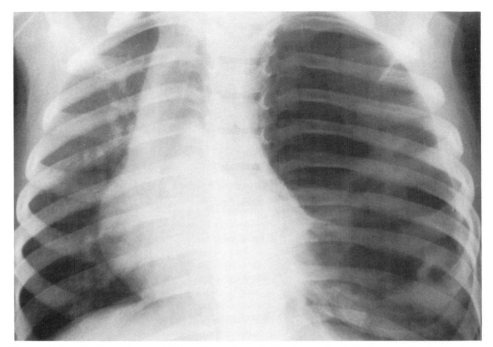

Figure 4–50. Cystic adenomatoid malformation of the lung. Frontal chest radiograph shows combination of hyperaeration and soft tissue density involving the left lung, with displacement of mediastinum to the right.

with anomalous systemic vessels supplying the pulmonary malformation (Fig. 4–53). Thoracotomy and resection of the involved area are usually necessary.

PHRENIC NERVE PARALYSIS AND EVENTRATION

Radiologic differentiation between phrenic nerve paralysis and eventration is frequently impossible. If there is associated Erb's palsy, with an elevated hemidiaphragm in an infant with respiratory distress, phrenic nerve paralysis is probably

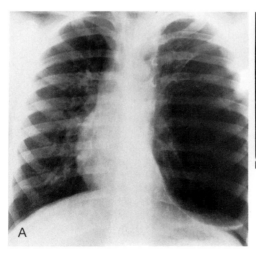

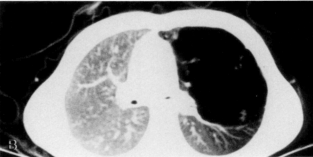

Figure 4–51. A, Cystic adenomatoid malformation presenting as a large solitary cyst of the left lung. B, Computerized tomography shows posterior displacement of the left pulmonary artery and the cystic characteristics of the cystic adenomatoid malformation.

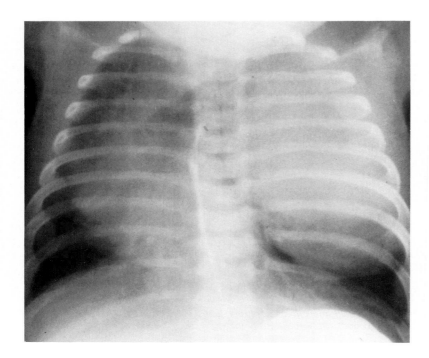

Figure 4–52. Solid cystic adenomatoid malformation in young infants. (Courtesy of V. Condon, Children's Hospital, Salt Lake City.)

Figure 4–53. A, Cystic adenomatoid malformation in a 3-year-old girl. Chest radiograph shows area of consolidation in the right lower lobe within which are several air-fluid levels.

Illustration continued on opposite page

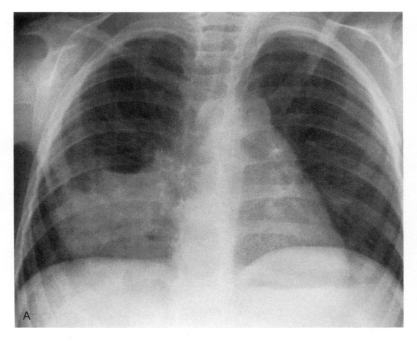

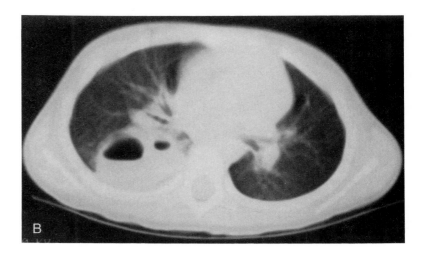

Figure 4–53. *B, Computerized tomography shows the posterior location of the lesion as well as the air-fluid levels. C, Digital subtraction arteriography shows systemic blood supply from the aorta to the right lower lobe lesion.*

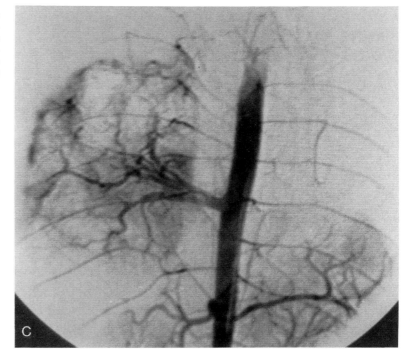

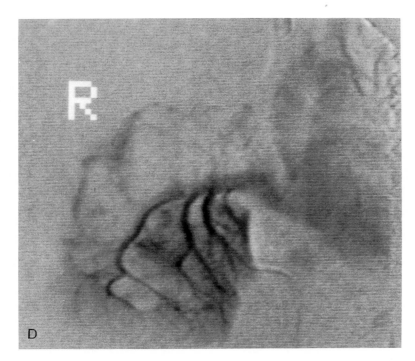

Figure 4–53. D, *Later phase of digital subtraction shows venous return to the right atrium. (Histologic diagnosis was type I cystic adenomatoid malformation.)*

present. An elevated diaphragm that does not show normal movement during respirations occurs in both eventration and phrenic nerve paralysis (Figs. 4–54 and 4–55). Semantic as well as radiologic differentiation of eventration and diaphragmatic hernia are confusing. Theoretically, if the partition between the chest cavity and abdomen contains striated muscle, even in scattered areas, it is an eventrated diaphragm; if it is a peritoneal sac without striated muscles, it is a hernia. Naturally, preoperative and even at times postoperative differentiation is impossible. Infants who appear to have an elevated diaphragm secondary to paralysis or eventration may benefit by surgical repair but recurrence is common. If possible, conservative management is advised. Respiratory problems become less prominent as the infant grows into childhood, presumably because an infant is more dependent on diaphragmatic breathing.

DIAPHRAGMATIC HERNIA

Many forms of congenital diaphragmatic hernia are readily recognized by chest radiographs. The most common type responsible for respiratory distress in the neonate is hernia of the pleuroperitoneal foramen, or foramen of Bochdalek. The hernia occurs more commonly on the left, but either side may be involved. The characteristic radiographic feature is that of multiple air- and fluid-filled loops of bowel having a cystic appearance in the affected hemithorax. Although the initial impression may be that of multiple pulmonary cysts, the absence of normal gas-containing bowel in the abdomen and the scaphoid appearance of the abdomen clinically are helpful features in diagnosis. Fetal ultrasound examination may detect this anomaly before birth (Fig. 4–56). Postoperative radiographs are useful in following the expansion of the usually hypoplastic lung (Fig. 4–57). Chest radiographs made prior to the passage of swallowed air into the herniated bowel will not show the radiolucent pattern but will show an opaque hemothorax. In rare instances during its early stage the appearance may be that of fluid density

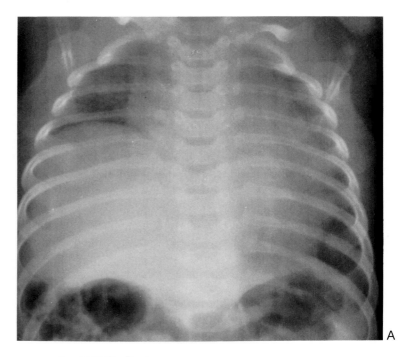

A

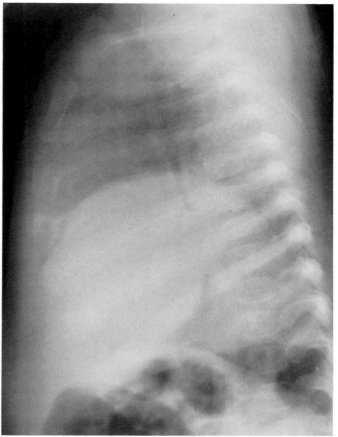

B

Figure 4–54. A, *Eventration of the diaphragm.* B, *Right hemidiaphragm is markedly elevated, and showed no movement during fluoroscopic examination.*

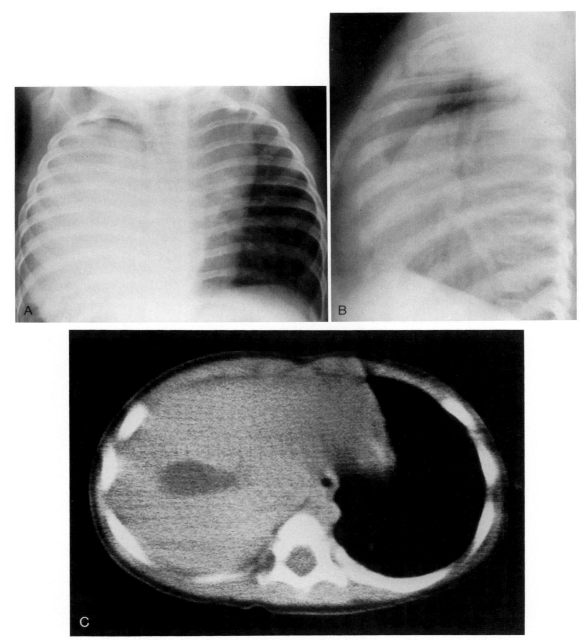

Figure 4–55. A, *Eventration of right hemidiaphragm. There was a 5-day history of cough and wheezing in a previously healthy 5-month-old girl. The frontal film demonstrates nearly completely opacified right hemithorax, with shift of heart and mediastinum to the left. B, Lateral view also demonstrates crescent of air in upper hemithorax. C, CT scan demonstrates the homogeneous density to be the liver, with the gallbladder within its midst.*

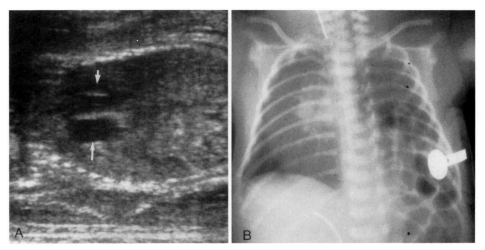

Figure 4–56. *Diaphragmatic hernia. A, Longitudinal fetal ultrasound shows that the heart is displaced to the right (short arrow) and the fluid-filled stomach (long arrow) is within the left side of the chest, displacing the heart to the right. B, Radiograph taken immediately after birth shows the left-sided diaphragmatic hernia and the heart mediastinum displaced to the right.*

within the chest, without the usually associated air-containing features (Fig. 4–58). Although an upper gastrointestinal tract study demonstrates the herniated bowel, it is rarely indicated (Fig. 4–59). Absence of gas within the abdomen may help to establish early recognition before air reaches the herniated bowel.

Paraesophageal hernias and esophageal hiatal hernias are usually associated with vomiting rather than with respiratory disturbance. Large paraesophageal hernias may be readily recognized on scout films of the chest and abdomen; they present as fluid- or air-filled cavities in the posterior right cardiophrenic region (Fig. 4–60). Upper gastrointestinal tract studies readily identify these lesions. Foramen of Morgagni hernias are extremely rare, and are not usually responsible for respiratory tract disturbances. They are also identified by upper gastrointestinal studies.

Delayed appearance of right diaphragmatic hernia should be suspected in the newborn with increasing respiratory distress accomplished by poor aeration of the right lower lobe, shift of the mediastinum to the left, elevation of the hepatic flexure, and apparent elevation of the diaphragm (Figs. 4–61 and 4–62).

ACCESSORY DIAPHRAGM

This rare anomaly is usually not responsible for respiratory distress, but is more often discovered as an incidental finding, particularly if the radiologist is familiar with its appearance. The condition is associated with hypoplasia of the lung, and, although either hemithorax may be involved, the condition is more common on the right side. The condition may be misinterpreted as lobar atelectasis or alveolar hypoplasia. The affected side is less radiolucent that the normal side, and mediastinal structures may be shifted to the side of the accessory diaphragm. The accessory diaphragm is complete anteriorly and incomplete posteromedially, and divides the pulmonary tissue into two compartments. The diaphragm extends from the normal anterior portion of the diaphragm, and inserts higher and more posteriorly along the fifth to seventh ribs. The lateral view shows a characteristic soft tissue density produced by loose areolar connective tissue paralleling the anterior chest wall (Fig. 4–63). Associated anomalies include congenital heart disease, anomalous pulmonary venous return, and diaphragmatic hernia.

Text continued on page 122

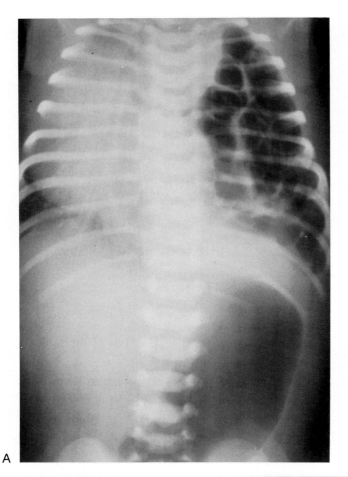

A

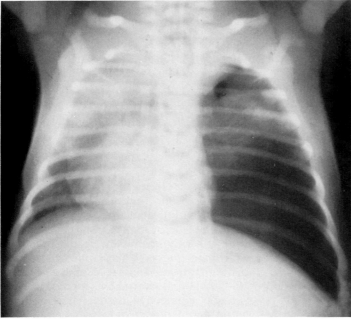

B

Figure 4–57. Foramen of Bochdalek diaphragmatic hernia. A, Preoperative examination shows multiple air-filled loops of bowel in the left hemithorax, displacing the mediastinum to the right. B, Postoperative examination 2 days later shows partial expansion of the left lung.

Illustration continued on opposite page

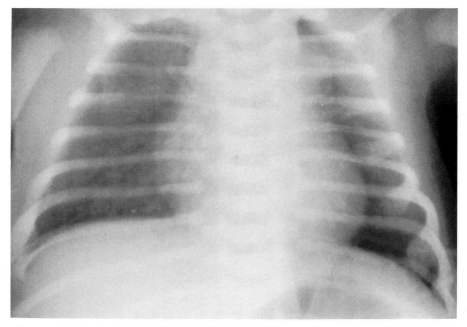

Figure 4–57. C, Examination 1 week after repair of the hernia shows complete expansion of the lung.

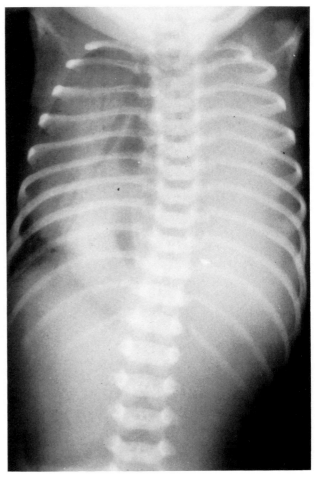

Figure 4–58. Foramen of Bochdalek hernia. The left hemithorax is opaque and there is absence of intestinal gas in the abdomen and in the herniated bowel. The examination was made in the first few minutes of life, before ingested air had entered the gastrointestinal tract.

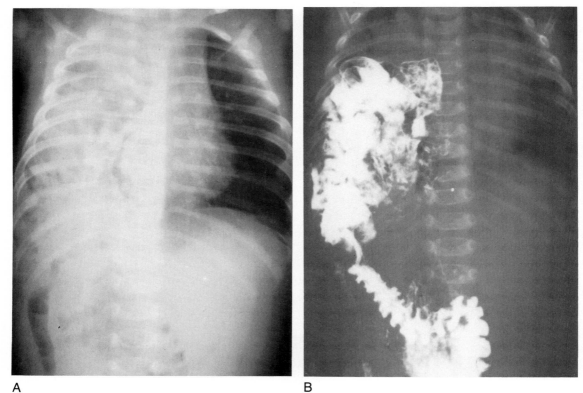

A   B

Figure 4–59. *Foramen of Bochdalek hernia. A, Loops of bowel are seen within the right hemithorax. B, Upper gastrointestinal tract examination outlines the herniated intestinal tract. The entire small bowel and most of the colon are in the right hemithorax.*

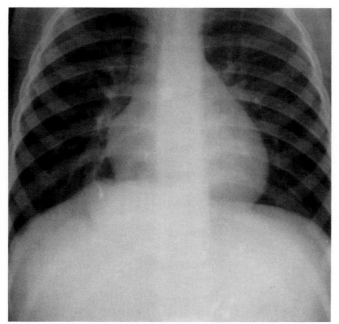

Figure 4–60. *Paraesophageal hiatus hernia. A, Frontal view of the chest shows air-fluid level in the herniated stomach.*

Illustration continued on opposite page

A

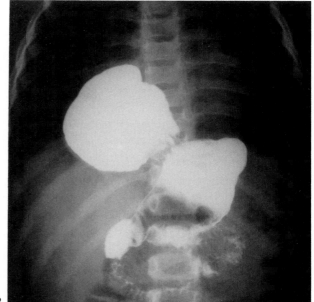

Figure 4–60. B, *Upper gastrointestinal tract examination outlines the herniated gastric fundus.*

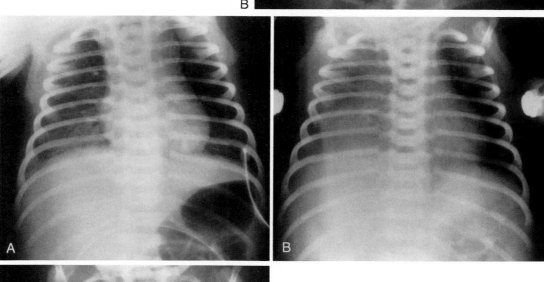

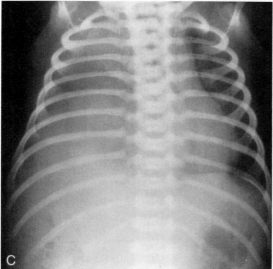

Figure 4–61. A, *Delayed presentation of right diaphragmatic hernia at 1 day of life. The initial chest radiograph demonstrates mild infiltration at both lung bases. B, Five days later the infiltration appears to be increasing, and the contour of the right hemidiaphragm is obscured. C, Three days later (ninth day of life) the right hemithorax is nearly completely opacified, and the heart and mediastinum are shifted to the left. This suggests a space-occupying lesion in right chest; however, the position of the hepatic flexure of colon is now elevated. The liver is protruding into the right hemithorax.*

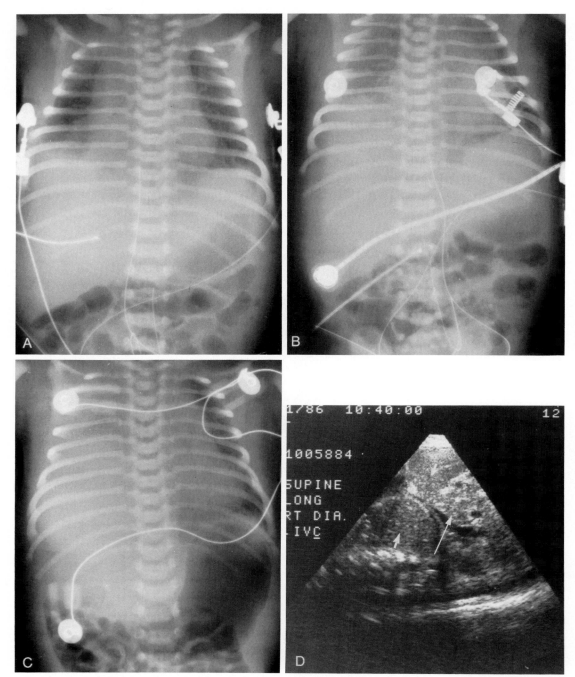

Figure 4–62. *Delayed presentation of right diaphragmatic hernia. A, Anteroposterior view of the chest at 1 day of age shows an ill-defined area of density at the right lung base. B, Anteroposterior view of the chest and abdomen at 2 days of age shows further increased density at the right lung base, and the heart and mediastinum are displaced slightly to the left side. C, At 4 days of age there is complete opacification of the right hemithorax, and the inferior margin of the liver is displaced upward. Gas-filled bowel loops extend upward into the right upper quandrant. D, Longitudinal real-time sector scan of the right upper quadrant shows liver parenchyma (small arrows) below and above the level of the right hemidiaphragm. The sector also includes a portion of the upper pole of the right kidney and inferior vena cava (long arrow).*

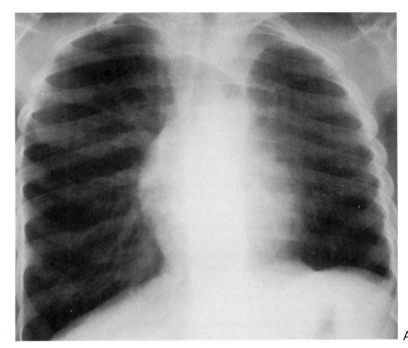

A

Figure 4–63. *Accessory diaphragm. A, Frontal chest radiograph shows that the normally sharp margin of the mediastinum is replaced by a hazy density, and the volume of the left hemithorax is diminished with elevation of the left hemidiaphragm. There is hyperaeration of the right lung, with herniation across the midline. B, A zone of homogeneous density parallels the sternum and blends with the diaphragm posterior to the xiphoid. (Courtesy of Dr. P. Allen.)*

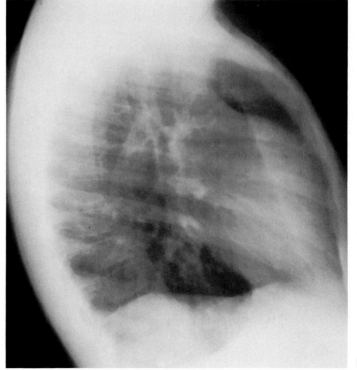

B

VASCULAR RING

There are a variety of vascular rings, most of which are responsible for inspiratory and expiratory stridor as well as for more severe forms of respiratory distress. Chronic or recurrent pneumonia, particularly on the right, is commonly associated with ring anomalies, and appropriate radiologic studies should be performed. The most common vascular anomalies that encircle the trachea and esophagus are a double aortic arch, with a common descending aorta usually on the left, and a right aortic arch with a ligamentum arteriosum or ductus arteriosus. A double arch is the type of ring most likely to cause symptoms in early infancy. Compression of the trachea by a large right aortic arch in patients with tetralogy of Fallot and truncus arteriosus may also occur.

Retroesophageal subclavian arteries are usually incidental findings, and are not commonly associated with respiratory problems. Routine fluoroscopic examination of the chest, as well as radiographs with the esophagus outlined with barium, are helpful in identifying vascular ring anomalies. There is compression on the anterior portion of the trachea and on the posterior portion of the barium-filled esophagus (Fig. 4–64). Changes in the size of the tracheal lumen during respirations may be recorded on cine film or videotape, with the tracheal lumen becoming markedly narrowed at the site of compression during expiration. Accurate differentiation of the types of ring anomalies is frequently impossible without angiograms and, although angiocardiography is useful in defining the type of vascular anomaly more clearly, it is unnecessary for surgical correction. Digital subtraction angiography represents a new and less invasive technique than arterial catheter arteriography (Fig. 4–65).

Left pulmonary artery sling anomaly is another vascular defect that may be responsible for respiratory disturbance or recurrent pneumonia. Routine radiographs and fluoroscopic studies may provide presumptive evidence of this defect,

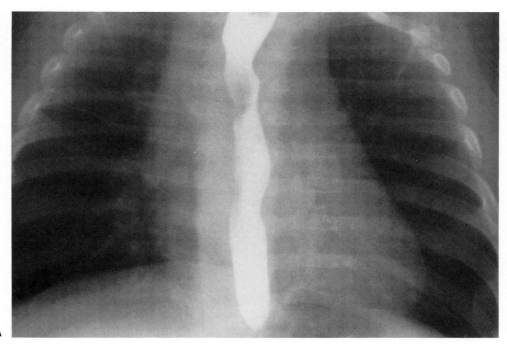

A

Figure 4–64. Vascular ring. A, Frontal view of the chest shows an indentation on the right side of the esophagus at the level of the aortic arch.

Illustration continued on opposite page

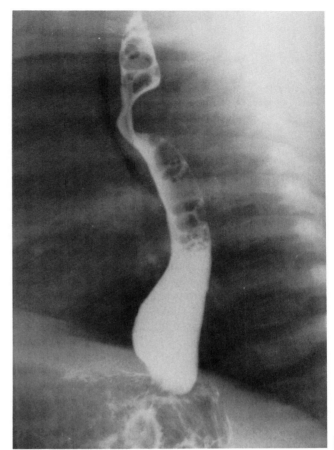

Figure 4–64. B, Lateral view shows an indentation on the esophagus caused by a large retroesophageal vessel and by constriction of the trachea. There is minimal infiltration in the right midlobe.

B

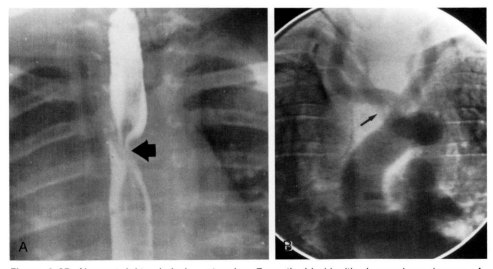

Figure 4–65. Aberrant right subclavian artery in a 7-month-old girl with abnormal esophagram. A, Prominent impression on left side of midesophagus (arrow). B, Digital subtraction angiogram using continuous mode technique shows aberrant right subclavian artery (arrow).

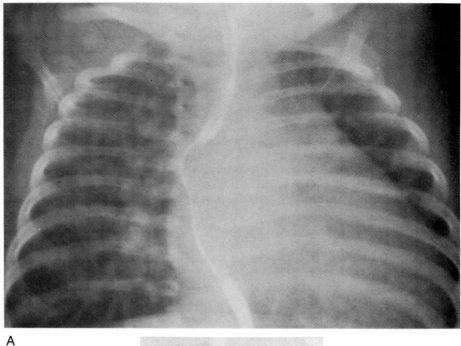

A

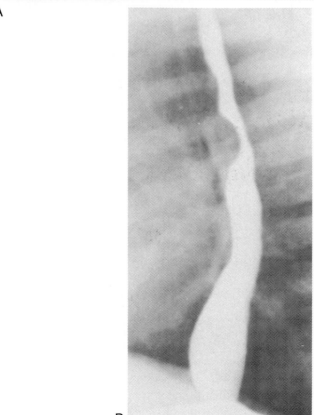

B

Figure 4–66. *Left pulmonary artery sling anomaly. A, Frontal chest radiograph shows local indentation on the left side of the barium column. B, Lateral radiograph shows anterior indentation of the esophagus by the aberrant left pulmonary artery.*

Illustration continued on opposite page

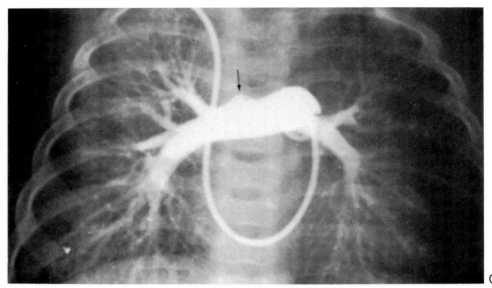

Figure 4–66. C, *Angiocardiogram shows ectopic origin of the left pulmonary artery (arrow).*

but pulmonary angiography is necessary for confirmation. In this condition the left pulmonary artery passes over the proximal aspect of the right main bronchus, behind the trachea, and in front of the esophagus. In so doing, it compresses the posterior tracheal wall or right main stem bronchus and the adjacent anterior wall of the esophagus. Routine films may show an increased distance between the esophagus and tracheal air column. The right lung is frequently overinflated as a result of partial obstruction by the ectopic left pulmonary artery. Occasionally, there will be hypoinflation of the right lung. The respiratory difficulty in these patients apparently is caused by complete or fragmented cartilaginous rings in the trachea above the carina rather than by external pressure by the aberrant artery. The trachea and major bronchi may have a dowser (Y-shaped) configuration, with both bronchi having the configuration of left major bronchus. Angiocardiography will demonstrate the lesion accurately (Fig. 4–66).

CHYLOTHORAX

Congenital chylothorax results from the leakage of chyle into the pleural space, and is presumably caused by congenital defects in the thoracic duct or by trauma, or may be iatrogenic following prolonged hyperalimentation. The radiographic features are those of massive pleural effusion, and diagnosis is made by thoracentesis (Fig. 4–67).

CONGENITAL DEFORMITY OF THE THORAX

Although many deformities of the thoracic cage constrict respiratory efforts, asphyxiating thoracic dystrophy, or Jeune's syndrome, represents an extreme example (Fig. 4–68). In this condition the small size of the thoracic cage severely restricts respiration, and early death is usually the result. Thanatophoric dwarfism is another related condition in which the size of the thoracic cage limits respirations to the extent that it is incompatible with life (Fig. 4–69).

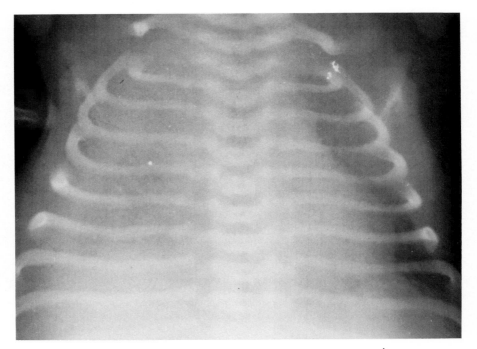

Figure 4–67. *Chylothorax. There is complete opacification of the right hemithorax by extensive pleural effusion. Diagnosis was made by thoracentesis. Several thoracenteses were necessary before spontaneous remission occurred.*

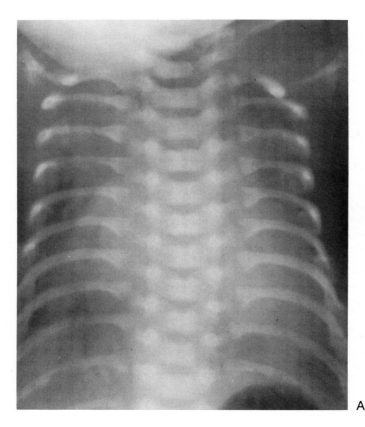

Figure 4–68. *Asphyxiating thoracic dystrophy. A, Frontal chest radiograph shows a small thoracic cage, with resulting limitation of pulmonary expansion.*

Illustration continued on opposite page

A

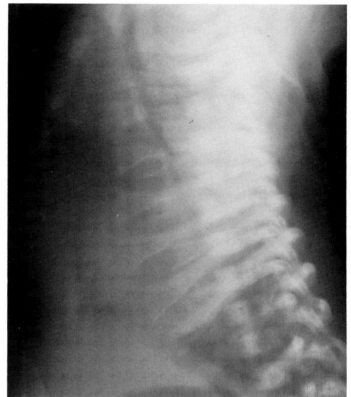

B

Figure 4–68. B, *Lateral view shows marked shortening of the ribs to better advantage.*

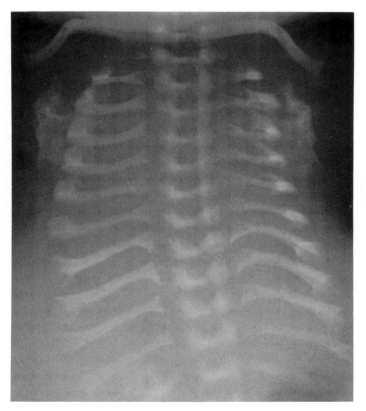

Figure 4–69. *Thanatophoric dwarf. Frontal chest radiograph shows the marked shortening of the ribs and the resulting deformity of the thoracic cage without pulmonary aeration.*

SUGGESTED READINGS

OBSTRUCTION OF UPPER AIR PASSAGES

Capitanio MA, and Kirkpatrick JA Jr: Upper respiratory tract obstruction in infants and children. Radiol Clin North Am, 6:265, 1968.

Capitanio MA, and Kirkpatrick JA Jr: Nasopharyngeal lymphoid tissue: Roentgen observations in 257 children two years of age or less. Radiology, 96:389, 1970.

Carswell F, Kerr MM, and Hutchinson JH: Congenital goiter and hypothyroidism produced by maternal ingestion of iodide. Lancet, 1:1241, 1970.

Currarino G, and Williams B: Lateral inspiration and expiration radiographs of the neck in children with laryngotracheitis. Radiology, 145:365, 1982.

Dunbar JS: Upper respiratory tract obstruction in infants and children. Caldwell Lecturer, 1969. Am J Roentgenol, 109:277, 1970.

Fagan CJ, and Swischuk LE: Juvenile laryngeal papillomatosis with spread to the lungs. Am J Dis Child, 123:139, 1972.

Fernbach SK et al.: Radiologic evaluation of adenoids and tonsils in children with obstructive sleep apnea: Plain films and fluoroscopy. Pediatr Radiol, 13:258, 1983.

Fujioka N, Young LD, and Girdany BR: Radiographic evaluation of adenoidal size in children: Adenoidal-nasopharyngeal ratio. Am J Roentgenol, 133:401, 1979.

Grunebaum M, and Moskowitz G: The retropharyngeal soft tissues in young infants with hypothyroidism. Am J Roentgenol, 108:543, 1970.

Han BK, Dunbar JS, and Striker TW: Membranous laryngotracheobronchitis (membranous croup). Am J Roentgenol, 133:53, 1979.

Hengerer AS, Strome M, and Jaffe BF: Injuries to the neonatal larynx from long-term endotracheal tube intubation and suggested tube modification for prevention. Ann Otol, 84:764, 1975.

Henry RL, Mellis CM, and Benjamin B: Pseudomembranous croup. Arch Dis Child, 58:180, 1983.

Iancu T, Boyanower U, and Laurin M: Congenital goiter due to maternal ingestion of iodide. Am J Dis Child, 128:528, 1974.

Jerald B, and Dungan WT: Cor pulmonale and pulmonary edema in children secondary to chronic airway obstruction. Radiology, 90:679, 1968.

Jeresaty RM, Huzar RJ, and Basu S: Pierre Robin syndrome. Cause of respiratory obstruction, cor pulmonale, and pulmonary edema. Am J Dis Child, 117:710, 1969.

Joseph PM et al.: Airway obstruction in infants and children. Radiology, 121:143, 1976.

Kanter RK, and Watchko JF: Pulmonary edema associated with upper airway obstruction. Am J Dis Child, 138:365, 1984.

Kushner DC, and Harris GBC: Obstructing lesions of the larynx and trachea in infants and children. Radiol Clin North Am, 16:181, 1978.

Landing BH, and Theadis RW: Tracheobronchial anomalies in children. Perspect Pediatr Pathol, 1:1, 1973.

Lofgren RH: Respiratory distress from congenital lingual cysts. Am J Dis Child, 106:610, 1963.

MacPherson R, and Leithiser RE: Upper airway obstruction in children: An update. Radiographics, 5:339, 1985.

Mahboubi S, Borden S, and Potsic W: Lingual cyst. Report of two cases. Am J Roentgenol, 133:751, October 1979.

McCook TA, and Felman AH: Retropharyngeal masses in infants and children. Am J Dis Child, 133:441, 1979.

McCook TA, and Kirks DR: Epiglottic enlargement in infants and children: Another radiologic look. Pediatr Radiol, 12:227, 1982.

Meine FJ et al.: Pharyngeal distension associated with upper airway obstruction. Radiology, 112:395, 1974.

Moskowitz PS, Sue JY, and Gooding CA: Tracheal coccidioidomycosis causing upper airway obstruction in children. Am J Roentgenol, 139:596, 1982.

Parkin JL, Stevens NH, and Jung AL: Acquired and congenital subglottic stenosis in the infant. Ann Otol, 85:573, 1976.

Rivero HJ, Young LW, and Flom L: Reliability of retropharyngeal soft tissue measurements in infants and children: New standards based on 586 normals. Presented to the Society of Pediatric Radiology, April 1986.

Rosen L, Hanafee W, and Nahum A: Nasopharyngeal angiofibroma, and angiographic evaluation. Radiology, 86:103, 1966.

Scott JR, and Kramer SS: Pediatric tracheostomy I: Radiographic features of normal healing. Am J Roentgenol, 130:887, 1978.

Scott JR, and Kramer SS: Pediatric tracheostomy II: Radiographic features of difficult decannulations. Am J Roentgenol, 130:893, 1978.

Slovis TL et al.: Choanal atresia: Precise CT evaluation. Radiology, 155:345, 1985.

Smith RJH, and Catlin FI: Congenital anomalies of the larynx. Am J Dis Child, 138:35, 1984.

Swischuk LE, Smith PC, and Fagan CJ: Abnormalities of the pharynx and larynx in childhood. Semin Roentgenol, 9:283, October 1974.

Taybi H: Congenital malformations of the larynx, trachea, bronchi and lungs. Progr Pediatr Radiol, 1:231, 1967.

Trail ML, Creely JJ Jr, and Landrum CE: Congenital choanal atresia. South Med J, 66:460, 1973.
Watts FD Jr, and Slovis TL: The enlarged epiglottis. Pediatr Radiol, 5:133, 1977.
Whitehouse WM, and Holt JF: Paradoxical expiratory ballooning of the hypopharynx in siblings with bilateral choanal atresia. Radiology, 59:216, 1952.
Williams HJ: Posterior choanal atresia. Am J Roentgenol, 112:1, 1971.
Wittenborg NH, Gyepes MT, and Crocker D: Tracheal dynamics in infants with respiratory distress, stridor and collapsing trachea. Radiology, 88:653, April 1967.

ASPIRATION OF FOREIGN BODIES

Baker DH, Berdon WE, and Grossman H: Physical and chemical injuries to the respiratory tract. Progr Pediatr Radiol, 1:326, 1967.
Berdon WE: Editorial comment (Foley catheter removal of esophageal foreign bodies). Pediatr Radiol, 13:119, 1983.
Campbell JB, Quattromani FL, and Foley RLC: Foley catheter removal of blunt esophageal foreign bodies: Experience with 100 consecutive children. Pediatr Radiol, 13:116, 1983.
Kassay D: Observation on 100 cases of bronchial foreign body. Arch Otolaryngol, 71:42, 1960.
Reed MH: Radiology of airway foreign bodies in children. J Can Assoc Radiol, 28:111, 1977.
Smith PD, Swischuk LD, and Fagan CJ: An elusive and often unsuspected cause of stridor or pneumonia (the esophageal foreign body). Am J Roentgenol, 122:178, 1974.

ESOPHAGEAL ATRESIA AND TRACHEOESOPHAGEAL FISTULA

Felman AH: The Pediatric Chest. Radiological, Clinical and Pathological Observations, pp 6–11. Springfield, IL, Charles C Thomas, 1983.
Filler RM, Rossello PJ, and Lebowitz RL: Life-threatening anoxic spells caused by tracheal compression after repair of esophageal atresia. Correction by surgery. J Pediatr Surg, 11:739, 1976.
Gray SW, and Skandalakis JE: Embryologic basis for the treatment of congenital defect. In Embryology for Surgeons, pp 69–79. Philadelphia, WB Saunders, 1972.
Haight C, and Towsley HA: Congenital atresia of esophagus with tracheoesophageal fistula, extrapleural ligation of fistula and end-to-end anastomosis of esophageal segments. Surg Gynecol Obstet, 76:672, 1943.
Holt JF, Haight C, and Hodges FJ: Congenital atresia of esophagus and tracheoesophageal fistula. Radiology, 47:457, 1946.
Kirkpatrick JA, Cresson SL, and Pilling GP: The motor activity of the esophagus in association with esophageal atresia and tracheoesophageal fistula. Am J Roentgenol, 86:884, 1961.
Kushner DC, and Harris GBC: Obstructing lesions of the larynx and trachea in infants and children. Radiol Clin North Am, 16:181, 1978.
Singleton EB, Wagner ML, and Dutton RV: Radiology of the Alimentary Tract in Infants and Children, 2nd ed., pp 55–65. Philadelphia, WB Saunders, 1977.

FOREGUT MALFORMATIONS

Effman E et al.: Tracheal agenesis. Am J Roentgenol, 125:767, 1975.
Felson B: The many faces of pulmonary sequestration. Semin Roentgenol, 7:3, 1972.
Gerle RD et al.: Congenital bronchopulmonary foregut malformations: Pulmonary sequestration communicating with the intestinal tract. N Engl J Med, 278:1413, 1968.

PNEUMOMEDIASTINUM AND PNEUMOTHORAX

Avery ME, Fletcher BD, and Williams R: Lung and Its Disorders in the Newborn Infant, 4th ed. Philadelphia, WB Saunders, 1981 p 284.
Berdon WE et al.: Localized pneumothorax adjacent to a collapsed lobe: A sign of bronchial obstruction. Radiology, 150:691, 1984.
Chernick V, and Avery ME: Spontaneous alveolar rupture at birth. Pediatrics, 32:816, 1963.
Dumas C et al.: Iatrogenic lesions of the upper airway in the newborn. J Can Assoc Radiol, 34:3, 1983.
Han SY, Rudolph AJ, and Teng CT: Pneumomediastinum in infancy. J Pediatr, 62:754, 1963.
MacEwan DW et al.: Pneumothorax in the neonate. Its recognition and its evaluation. Ann Radiol, 7:459, 1964.
Morrow G, Hope JW, and Boggs TR: Pneumomediastinum, a silent lesion in the newborn. J Pediatr, 70:354, 1967.
Singleton EB: Radiological considerations of intensive care in the premature infant. Radiology, 140:291, 1981.
Stern L et al.: Pneumothorax and pneumomediastinum associated with renal malformations in newborn infants. Am J Roentgenol, 116:785, 1972.

CONGENITAL LOBAR EMPHYSEMA

Allen RP, Taylor RL, and Reiquan CW: Congenital lobar emphysema with dilated septal lymphatics. Radiology, 86:929, May 1966.
Campbell PE: Congenital lobar emphysema. Aust Paediatr J, 5:226, 1969.
Capitanio MA, and Kirkpatrick JA Jr: Roentgen examination in the evaluation of the newborn infant with respiratory distress. J Pediatr, 75:896, 1969.
Franken EA, and Buehl I: Infantile lobar emphysema. Report of two cases with unusual roentgen manifestations. Am J Roentgenol, 98:354, 1966.
Griscom NT et al.: Fluid-filled lung due to airway obstruction in the newborn. Pediatrics, 43:383, 1969.
Hendren WH, and McKee DM: Lobar emphysema of infancy. J Pediatr Surg, 1(1):24, 1966.
Hislop A, and Reid L: New pathological findings in emphysema of childhood. I. Polyalveolar lobe with emphysema. Thorax, 25:682, 1970.
Jones, JC, et al.: Lobar emphysema and congenital heart disease in infancy. J Thorac Cardiovasc Surg, 49:1, 1965.

CONGENITAL CYSTIC ADENOMATOID MALFORMATION

Birdsell BC et al.: Congenital cystic adenomatoid malformation of the lung. A report of eight cases. Can J Surg, 9:350, 1966.
Craig JM, Kirkpatrick JA Jr, and Neuhauser EBD: Congenital cystic adenomatoid malformation of lungs in infants. Am J Roentgenol, 76:516, 1956.
Madewell JE et al.: Cystic adenomatoid malformation of the lung. Am J Roentgenol, 124:436, 1972.
Moccia WA, Kaude JV, and Felman AH: Congenital eventration of the diaphragm. Diagnosis by ultrasound. Pediatr Radiol, 10:197, 1981.
Stocker JT, Drake RM, and Madewell JE: Cystic and congenital lung disease in the newborn. Perspect Pediatr Pathol, 4:93, 1978.
Stocker JT, Madewell JE, and Drake RM: Congenital cystic adenomatoid malformation of the lung: Classification and morphologic spectrum. Hum Pathol, 8:155, 1977.

PHRENIC NERVE PARALYSIS AND EVENTRATION

Lundstrom CH, and Allen RP: Bilateral congenital eventration of the diaphragm. Case report with roentgen manifestations. Am J Roentgenol, 97:216, 1966.
McNamara JJ et al.: Eventration of the diaphragm. Surgery, 64:1013, 1968.

DIAPHRAGMATIC HERNIA

Berdon WE, Baker DH, and Amoury R: The role of pulmonary hypoplasia in the prognosis of newborn infants with diaphragmatic hernia and eventration. Am J Roentgenol, 103:413, 1968.
Chin DH et al.: Congenital diaphragmatic hernia diagnosed prenatally by ultrasound. Radiology 148:119, 1983.
Hobbins JC et al.: Ultrasound in a diagnosis of congenital anomalies. Am J Obstet Gynecol, 134:331, 1979.
Kenny JD et al.: Right-sided diaphragmatic hernia of delayed onset in the newborn infant. South Med J, 70:373, 1977.
Kirchner SG et al.: Delayed radiographic presentation of congenital right diaphragmatic hernia. Radiology 115:155, 1975.
McCarten KM et al.: Delayed appearance of right diaphragmatic hernia associated with group B streptococcal infection in newborns. Radiology, 139:385, 1982.
Merten DF et al.: Anteromedian diaphragmatic defects in infancy: Current approachs to diagnostic imaging. Radiology, 142:361, 1982.
Shkolnik A et al.: New application of real-time ultrasound in pediatrics. RadioGraphics, 2:422, 1982.
Silverman FN (ed.): Caffey's Pediatric X-Ray Diagnosis, 8th ed, pp 1785–1791. Chicago, Year Book Medical Publishers, 1985.
Singleton EB, Wagner ML, and Dutton RV: Radiology of the Alimentary Tract in Infants and Children, 2nd ed, pp 377–389. Philadelphia, WB Saunders, 1977.

ACCESSORY DIAPHRAGM

Davis WS, and Allen RP: Accessory diaphragm. Radiol Clin North Am, 6:253, 1968.
Felson, B: Pulmonary agenesis and related anomalies. Semin Roentgenol, 7:17, 1972.
Hashida Y, and Sherman FE: Accessory diaphragm associated with neonatal respiratory distress. J Pediatr, 59:529, 1961.
Kenanoglu A, and Tunchilek E: Accessory diaphragm on the left side. Pediatr Radiol, 7:172, 1978.
Nigogosyan G, and Ozardo A: Accessory diaphragm. A case report. Am J Roentgenol, 85:309, 1961.
Slovis TL et al.: Choanal atresia: Precise CT evaluation. Radiology, 155:345, 1985.

VASCULAR RING

Berdon WE, and Baker DH: Vascular anomalies and the infant lung: Rings, slings and other things. Semin Roentgenol, 7:39, 1972.

Berdon WE et al.: Innominate artery compression of trachea in infants with stridor and apnea. Radiology, 92:272, 1969.

Capitanio MA, Ramos R, and Kirkpatrick JA Jr: Pulmonary sling roentgen observation. Am J Radiol, 122:28, 1971.

Capitanio MA et al.: Obstruction of the airway by the aorta: An observation in infants with congenital heart disease. Am J Roentgenol, 140:675, 1983.

Clarkson PM et al.: Aberrant left pulmonary artery. Am J Dis Child, 113:373, 1967.

Hallman GL, Cooley DA, and Gutgesell HP: Surgical Treatment of Congenital Heart Disease, 3rd ed. Philadelphia, Lea & Febiger, 1987.

Jue KL et al.: Anomalous origin of the left pulmonary artery from the right pulmonary artery. Report of two cases and review of the literature. Am J Roentgenol, 95:598, 1965.

Shuford WH, Sybers RG, and Edwards FK: The three types of right aortic arch. Am J Roentgenol, 109:67, 1970.

Silverman FN (ed.): Caffey's Pediatric X-Ray Diagnosis, 8th ed, pp 1045–1057. Chicago, Year Book Medical Publishers, 1985.

Stewart JR, Kincaid OW, and Edwards JE: An Atlas of Vascular Rings and Related Malformations of the Aortic Arch System. Springfield, IL, Charles C Thomas, 1964.

CHYLOTHORAX

Avery ME, Fletcher BD, and Williams RG: The Lung and Its Disorders in the Newborn Infant, 4th ed., pp 197–199. Philadelphia, WB Saunders, 1981.

Decancq HG: Treatment of chylothorax in children. Surg Gynecol Obstet, 121:509, September 1965.

Knight L, Tobin J Jr, and L'Heureaux P: Hydrothorax: A complication of hyperalimentation with radiologic manifestations. Radiology, 111:693, 1974.

Kramer SS, Taylor GA, and Simmons MA: Lethal chylothoraces due to superior vena caval thrombosis in infants. Am J Roentgenol, 137:559, 1981.

CONGENITAL DEFORMITY OF THE THORAX

Barnes ND, Hull D, and Soimons JS: Thoracic dystrophy. Arch Dis Child, 44:11, 1969.

Herdman RC, and Langer LO: Thoracic asphyxiant dystrophy and renal disease. Am J Dis Child, 116:192, 1968.

Keats TE, Riddervold HO, and Michaelis LL: Thanatophoric dwarfism. Am J Roentgenol, 108:473, 1970.

Parienty R, and Maroteaux P: Pulmonary effects of skeletal diseases. Progr Pediatr Radiol, 1:218, 1967.

Prinar T, and Neuhauser EB: Asphyxiating thoracic dystrophy of the newborn. Am J Roentgenol, 98:358, 1966.

Stokes DC, et al.: Respiratory complications of achondroplasia. J Pediatr, 102:534, 1983.

5 PULMONARY INFECTIONS OF NEWBORNS, INFANTS, AND CHILDREN

NEONATAL PNEUMONIA
Group B Streptococcal Pneumonia
Listeria Monocytogenes
Chlamydia Pneumonia
TORCH
Pneumonia Alba
Tuberculosis
ACUTE DISORDERS
Bronchiolitis
Bronchitis
Pneumonia
    Bacterial Pneumonias
    Viral Pneumonias
    Primary Atypical Pneumonia
Hydrocarbon Pneumonia
Near Drowning
CHRONIC OR RECURRENT
  DISORDERS
Allergic Pneumonitis
Reactive Airway Disease (Asthma)
Cystic Fibrosis
Pneumonia Complicating Congenital
  Heart Disease
Aspiration Pneumonia
Bronchiectasis
Pulmonary Sequestration

Esophageal Bronchus
Hypoimmune Diseases
    Congenital Immune Deficiency
    Acquired Immune Deficiency
      Syndrome
Chronic Granulomatous Disease of
  Childhood
Pneumocystis Carinii Pneumonia
Cytomegalic Inclusion Disease
  Pneumonia
Childhood Tuberculosis
Pulmonary Mycoses
Sarcoidosis
Parasitosis
Other Interstitial Pneumonias
    Idiopathic or Usual Interstitial
      Pneumonia (UIP)
    Desquamative Interstitial
      Pneumonia (DIP)
    Lymphocytic Interstitial Pneumonia
      (LIP)
Lymphomatoid Granulomatosis
Ectodermal Dysplasia
Shwachman Syndrome
Inflammatory Pseudotumor

NEONATAL PNEUMONIA

Infectious agents causing neonatal lung infections are contracted either in the uterus or during passage through the birth canal. The clinical symptoms are usually recognized during the first few days of life, although the less virulent infections may not become evident until several weeks have passed.

Group B Streptococcal Pneumonia

Group B streptococcal pneumonia may be present at birth, or during the first days of life, and may resemble hyaline membrane disease clinically and radiographically. Frequently there is a history of premature and prolonged rupture of the membranes. Affected infants are often of low birth weight. Signs of sepsis and positive blood cultures establish the diagnosis. Radiographically the lungs show a granular pattern and air bronchogram similar to those of hyaline membrane disease (Fig. 5–1). The reason for this is unclear, especially because infants who do not live may show histologic changes of atypical hyaline membrane disease. Other neonates with group B streptococcal pneumonia may show areas of consolidation similar to those of bacterial pneumonias seen in older infants (Fig. 5–2). Associated osteomyelitis is a common complication.

Listeria Monocytogenes Pneumonia

Listeria monocytogenes is a gram-positive rod that may produce pneumonia in the neonate. Chest radiographs may resemble meconium aspiration pneumonia and show disseminated, coarse pulmonary infiltrates with pulmonary hyperinflation (Fig. 5–3). The clinical course of sepsis, history of maternal febrile illness prior to birth, and a chocolate-colored amniotic fluid help to establish the diagnosis. The diagnosis is confirmed by isolation of the agent from blood. If there is generalized septicemia, with meningitis, the condition may be described as granulomatosis infantiseptica.

Chlamydial Pneumonia

Chlamydial pneumonia, previously named pertussoid eosinophilic pneumonia, occurs in infants usually between 1 and 4 months of age. It is the result of infection by Chlamydia trachomatis, an obligate intracellular parasite similar to viruses that are susceptible to certain antibiotics such as erythromycin and tetracycline. The infant is infected during the birth process if the mother has chlamydial urethritis or cervicitis. Clinically the infants are usually afebrile, have a pertussislike cough, conjunctivitis, eosinophilia, and elevated IgM, IgG, and IgA levels. The most significant of these is the increased IgM concentration. Radiographically the lungs generally show a pattern of bronchopneumonia, with ill-defined small nodular densities scattered symmetrically throughout both lungs (Fig. 5–4). The identifi-

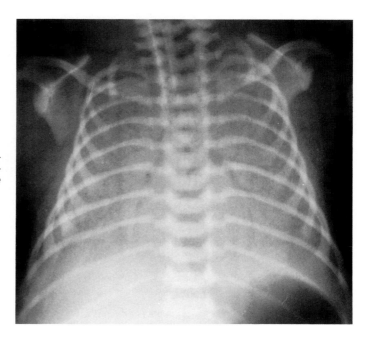

Figure 5–1. Group B streptococcal pneumonia in a 2-day-old infant. The diffuse granularity and air bronchogram resemble those of hyaline membrane disease.

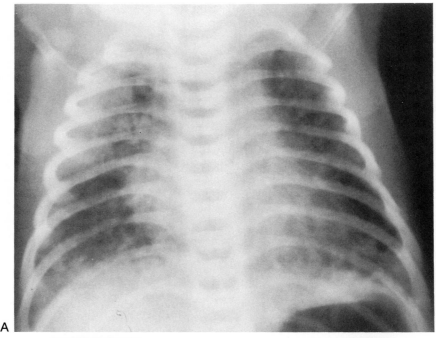

A

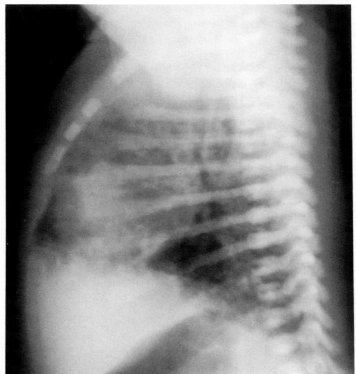

B

Figure 5–2. *Intrauterine infectious pneumonia. A, Chest radiograph shows segmental areas of atelectasis and air trapping, as well as coarse linear densities occupying both lungs. B, Lateral view shows flattening of the diaphragm and increase in anteroposterior diameter of the chest (bacteriologic evidence of streptococcal pneumonia).*

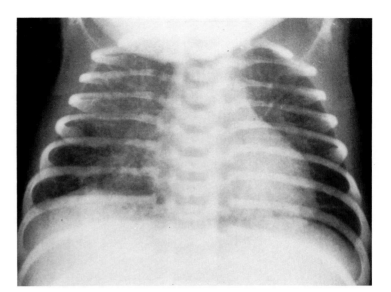

Figure 5–3. Listeria monocytogenes pneumonia in a neonate. Inflammatory infiltrates involve both lungs.

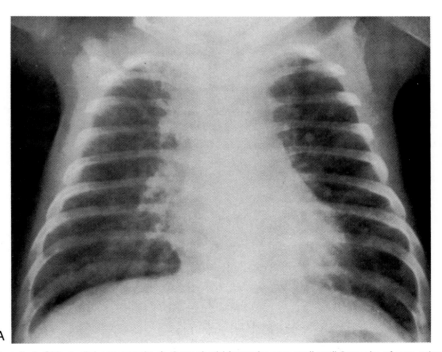

A

Figure 5–4. Chlamydial pneumonia. A, 8-week-old boy who was well until 3 weeks of age, when he developed a paroxysmal cough, conjunctivitis, eosinophilia, and elevated immunoglobulin levels. The initial chest radiograph shows bilateral bronchopneumonia with a reticular nodular pattern.

Illustration continued on following page

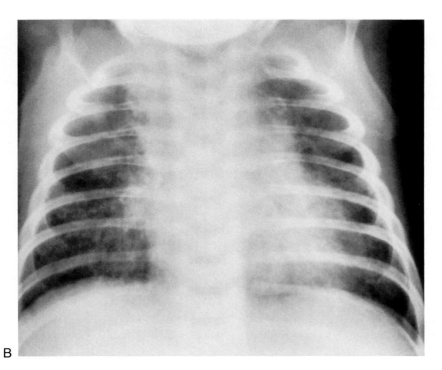

B

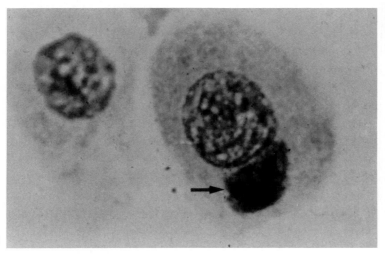

C

Figure 5–4. B, *A 1-month-old infant with a similar clinical course as the patient described in A. C, Conjunctival scrapings show characteristic cytoplasmic inclusion bodies of chlamydia.*

cation of the organism from conjunctival scrapings or tracheal aspirations is diagnostic. The organisms may also be grown in cell cultures.

TORCH

TORCH is an abreviation for several intrauterine infections—toxoplasmosis, syphilis, (other,) rubella, cytomegalovirus (Fig. 5–5), and herpes. The latter is usually acquired during delivery. Any of these conditions may occasionally cause pneumonia. Differentiation is made by clinical laboratory tests. Typical intracranial calcifications may help in the diagnosis of toxoplasmosis and cytomegalovirus, and radiographic changes of the long bones may be helpful in the diagnosis of rubella and cytomegalovirus infections.

Syphilitic pneumonia (pneumonia alba) is diagnosed by the positive serology and luetic bone changes, if present. The pulmonary changes are nonspecific (Fig. 5–6).

Tuberculosis

Although rare, primary tuberculosis in the neonate can occur, and is either the result of infected amniotic fluid being aspirated or hematogenously passed through an infected placenta.

The radiographic changes in neonatal tuberculosis are usually overwhelming and, in the case of transplacental infection, these changes assume a miliary disseminated distribution throughout both lungs (Fig. 5–7). In the case of aspiration they may selectively involve one or more lobes.

ACUTE DISORDERS

Bronchiolitis

Bronchiolitis is a disease of infancy, usually occurring during the first year of life. Common clinical manifestations include an abrupt onset of tachypnea,

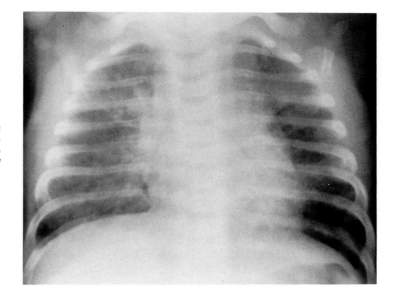

Figure 5–5. Cytomegaloviral pneumonia in a 2-week-old boy. The perihilar infiltrates are nonspecific, and are similar to those found in a number of other viral pneumonias.

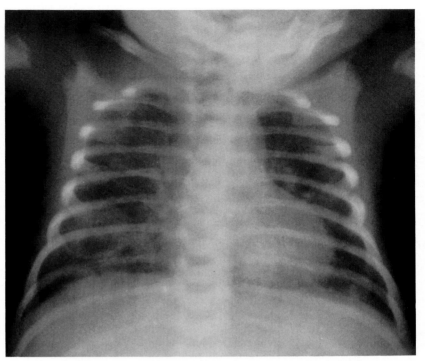

Figure 5–6. Syphilitic pneumonia (pneumonia alba) in neonate. Abnormal densities are seen in the right lower lobe. Luetic bone changes are seen in the proximal humeri. (Courtesy of D. P. Goodman, Driscoll Chldren's Hospital, Corpus Christi, Texas.)

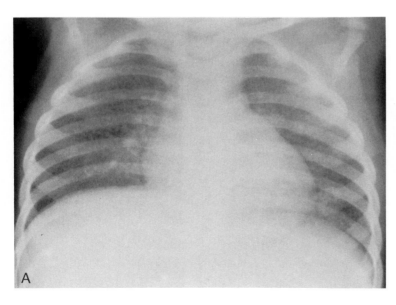

Figure 5–7. Miliary tuberculosis acquired in utero. A, Two-week-old infant with very early miliary tuberculosis.

Illustration continued on opposite page

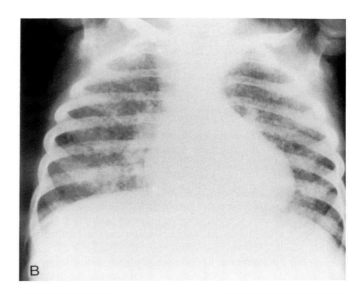

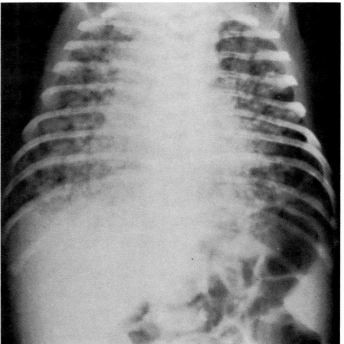

Figure 5–7. B, Three-week-old infant with more advanced miliary tuberculosis. C, Transplacental tuberculosis in a 2-week-old infant. Frontal chest radiograph shows disseminated miliary lesions scattered throughout both lungs, with early coalescence in several areas. There is associated hepatomegaly.

dyspnea, low-grade fever, tachycardia, and physical signs of wheezing and pulmonary hyperinflation.

A number of viruses have been isolated in infants with bronchiolitis, including the respiratory syncytial virus, parainfluenza viruses, influenza viruses, and adenovirus.

There is normally an increase in luminal diameter of the tracheobronchial tree in inspiration and a decrease in expiration, but inflammatory disease of the small bronchi and bronchioles of the young infant may severely restrict the caliber of these structures, allowing the passage of air into the alveoli during inspiration, and restricting the egress of air during expiration.

Radiographically the lungs are hyperlucent, the anteroposterior diameter of the chest increased, and the diaphragm flattened or even inverted (Fig. 5–8). Segmental atelectasis is common in bronchiolitis associated with the respiratory syncytial virus. Intercostal bulging of the lungs may be prominent, and the heart may appear unusually small because of the hyperinflation. Because the rib cage in this age group is quite flexible, subcostal retraction may also be seen, and fluoroscopically there is limited excursion of the rib cage and diaphragm.

Chest radiographs showing pulmonary hyperinflation may also occur in infants with acidosis and dehydration. The radiographic findings in such cases may be indistinguishable from those of bronchiolitis (Fig. 5–9).

Bronchopneumonia is a common complication of bronchiolitis, and is manifested radiographically by an increase in the prominence of the peribronchial markings (Fig. 5–10). Radiographic differentiation between bronchiolitis and asthma in this age group is usually impossible. Any case of an infant with recurrent attacks of either bronchiolitis or reactive airway disease (asthma) should alert the pediatrician to the possibility of fibrocystic disease.

Bronchitis

Bronchitis is usually a complication of diseases of the upper respiratory tract. Viruses predominate as the major cause, while bacterial bronchitis is generally a secondary infection.

Clinical symptoms consist mainly of cough and fever but, in the infant age group, especially in those under the age of 1 year, the symptom complex of bronchiolitis or croup may be predominant.

A fundamental principle has been that bronchitis is not radiographically discernible. Although the chest radiograph may be normal, suggestive radiographic findings are frequently present in the pediatric patient, consisting of prominent linear markings extending peripherally from the hilus; these are undoubtedly caused by edema of the bronchial walls (Fig. 5–11). Radiographic distinction between bronchitis and mild interstitial pneumonia may be impossible.

Pneumonia

Acute pneumonitis is the most common lung disease of the pediatric patient. It may be alveolar or interstitial in distribution, and may be viral, bacterial, fungal, chemical, or protozoan in etiology. The varieties of pneumonia in infants and children are more common than those seen in the adult patient, and a number of unusual conditions found only in children must be considered in the differential diagnosis. Special diagnostic radiographic patterns are rarely present; consequently, an accurate diagnosis depends on careful correlation of the radiographic studies and the clinical and laboratory findings.

Mycoplasm pneumoniae, in addition to the common viruses (respiratory syncytial virus, influenza virus, parainfluenza virus, and enterovirus), account for

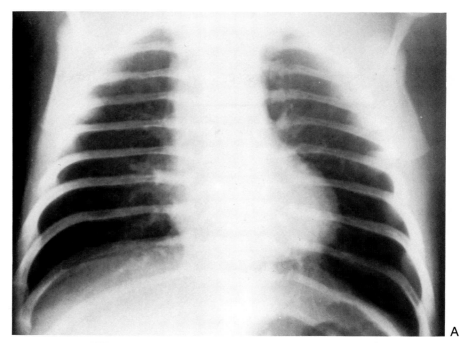

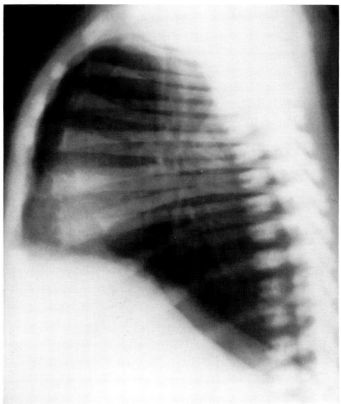

Figure 5–8. Bronchiolitis. A, The lungs are hyperinflated, and the heart is small. B, Lateral projection shows increase in the anteroposterior diameter of the chest, with flattening of the diaphragm and inversion of the posterior portion of each hemidiaphragm.

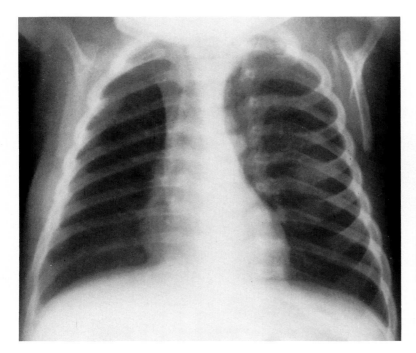

Figure 5–9. Hyperinflation associated with acidosis in infant with acute enteritis. Frontal projection shows hyperinflation of the lungs, with a small cardiac silhouette similar to that seen in bronchiolitis.

Figure 5–10. Bronchiolitis with associated bronchopneumonia. The lungs are hyperlucent and the diaphragm is in an abnormally low position. Linear areas of interstitial pneumonia are identified in the perihilar areas, and are seen to best advantage superimposed on the cardiac silhouette.

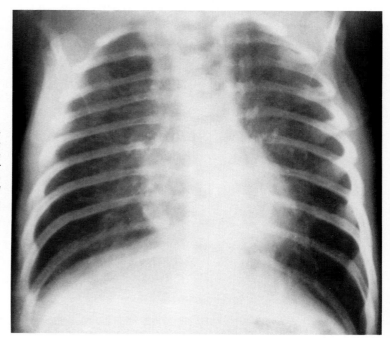

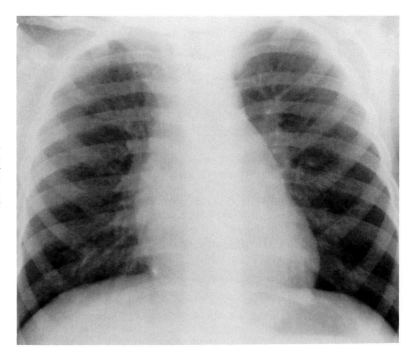

Figure 5–11. Bronchitis in a 3-year-old child. There is a faint increase in the peribronchial markings that is not sufficiently prominent to be diagnosed as interstitial pneumonia, but is more prominent than that expected in the normal chest.

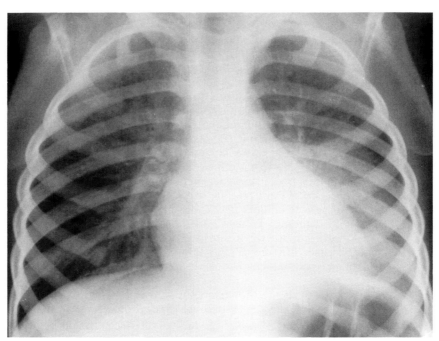

Figure 5–12. Left lower lobe lobar pneumonia in a 4-year-old child who clinically was thought to have acute appendicitis. The sharp definition of the left cardiac border indicates that the left lower lobe is involved, rather than the lingula.

the great majority of respiratory infections (including pneumonia) in childhood. Only 5 to 10% are primarily bacterial in origin.

However, radiographic differentiation between interstitial and alveolar pneumonias is frequently possible. Viral infections usually produce an interstitial pneumonia or bronchopneumonia, and consist of an inflammatory reaction of the peribronchial tissues with increased densities conforming to the radiating pattern of the bronchial tree. Alveolar pneumonias are usually caused by bacterial infections, and produce a more diffuse homogeneous density involving a lobe or segment of a lobe. Mixed types are common. It should be clearly understood that the radiographic differentiation of pneumonia does not always conform to the pathologist's description of interstitial and alveolar pneumonia. An inflammatory process that histologically is interstitial in location may by extending into the adjacent alveoli or by obstructing alveolar ducts produce the radiographic appearance of alveolar pneumonia. Bronchopneumonia to the pathologist implies a more localized involvement with areas of necrosis but, to the radiologist, it usually means a form of interstitial pneumonia that affects the larger branches of the bronchial tree. An awareness of the discrepancy in the radiographic morphology and histopathology is important to avoid the semantic conflicts that frequently confuse this subject.

BACTERIAL PNEUMONIAS

Although bacterial pneumonias usually produce an alveolar pattern of consolidation, interstitial or mixed forms may occur. Many organisms may infect the lungs, with the most common being gram-positive cocci—namely, Streptococcus pneumoniae, Haemophilus influenza type B, and Staphylococcus aureus. Less common organisms are the gram-negative bacilli, including Klebsiella and Pseudomonas. In hospitalized children between the ages of 6 months and 2 years, Haemophilus influenza type B is the most common cause of bacterial pneumonia.

Why the disease presents as lobar pneumonia in one patient and as bronchopneumonia in another is unclear. Clinically pneumonia is frequently preceded by an upper respiratory tract infection, and is characterized in the infant by an abrupt onset of fever, rapid respirations, and tachycardia. Headaches, malaise, chills, and chest pain are other findings seen in the older child. Abdominal pain frequently mimicking that of appendicitis may also occur. Consequently, chest radiographs are important in the differential diagnosis. Although right lower lobe pneumonia with diaphragmatic irritation should theoretically be more commonly associated with clinical signs mimicking those of appendicitis, in our experience the left lower lobe is more commonly involved (Fig. 5–12).

Radiographically lobar pneumonia may vary in size from subsegments (Figs. 5–13 and 5–14) to an entire lobe. However, complete involvement of an entire lobe in the pediatric age group is unusual, except in middle lobe involvement (Fig. 5–15). Peripheral air bronchograms are not usually seen in acute alveolar pneumonia in infants and children, presumably because the bronchial segments fill with exudate. Pleural effusion is a common complication (Fig. 5–16). Parenchymal breakdown with abscess formation is usually not found in the uncomplicated case, but may result if bronchial drainage is impaired or if aspiration of foreign material has occurred. Hilar adenopathy is less common than in viral infections.

Uncomplicated lobar pneumonia usually resolves within 2 weeks, depending on the severity of the parenchymal component and on the degree of pleural involvement. It should always be remembered that radiographic manifestations lag behind clinical findings during both the consolidating and the resolving phases of pneumonia. If resolution is inordinately delayed, underlying lesions such as atelectasis, foreign bodies, or granulomatous processes should be considered. Atelectasis and empyema are the major complications of staphylococcal and pneumococcal pneumonia (Fig. 5–17).

Text continued on page 150

Figure 5–13. Lobar pneumonia caused by Streptococcus pneumoniae in 18-month-old infant. The frontal projection shows homogeneous consolidation sharply demarcated inferiorly by a minor interlobar fissure, indicating its anterior location.

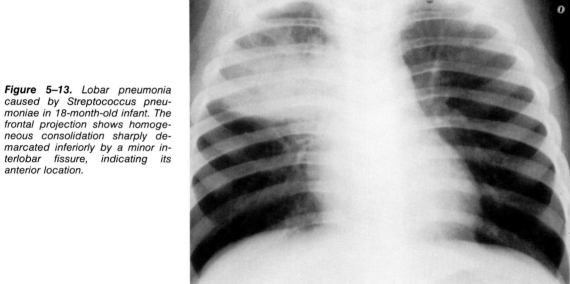

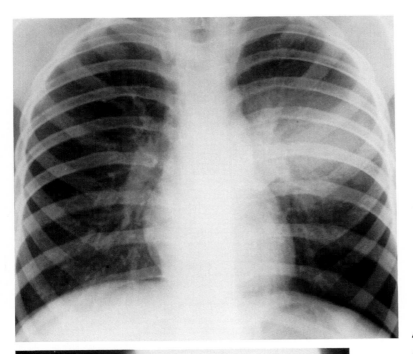

A

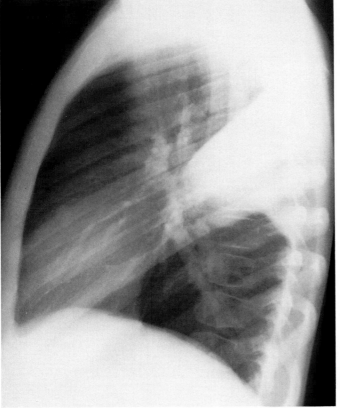

B

Figure 5–14. Acute pneumococcal pneumonia in a 12-year-old child. A, Frontal projection shows consolidation that, by its location and the sharpness of the adjacent mediastinal border, identifies the lesion as being in the apical segment of the left lower lobe. B, Lateral view confirms the left lower lobe apical localization.

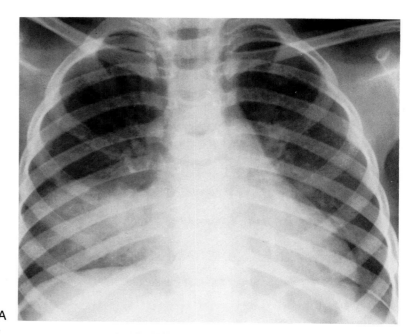

A

Figure 5–15. Middle lobe lobar pneumonia in 4-year-old child. A, Frontal projection shows the typical middle lobe distribution, with characteristic obliteration of the right cardiac border. B, Lateral view shows complete lobar consolidation, with associated convexity of the minor and major interlobar fissures.

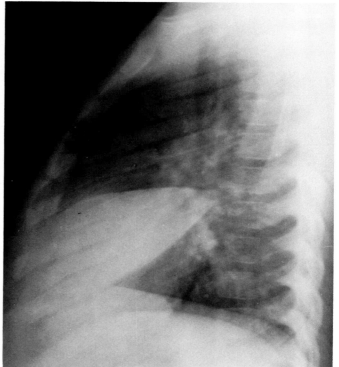

B

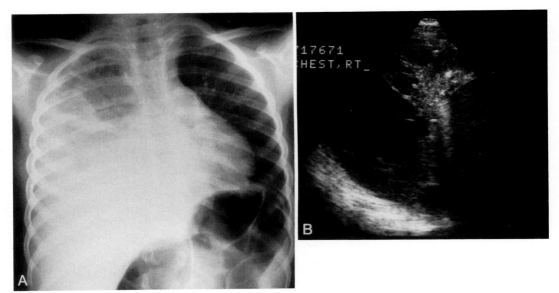

Figure 5–16. Pneumococcal pneumonia and empyema in a 6-year-old boy. A, Extensive pulmonary consolidation of the right middle and lower lobes is noted, as well as right pleural effusion. The initial clinical impression was appendicitis because of the patient's right lower quadrant pain. B, A 12-year-old with acute pneumococcal pneumonia and empyema. Intercostal real-time scan shows a large pleural effusion, which was aspirated.

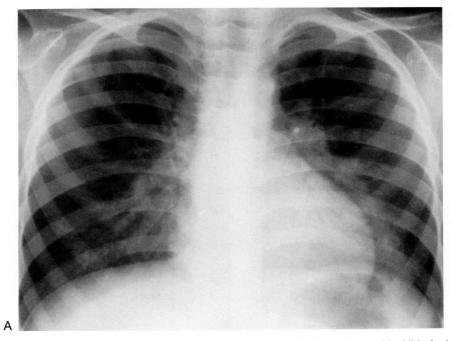

Figure 5–17. Alveolar and intestitial pneumococcal pneumonia in a 4-year-old child. A, Initial examination shows mixed alveolar and interstitial distribution bilaterally, more severe in the left lower lobe.

Illustration continued on opposite page

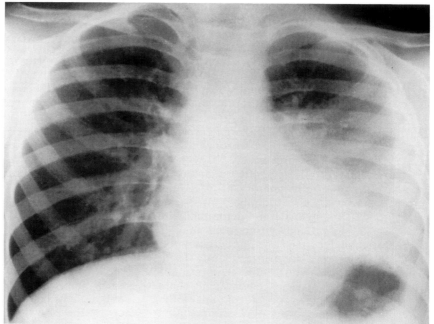

B

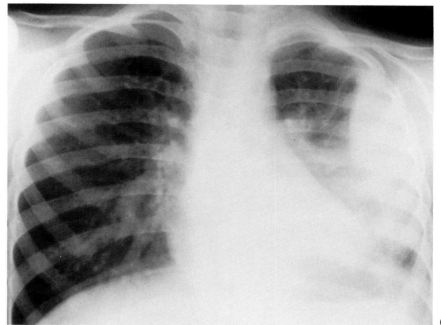

C

Figure 5–17. B, *Repeat examination 4 days later shows left pleural effusion, with increased consolidation of the left lung and scoliosis of the dorsal spine secondary to splinting of the left hemithorax. C, Repeat chest radiographs 2 weeks later show loculated empyema with persistent pneumonia.*

The bronchopneumonic or interstitial forms of bacterial pneumonias appear radiographically as linear, streaky densities paralleling the bronchovascular markings, obliterating the sharply defined edges of the vascular structures and indistinguishable from the usual viral pneumonias. Commonly there are areas of coalescence that produce small patchy densities (Fig. 5–18). The involvement is usually bilateral, but one side or one lobe may be more severely affected than the other(s). Segmental areas of air trapping and atelectasis are commonly present. Although coalescence of areas of bronchopneumonia may lead to suppuration, it is uncommon in the pediatric patient.

Round Pneumonia. Round pneumonia is a well-defined oval or round area of consolidation within the lung, frequently found in the superior dorsal segment of the right or left lower lobes. The usual causative organism is Pneumococcus. Because of the round configuration in the sharply demarcated margins, the lesion may be mistaken for a bronchial cyst or metastatic neoplasm (Fig. 5–19). Clinically the patients are acutely ill, with elevated temperature, cough, and leukocytosis similiar to those of other pneumococcal infections. Experimental evidence suggests that the inflammatory process spreads centrifugally through the pores of Kohn and channels of Lambert, producing the round area of consolidation.

Staphylococcal Pneumonia. Staphylococcal pneumonia is most common in the infant age group, and may be rapidly fatal in young infants. Although staphylococcal pneumonia may be a complication of viral infections of the respiratory tract, it frequently has a sudden onset without concomitant disease.

The radiographic features, although not always diagnostic, are frequently suggestive. One radiographic characteristic of staphylococcal pneumonia is its rapid progression, developing within a few hours. Initially hyperaeration of the lungs may be the only manifestation, as may be the case in nearly all diseases of the lower respiratory tract in infancy. This is followed by patchy infiltration, usually unilateral, which becomes confluent, involving one or more lobes. The presenting radiographic findings may be marked pleural effusion or pneumothorax, or a combination of these (Figs. 5–20, 5–21, 5–22, and 5–23). Local bulging of the intercostal spaces with tumefaction of the overlying skin (empyema necessi-

Text continued on page 156

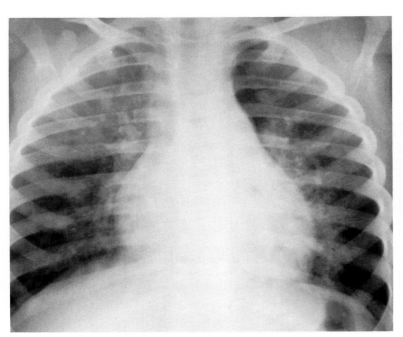

Figure 5–18. *Diphtheria pneumonia in 2-year-old boy. The frontal chest radiograhs show bilateral interstitial pneumonia, with small patchy areas of alveolar involvement. Clinically, the infant had diphtheria with proven pulmonary involvement.*

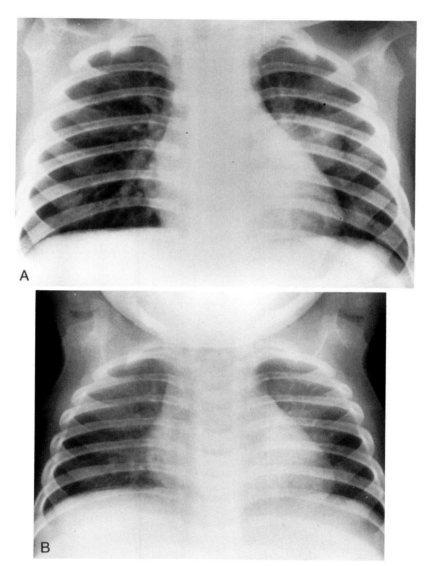

Figure 5–19. *Round pneumonia. A, Sharply demarcated round density occupies the region of the superior dorsal segment of the left lower lobe. B, Repeat examination in 3 days shows nearly complete resolution. Pneumococcal organisms were identified as the causative agent.*

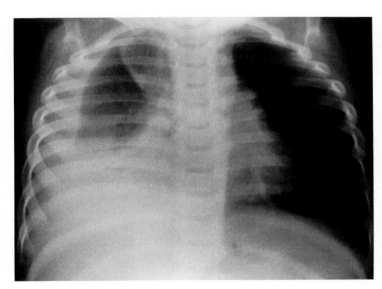

Figure 5–20. Staphylococcal empyema in an infant presenting with right lower lobe pneumonia and right pleural effusion, with fluid extending into the azygous lobe fissure.

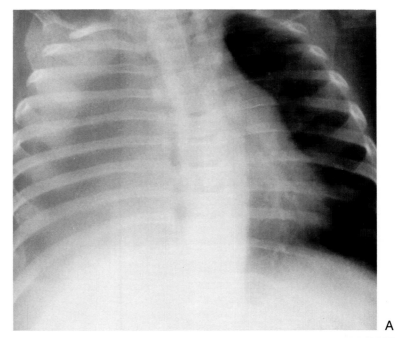

A

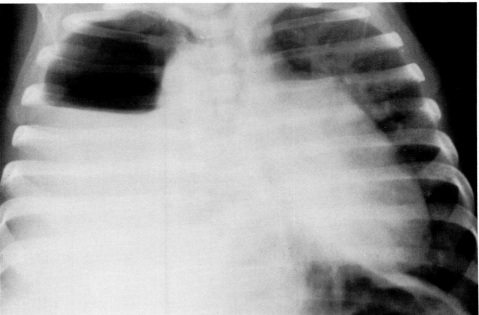

B

Figure 5–21. Staphylococcal pneumonia in a 5-month-old infant presenting with combination of air and fluid in the right hemithorax. A, Although air-fluid levels are not seen in this supine portable film, the shift of mediastinal structures to the left and the combination of radiolucency and increased density in the right hemithorax indicate that both air and fluid are present. B, Upright film shows air-fluid level representing presumptive evidence of staphylococcal infection.

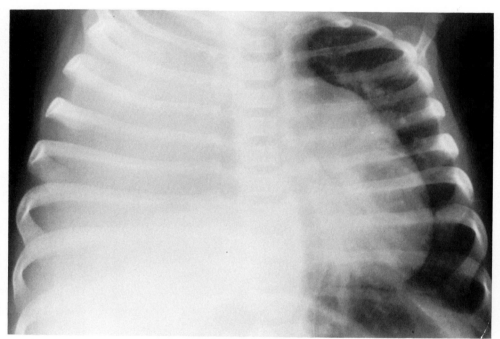

Figure 5–22. *Staphylococcal pyopneumothorax in a 4-month-old girl. The supine film shows opacification of the right hemithorax with separation of the ribs and shift of mediastinal structures to the left. Associated interstitial pneumonia is seen in the left lung.*

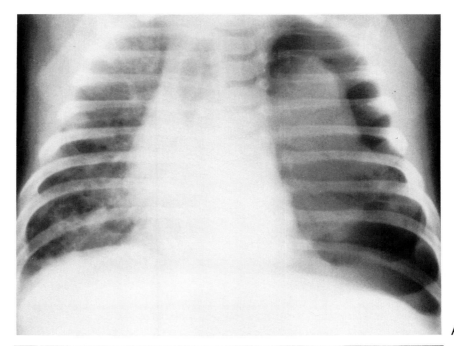

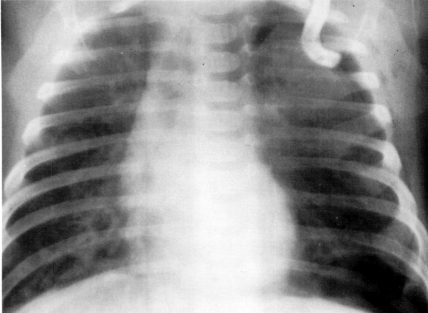

Figure 5–23. *Spontaneous pneumothorax in infant with staphylococcal pneumonia. A, Frontal view of the chest shows pneumothorax on the left, with collapse of the left lung and herniation of air across the anterior mediastinum. Associated interstitial pneumonia is seen on the right. B, After intubation there is partial expansion of the left lung.*

Illustration continued on following page

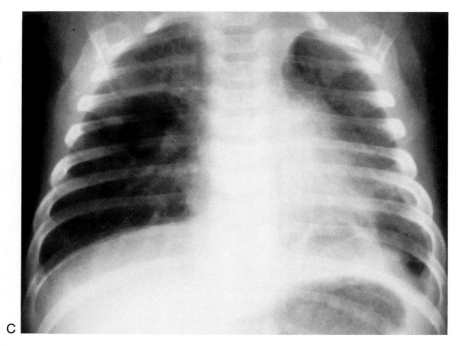

C

Figure 5–23. *C, Repeat radiograph 1 week later shows nearly complete resolution of the pneumonia, with increase in size of numerous small pneumatoceles.*

tatis) may occur if thoracic intubation is not performed (Fig. 5–24). Either situation usually obscures the underlying lung disease, but should alert the radiologist and clinician to the probability that staphylococcal pneumonia is present, and appropriate antibiotic and supportive measures should be given without waiting for bacteriologic confirmation. Computerized tomography is frequently helpful in differentiating the extent of the pleural effusion and consol-

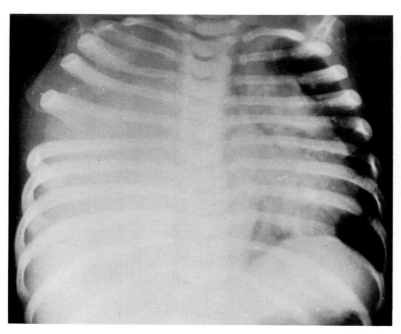

Figure 5–24. *Staphylococcal empyema with local bulging of the intercostal spaces and extension into the overlying soft tissues.*

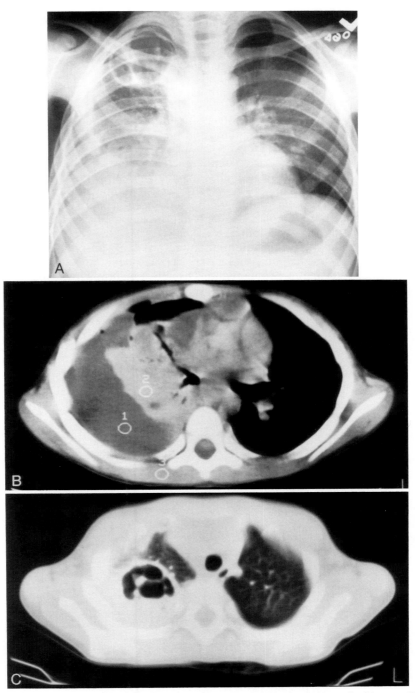

Figure 5–25. *Staphylococcal pneumonia and empyema in a 6-year-old boy. A, Chest radiograph shows a large right pleural effusion as well as pneumonia involving most of the right lung and pneumatoceles in the right apex. B, Computerized tomography shows the extensive empyema (1), as well as the consolidation of the lung (2). C, Computerized tomography of the upper lobe shows multiple pneumatoceles in the right apex.*

idation (Fig. 5–25). Frequent follow-up radiographic studies are mandatory to follow the expansion of the lung and progression or resolution of the infectious process.

Concomitant osteomyelitis with pneumonia commonly indicates staphylococcal infection (Fig. 5–26). Periosteal new bone formation of the ribs in a patient with pleural effusion is presumptive evidence of empyema, but this is usually not recognized until treatment has been started (Fig. 5–27). Parenchymal breakdown may occur, forming an abscess cavity. Most of the radiolucent areas that develop are pneumatoceles, however, which may persist for months after complete resolution of the pneumonia. They should not be mistaken for congenital cysts or persistent areas of infection (Fig. 5–28). Follow-up studies show complete resolution of the surrounding infiltration, with the thin-walled pneumatoceles becoming gradually smaller and ultimately disappearing (Fig. 5–29). Fluid levels may occasionally be seen in pneumatoceles but, with adequate treatment, these usually disappear, leaving the clear pneumatoceles (Figs. 5–30 and 5–31). Residual fluid levels presumably represent persistent infection. Rupture of the pneumatocele occurs rarely, producing pneumothorax (Fig. 5–31C). In our experience this has been a complication only in incompletely treated cases. Surgical resection, although once commonly employed, is now recognized as unnecessary. Initially, radiographic differentiation between an abscess and a pneumatocele may be impossible but, in our experience, pneumatocele formation is accompanied by clinical improvement and is usually a favorable prognostic sign. Abscess formation is generally associated with a persistence of clinical symptoms, and is much less common than pneumatocele formation.

Staphylococcal pneumonia may result from septic emboli secondary to staphylococcal disease in other portions of the body. The radiographic features consist of multiple, small, fluffy densities disseminated throughout both lungs. Rapid

Text continued on page 164

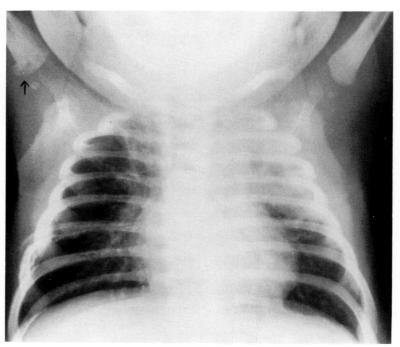

Figure 5–26. *Staphylococcal pneumonia with associated osteomyelitis of the right sixth rib and of the right proximal humeral metaphyses in 1-month-old infant. The small radiolucent areas in the consolidated left upper lobe represent small pneumatoceles.*

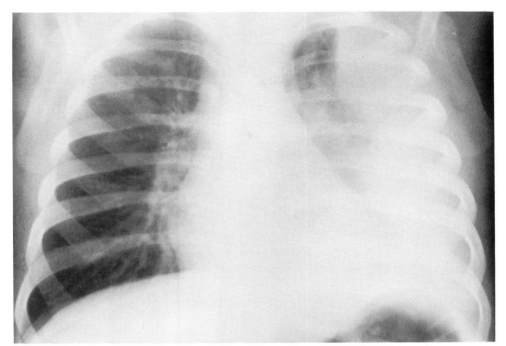

A

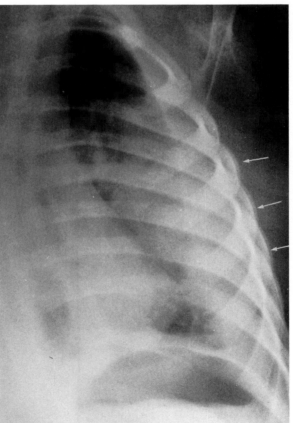

B

Figure 5–27. Periosteal new bone formation involving ribs in a child with staphylococcal empyema. A, Frontal chest film shows empyema with underlying parenchymal infection. B, Repeat radiograph 3 weeks later shows residual pleural change and periosteal new bone formation after the patient has become asymptomatic (arrows).

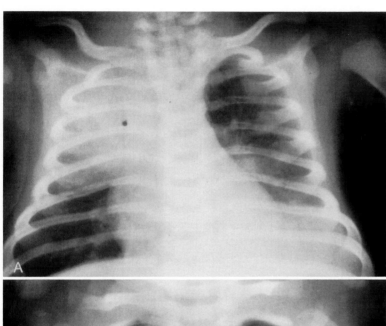

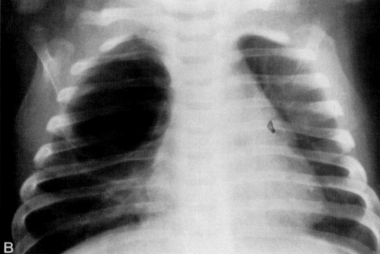

Figure 5–28. Staphylococcal pneumonia in a 6-month-old child. A, Lobar consolidations identified in the right upper lobe and in a portion of the left lower lobe. B, Repeat radiograph 3 weeks later shows a large pneumatocele occupying the right upper lobe. This eventually became smaller, and disappeared after approximately 6 months.

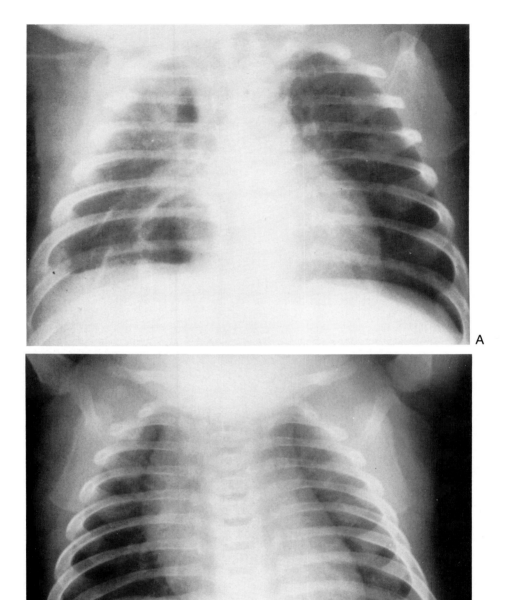

Figure 5–29. Staphylococcal pneumonia in infant with resolution of pneumatocele. A, Chest radiograph made after infant was clinically well shows pneumatoceles in right lung. B, Repeat chest examination 4 months later shows normal chest.

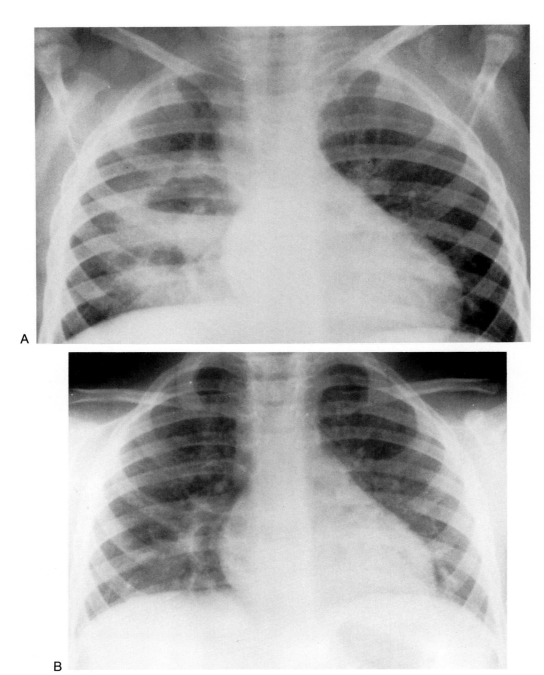

Figure 5–30. Staphylococcal pneumonia containing fluid. A, Air-fluid levels in pneumatoceles in patient with resolving staphylococcal pneumonia. The frontal projection of the chest shows air-fluid levels within pneumatoceles, which developed during clinical improvement after antibiotic therapy. B, Repeat chest radiographs 3 weeks later show that the fluid within the pneumatoceles has disappeared, and that there is nearly complete resolution of the surrounding pneumonia.

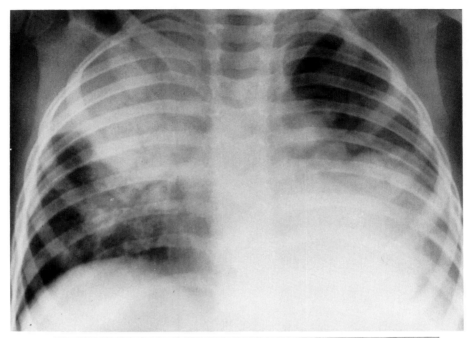

A

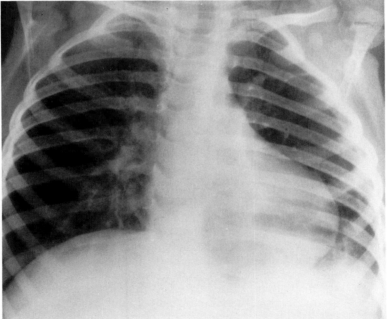

B

Figure 5–31. *Staphylococcal pneumonia with clearing and complicating pneumothorax. A, Extensive staphylococcal pneumonia involving right upper lobe, left lower lobe, and left lingula of 4-year-old child. B, Repeat radiograph 2 weeks later shows complete resolution of the inflammatory process, with multiple residual pneumatoceles in the left lung.*

Illustration continued on following page

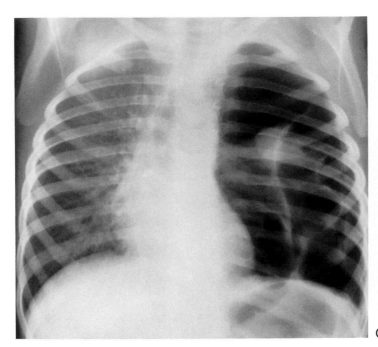

Figure 5–31. C, Tension pneumothorax developed 2 weeks later, presumably from rupture of a pneumatocele. The mediastinum is displaced to the right. The patient had clinical evidence of recurrent infection, which was thought to be responsible for this rare complication.

C

increase in size of the lesions over a 24- to 48-hour period occurs, accompanied by coalescence of some of the areas of involvement. Early excavation is common and presents typical multiple small cavities (Fig. 5–32). The radiographic appearance, accompanied by high fever and a septic clinical course, should initiate investigation for the original source of infection.

Streptococcal pneumonia may occur as a primary infection, but it frequently complicates viral or other bacterial diseases. The radiologic features are not diagnostic, and the appearance may be that of lobar or bronchial pneumonia. Although pleural effusion is not uncommon, pneumatoceles rarely occur. The accompanying pleural disease may result in a persistent, thickened "rind."

Pneumonias, caused by Haemophilus influenzae and Klebsiella pneumoniae (Friedländer's bacillus) produce radiographic changes indistinguishable from those of the other previously described bacterial infections. Both lobar and bronchopneumonic distributions can be seen. However, when Klebsiella pneumoniae is responsible for lobar involvement, the infection is frequently extensive, affecting an entire lobe. It may produce marked bulging of the fissures, presumably from the abundant secretions that result from infections by this organism.

Haemophilus aphrophilus is a gram-negative coccobacillus that may produce pneumonia, similar to haemophilus influenzae pneumonia, but more commonly is the cause of endocarditis, brain abscesses, and other infections. A history of canine contact may or may not be present.

Pneumonias caused by coliform group, Pseudomonas, and Proteus organisms are uncommon, and are usually found as complications of other debilitating diseases. The pulmonary distribution resulting from this type of infection is usually lobar, and the incidence of abscess formation and empyema is high.

Pertussis Pneumonia. Since the introduction of prophylactic vaccination the incidence of whooping cough has diminished, along with the ensuing complications of this disease. It is difficult to determine the true incidence of pertussis pneumonia because of the frequency of a superimposed bacterial pneumonia. The severity of the pneumonia is greatest in the infant age group, especially in those under 6 months.

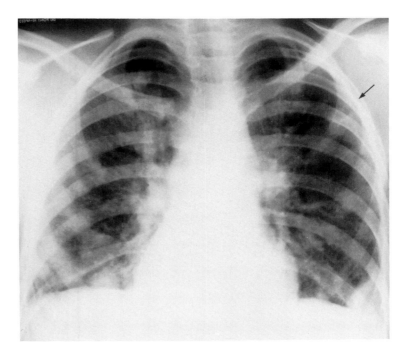

Figure 5–32. *Staphylococcal emboli. Multiple nodular densities are scattered throughout both lungs, with several of the nodules showing early cavitation (arrow). The patient had a bacteremia resulting from osteomyelitis of the left femur.*

The roentgenographic findings in pertussis pneumonia are nonspecific. The most common findings in infants are hyperaeration, with diffuse bilateral interstitial bronchopneumonia. The interstitial involvement may be very extensive, radiating out from the hila and obliterating the cardiac borders (Fig. 5–33). This has been described as the "shaggy heart" sign and, although undoubtedly seen in pertussis, is no different from severe interstitial pneumonia produced by other organisms (Fig. 5–34). Widespread areas of segmental atelectasis may occur, but lobar consolidation is usually secondary to other bacterial invaders. The milder radiographic findings generally clear in 2 weeks, but atelectasis may persist for several weeks after the patient is clinically well. Bronchiectasis may be a complication, particularly in those patients who show delay in resolution of the interstitial pneumonia or of the atelectasis.

VIRAL PNEUMONIAS

Most acute pneumonias found in infants and young children are viral, and are usually preceded by an upper respiratory tract infection. Although a number of viruses may cause pneumonia in this age group the respiratory syncytial virus, parainfluenza viruses, influenza viruses, and adenovirus seem to predominate.

Radiographically the inflammatory distribution is of an interstitial type, consisting of radiating areas of increased density extending out from the hilar areas and paralleling the bronchial tree (Fig. 5–35). The distribution is usually bilateral, but one or more lobes or pulmonary segments may predominate. The lungs are invariably hyperinflated, and patchy areas of confluent pneumonia or atelectasis are commonly present. Adenoviral pneumonia may produce chronic changes of bronchiectasis, and present a clinical and radiographic course simulating that of cystic fibrosis.

Measles Pneumonia. Respiratory tract infections varying from laryngitis to tracheobronchitis, bronchiolitis, or pneumonia commonly occur in a child with

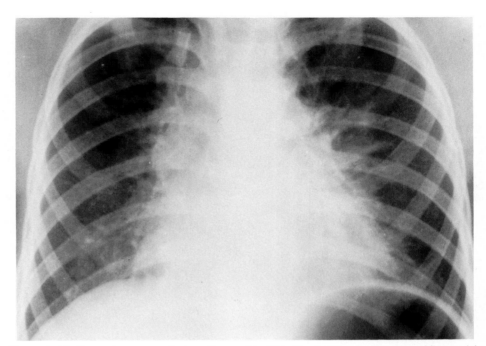

Figure 5–33. *Pertussis pneumonia in a 5-year-old child. The cardiac borders are obliterated by extensive interstitial inflammatory disease.*

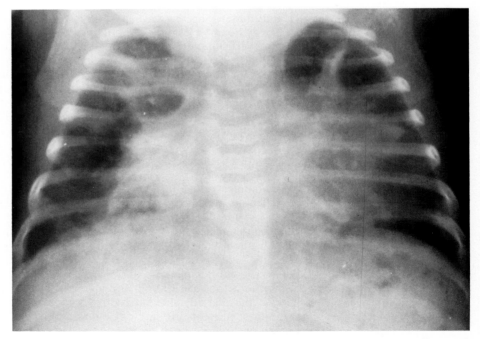

Figure 5–34. *Severe viral interstitial and alveolar pneumonia in a 9-week-old infant. The cardiac borders are obliterated, producing an irregular contour.*

Figure 5–35. Characteristic viral bronchopneumonia in a 4-year-old child. A, Bilateral interstitial lung disease is identified in the perihilar and lower lobe areas of both lungs. Bilateral hilar adenopathy is also present. B, Follow-up radiograph 3 weeks later shows a normal chest.

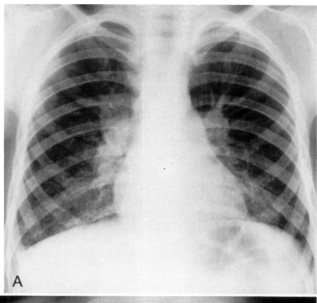

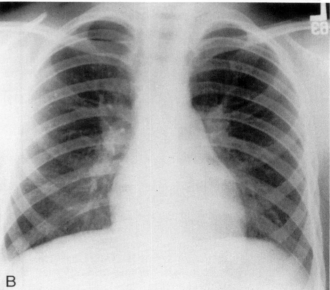

measles. It is usually impossible to determine whether the infection is due to the measles virus or to some other viral or bacterial invader.

The radiographic features in either case are those of interstitial pneumonia or bronchopneumonia, with radiating areas of increased density extending peripherally from the hilar areas. Hilar adenopathy is commonly present. Coalescence of the areas of infection and areas of atelectasis frequently develops (Fig. 5–36). Uncomplicated viral measles pneumonia usually clears with the clinical remission, but complications of bacterial pneumonia may prolong the recovery period.

Measles may cause reactivation of tuberculosis. Consequently, a child who has clinical or radiographic evidence of tuberculosis, or a child who has a positive tuberculin test, should have frequent follow-up chest radiographs during and after the recovery period. Undoubtedly present utilization of measles vaccine will eventually eliminate this condition. However, the use of the vaccine, which formerly consisted of inactivated virus, has resulted in a number of bizarre conditions in children who were later exposed to measles. An example of the pulmonary manifestations of this atypical type of reaction is the development of pneumonia with a residual solitary pulmonary nodule (Fig. 5–37).

Although the etiology of giant cell pneumonia (Hecht's pneumonia) has been disputed for years, the current belief is that the measles virus is the responsible organism. Patients affected with giant cell pneumonia usually do not develop the clinical manifestations of measles, but commonly have underlying chronic debilitating diseases such as leukemia or hypoimmune disorders.

The radiographic findings of giant cell pneumonia are generally those of a bilateral, confluent, interstitial, and alveolar infiltration, concentrated mainly in the perihilar areas of the lung (Fig. 5–38). Pneumothorax and pneumomediastinum may be serious complications. The mortality rate is extremely high because of the poor host resistance.

Varicella and Herpetic Pneumonia. Varicella pneumonia in normal patients with chickenpox is uncommon; however, other viral or bacterial pneumonias may occur in a normal child with chickenpox. When varicella pneumonitis occurs in children, it is more commonly seen in the immunocompromised patient or in a child who is receiving steroid therapy. In addition, bacterial and viral pneumonia may complicate these immunocompromised individuals. Although congenital varicella has been reported, it is extremely rare.

In the adult with true varicella, pneumonia secondary to the varicella virus is more common than in children, and is often responsible for an extremely ill patient with a critical clinical course.

The radiographic findings in varicella pneumonia usually show widespread, ill-defined miliary and nodular densities, varying in size from a few millimeters to a centimeter in diameter (Figs. 5–39 and 5–40). If the clinical story is unknown, the pulmonary findings may be mistaken for those of septic emboli. The lesions frequently appear more numerous in the perihilar and basilar areas of the lungs. The peribronchial markings are also increased, and represent an interstitial component of the infection. Coalescence of the nodular lesions produces small areas of consolidation. Frequently the nodules show concomitant clearing in some areas, with new nodular lesions developing in other pulmonary segments. Resolution occurs slowly, often requiring several weeks for complete disappearance. Identical radiographic findings may be seen in herpes zoster and herpes simplex pneumonia (Fig. 5–41). Occasionally the nodules may persist and eventually calcify, producing a radiographic picture similar to that of calcified histoplasmosis.

PRIMARY ATYPICAL PNEUMONIA

With the discovery of the Eaton agent (Mycoplasma pneumoniae), the etiology of primary atypical pneumonia has been resolved. The clinical features include an abrupt onset of cough accompanied by chills, fever, and malaise.

Text continued on page 174

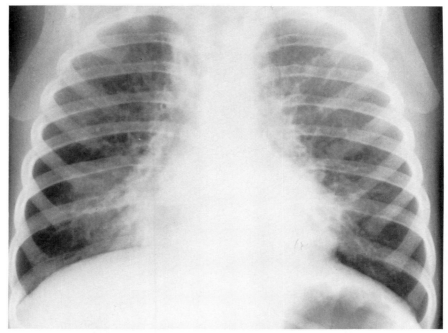

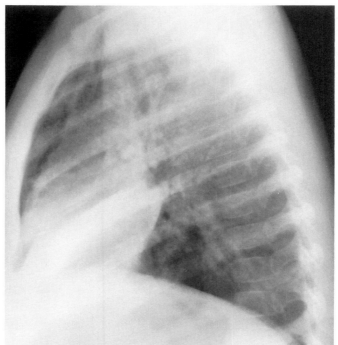

Figure 5–36. *Viral interstitial pneumonia in a 3-year-old child with measles. A, Frontal chest radiograph shows radiating areas of interstitial pneumonia extending laterally from the hilar areas. B, Lateral view shows consolidation in the right middle lobe area, as well as complicating mediastinal emphysema.*

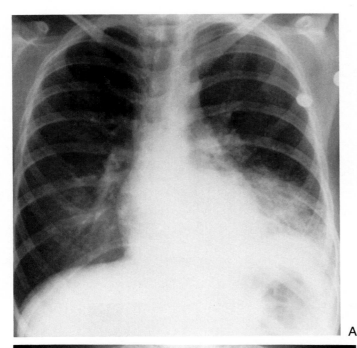

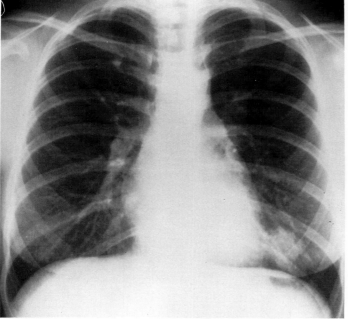

Figure 5–37. *Atypical measles pneumonia in a 9-year-old girl who had received inactivated vaccine 3 years prior to a recent exposure to measles. A, Chest radiograph shows left lower lobe consolidation, with associated hilar adenopathy. B, Repeat chest radiograph 20 months later shows a 5-cm nodular lesion in the left lower lobe. (Courtesy of Dr. L. Young.)*

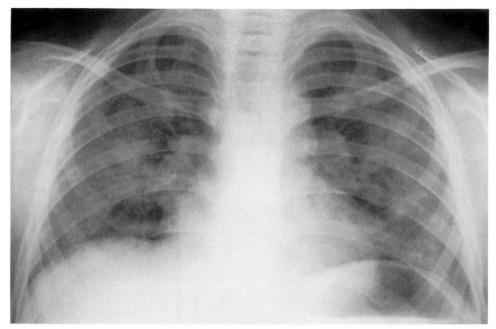

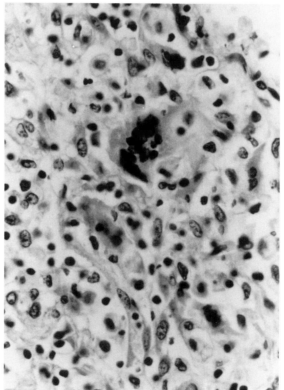

Figure 5–38. A, *Giant cell pneumonia, proven by autopsy, in an 8-year-old girl with leukemia. Hepatosplenomegaly has restricted the usual low position of the diaphragm. B, Photomicrograph of lung biopsy shows large multinuclear giant cells (40 ×).*

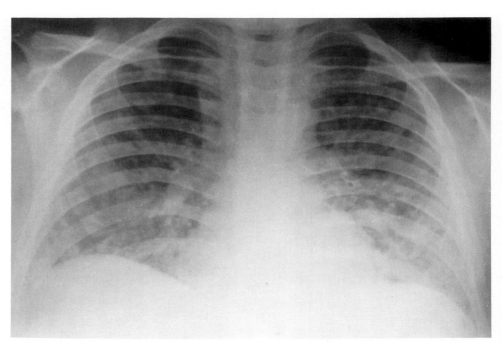

Figure 5–39. Varicella pneumonia in a 6-year-old child with nephrotic syndrome treated with steroids. Portable chest radiograph shows multiple ill-defined nodular lesions scattered throughout both lungs.

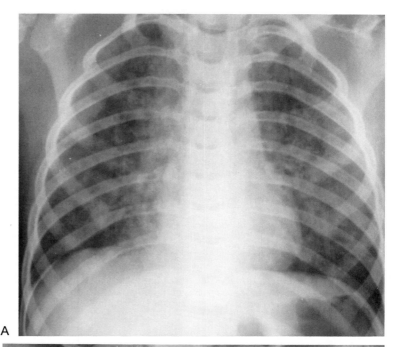

A

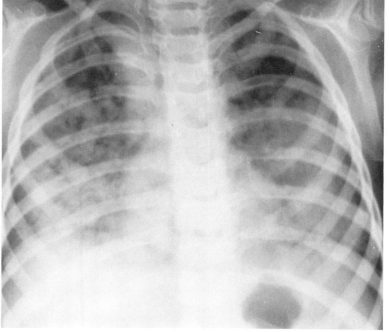

B

Figure 5–40. Varicella pneumonia in a 4-year-old child with leukemia. A, Frontal chest radiograph shows multiple ill-defined nodular lesions scattered throughout both lungs. B, Repeat chest radiograph 2 days later shows coalescence of many of the lesions.

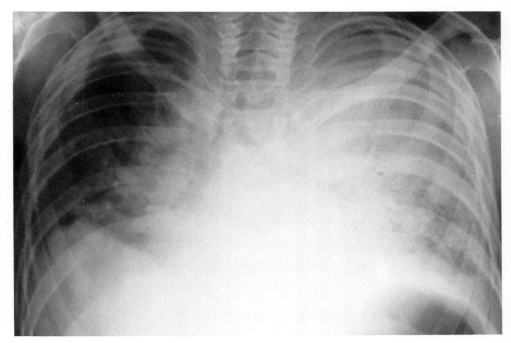

Figure 5–41. *Herpes zoster pneumonia in child with terminal leukemia. Frontal chest radiograph shows diffuse densities occupying most of the left lung and the right perihilar area. Earlier films showed more discrete nodular lesions. The large liver and spleen produce the high position of the diaphragm.*

Preceding upper respiratory tract symptoms are uncommon. The blood count is usually within normal range, and the bacterial cultures are uninformative. Although any age group may be affected, the peak incidence occurs most often in school-age children (5–19 years of age). The clinical course is more severe and protracted in children with sickle cell disease.

The diagnosis is made by the usual clinical findings, radiographic evidence of pneumonia, elevated cold agglutinin levels, and appropriate antibody studies.

The radiographic features are nonspecific and may involve one or more lobes (Fig. 5–42). The infiltration may be interstitial, alveolar, or mixed. Resolution is commonly slow, requiring several weeks for complete disappearance. Hilar adenopathy is common, particularly in the young age group, but pleural effusion is rare.

Hydrocarbon Pneumonia

Hydrocarbon pneumonia is well known to both the pediatrician and the radiologist and, although the incidence has decreased, it is still a common cause of pneumonia in young children. The main offenders are kerosene, furniture polishes, lighter fluid, and insecticides.

Approximately 60 to 80% of children who ingest hydrocarbons develop pneumonia, and there is a fairly good correlation between the severity of the clinical and radiographic findings and the amount of material ingested. The controversy as to whether the pneumonia is produced by direct aspiration of the hydrocarbon material or is secondary to absorption from the gastrointestinal tract, with secondary deposition into the lungs, seems to be resolved. Direct aspiration or aspiration secondary to emesis or lavage therapy is the cause of the parenchymal infiltration. If aspiration pneumonia occurs it is usually demonstrable almost immediately, and well within 6 hours after ingestion.

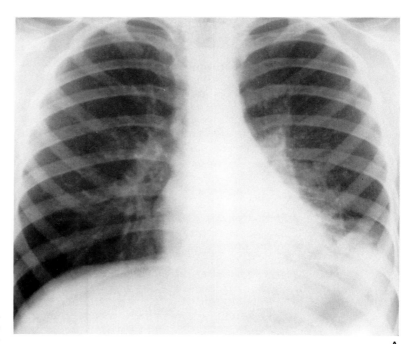

A

Figure 5–42. *Mycoplasma pneumonia in a 7-year-old child. A, Frontal chest examination shows infiltration in the left lower lobe with mixed alveolar and interstitial characteristics. B, Repeat radiograph 2 weeks later shows minimal residual pneumonia.*

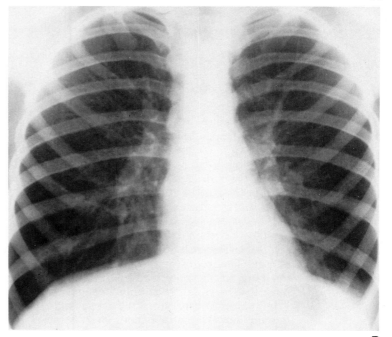

B

The radiographic findings are usually characteristic. Generally the infiltrates are linear, with a predilection for the lower lobes, especially the right lower lobe, and with patchy areas of coalescence. The peripheral portions of the lungs are usually spared. Overaeration occurs mainly in the younger age group but is not necessarily a prominent feature of the disease. Perihilar densities resembling those of pulmonary edema may occur, but this pattern of involvement is less common than lower lobe involvement. Usually follow-up radiographs show an increase in severity over a period of 12 to 24 hours. Gradual resolution begins after 3 to 4 days, generally with complete clearing in 2 to 3 weeks (Fig. 5–43).

Pneumomediastinum and pneumothorax are uncommon but serious complications, which can be easily recognized during follow-up radiographic studies (Fig. 5–44). Pneumatoceles may develop and, as in cases of staphylococcal pneumonia, occur during the process of resolution and may persist for many weeks after complete resolution of the inflammation (Fig. 5–45).

Near Drowning

Patients who have undergone near drowning may show various pulmonary changes as a result of a combination of aspiration and physiologic changes producing pulmonary edema. The most common radiographic pattern consists of perihilar hazy densities, with sparing of the lung periphery (Fig. 5–46). Other cases may show areas of consolidation or fluffy ill-defined densities scattered throughout the lungs.

Progression of the process usually occurs during the first few days, followed by rapid resolution unless there is superimposed infection. Unfortunately, many of these infants and children have severe central neurologic damage because of hypoxia.

CHRONIC OR RECURRENT DISORDERS

Allergic Pneumonitis

Although pulmonary consolidation or patchy infiltrations may represent an allergic response to various conditions, a diagnosis of allergic pneumonia is frequently made when all other explanations for chronic or repeated pneumonia have been excluded. However, an allergic response of the lungs to many antigenic substances is common in all pediatric age groups. In the young infant the clinical and radiographic manifestations may be those of bronchiolitis or pneumonitis. In the older child, clinical and radiographic manifestations of asthma or pneumonia, or of both, may be the allergic response. Regardless of the age the patient should have a complete evaluation, including appropriate skin tests, sweat testing for fibrocystic disease, and electrophoretic studies of serum protein levels to determine whether a hypoimmune syndrome is present.

Recurrent or chronic pneumonia in young infants may be secondary to milk allergy. Theoretically this may result from the aspiration of milk, which sensitizes the lung to an allergic response. Radiographically there is evidence of chronic lung disease that frequently changes in pattern and distribution (Fig. 5–47). Elimination of milk from the diet results in cure. The possibility of milk allergy pneumonia (Heiner's pneumonia) being a precursor of idiopathic pulmonary hemosiderosis is questionable because of the anemia accompanying this type of allergic response.

The radiographic changes of pulmonary allergy are primarily those of hyperinflation of the lungs. The diaphragm is depressed, the anteroposterior diameter of the chest is increased, the ribs are elevated, the intercostal spaces may bulge,

Text continued on page 182

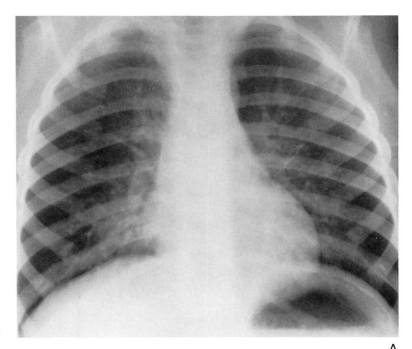

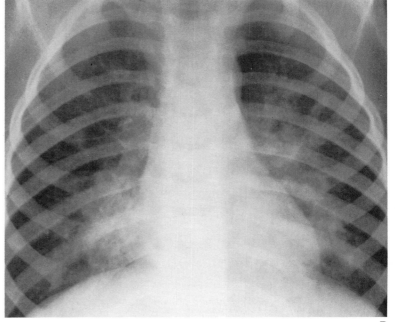

Figure 5–43. Hydrocarbon pneumonia in a 21-month-old child. A, Initial chest radiograph made approximately 30 minutes after ingestion of the hydrocarbon shows ill-defined pneumonia in the right lower lobe, with less extensive involvement in the left lower lobe. B, Repeat radiograph 24 hours later shows increase in the extent of parenchymal involvement. Complete resolution occurred within 2 weeks.

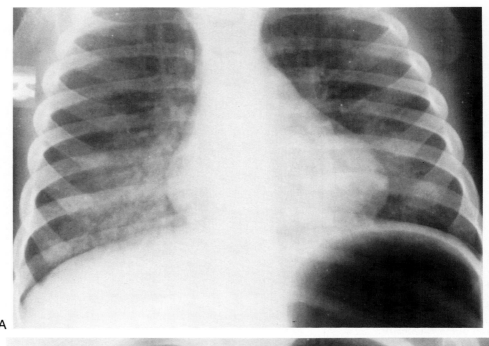

A

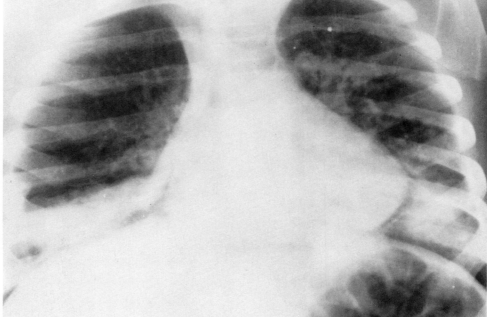

B

Figure 5–44. *Furniture polish ingestion in a 12-month-old child. A, Initial chest radiograph shows bilateral lower lobe infiltration. B, Repeat chest radiograph 2 days later shows increase in the degree of consolidation, as well as complicating pneumomediastinum.*

Illustration continued on opposite page

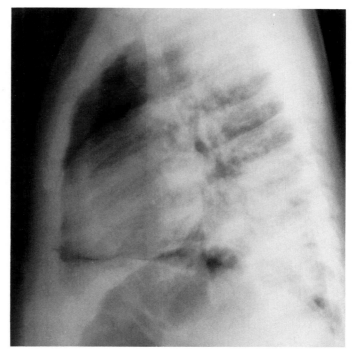

Figure 5–44. *C, Lateral view shows air in mediastinal structures to better advantage.*

C

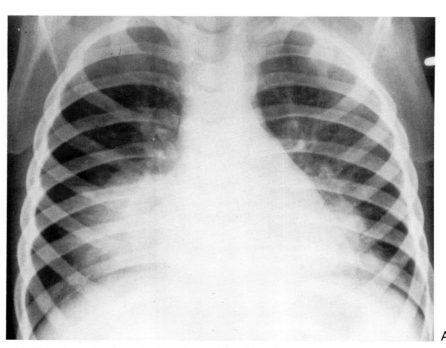

A

Figure 5–45. *Hydrocarbon ingestion in a 2-year-old child. A, Chest radiograph made approximately 12 hours after ingestion of lighter fluid shows bilateral consolidation involving lower lobes and right middle lobe.*

Illustration continued on following page

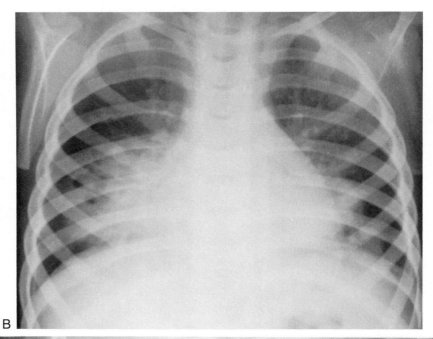

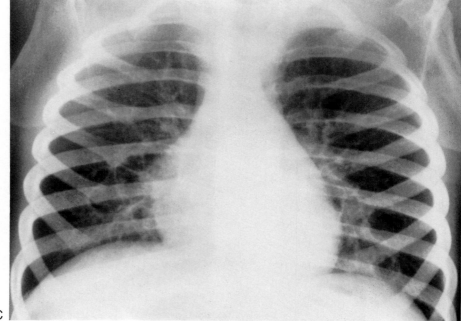

Figure 5–45. *B, Repeat radiograph 5 days later, after the infant was asymptomatic, shows early pneumatocele formation bilaterally. C, Repeat chest radiograph 2 weeks later shows nearly complete resolution of the pneumonia, with residual pneumatoceles. Follow-up studies showed a gradual decrease in size of the pneumatoceles, with ultimate complete disappearance.*

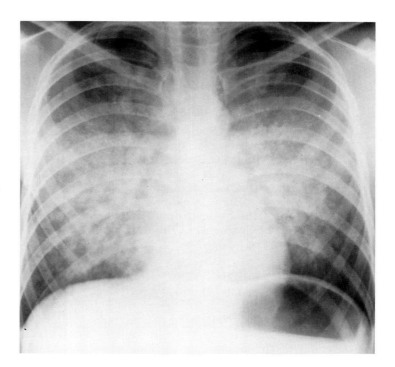

Figure 5–46. Massive aspiration in a near-drowned child. Resuscitation was accomplished with complete clearing of the lungs in 3 days.

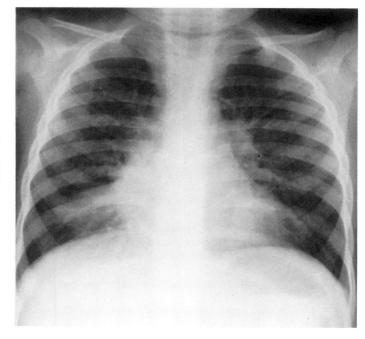

Figure 5–47. Milk allergy pneumonia in a 3-year-old child. There is bilateral broncho-pneumonia with consolidation of the right middle lobe. The patient had recurrent pneumonia, but after milk was eliminated from the diet, remained well.

and the heart appears unusually small. Interstitial pneumonia frequently accompanies the allergic episodes in both infants and children. The inflammatory process usually assumes the form of an interstitial pneumonia, which is usually bilateral, involving predominantly the lower lobe areas. The diagnosis in all age groups is made on the basis of a history of repeated attacks of hyperinflation of the lungs, with or without associated interstitial pneumonia, and after appropriate laboratory tests have excluded other causes.

Löffler's pneumonia is a manifestation of allergy that may occur in the pediatric patient but is more common in the adult. It is extremely rare in the infant age group. The characteristic radiographic findings are those of pulmonary infiltrates, usually alveolar in distribution, which vary in extent and distribution on successive x-ray examinations (Fig. 5–48). These fleeting infiltrates may or may not be associated with pulmonary hyperaeration. Adenopathy and pleural effusion rarely occur. There is frequently eosinophilia, and the possibility of intestinal parasites such as Ascaris lumbricoides and Toxocara canis being etiologically related should be considered.

An unusual form of allergic pneumonia is due to exposure to pet birds (bird fancier's disease). The radiographic findings usually consist of a reticulonodular pattern.

Reactive Airway Disease (Asthma)

The clinical and radiographic manifestations of asthma in the child are similar to those recognized in the adult. Differentiation between bronchiolitis and asthma in the infant is usually impossible.

The etiologic causes of asthma in the child are the same as those considered in the adult—namely, an underlying allergic response to a specific antigen, asthmatic attacks resulting from some underlying psychosomatic basis, or a combination of the two. In the pediatric patient the psychological considerations seem to play a more important etiologic role than in the adult.

The radiographic findings consist primarily of hyperaeration of the lungs. Chest radiographs show a more horizontal position of the ribs than is usually seen, flattening of the diaphragm, and an increase in the anteroposterior diameter of the chest (Fig. 5–49). The heart appears unusually small, depending on the degree of hyperaeration. Associated bronchopneumonia may occasionally accompany the asthmatic attacks (Fig. 5–50). Frequently, segmental areas of atelectasis may be identified as a result of mucus plugs. Pneumomediastinum may be a complication, and results from rupture of alveoli with dissection of air medially along the perivascular sheaths (Fig. 5–51). Pneumothorax may also occur if air extends from the mediastinum to the pleural space. Chronic asthma ultimately results in pulmonary hypertension, with increased prominence of the pulmonary arteries in the hilar areas.

Cystic Fibrosis

Cystic fibrosis, as originally described, was thought to be a disease limited to the pancreas. It is now known, however, that the mucus-secreting glands in general, as well as sweat glands, are involved. The etiology remains obscure but is known to be autosomal recessive. Although cystic fibrosis on rare occasions affects a black or Asiatic child, it is predominantly a white disease. Varying mild forms of cystic fibrosis may occur, but the morbidity is usually severe and the mortality is high. Cystic fibrosis is one of the major chronic incurable diseases of children and young adults.

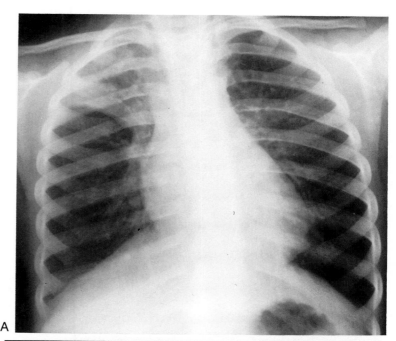

Figure 5–48. Löffler's pneumonia in a 2-year-old child with eosinophila. A, Initial chest radiograph shows atelectasis and pneumonia involving the right upper lobe. B, Repeat chest examination 2 days later shows change in distribution, with right middle lobe infiltration.

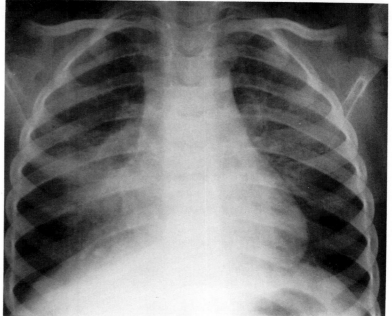

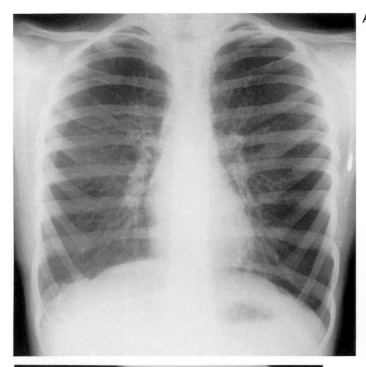

A

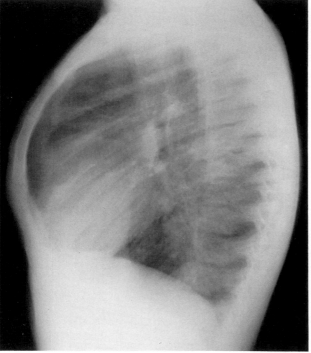

B

Figure 5–49. Asthma in a 7-year-old child. A, Frontal chest radiograph shows low position of the diaphragm, with diaphragmatic costal attachments seen at the right base. The ribs are more horizontal than normal, the heart is small, and the lungs are hyperlucent. B, Lateral view shows marked increase in the anteroposterior diameter of the chest, with increased convexity of the sternum.

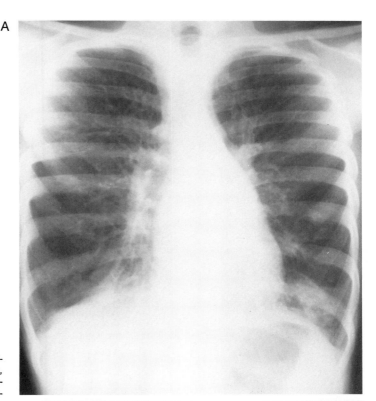

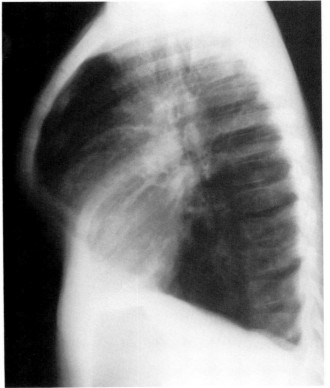

Figure 5–50. Chronic asthma with associated pneumonia in a 7-year-old child. A, Frontal chest radiograh shows hyperinflation of the lungs, with associated bronchopneumonia. Density in the left base probably represents segmental atelectasis. Radiolucency in the suprasternal notch area is secondary to contraction of the accessory muscles of respiration, the sternocleidomastoid muscles. B, Lateral view shows marked pectus carinatum deformity.

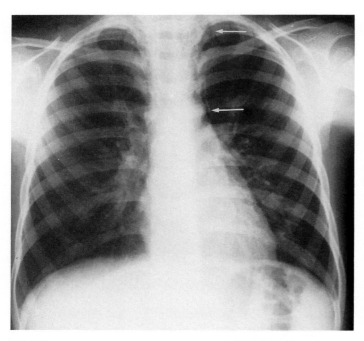

A

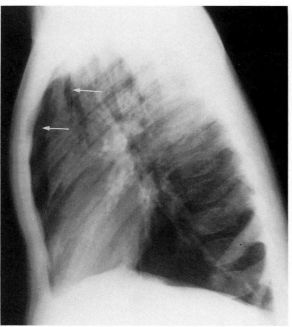

B

Figure 5–51. Pneumomediastinum complicating asthma in a 5-year-old child. A, Frontal chest radiograph shows hyperaeration
of the lungs, with air in the left superior
mediastinum and in the soft tissues of the
neck (arrows). B, Lateral view shows air in
the anterior mediastinum to better advantage, as well as streaky radiolucent areas
of air in the mediastinal structures (arrows).

There are various clinical manifestations. The earliest and perhaps most severe form is meconium ileus, which occurs in the newborn infant and is the result of thick tenacious meconium obstructing the terminal ileum and colon. The obstruction is usually severe, and immediate surgical intervention is generally necessary. Unfortunately, even if the obstruction is successfully corrected, the child invariably develops either the pulmonary complications or intestinal tract manifestations of cystic fibrosis.

The major clinical changes reflect the involvement of the pancreas, the lungs, the liver, and the intestinal tract. Fatty infiltration of the liver and chronic disease of the gallbladder with cholelithiasis frequently occur. Although there are no mucous glands in the biliary tree the thick tenacious bile is part of the mucoviscidosis picture, and the ensuing cirrhosis may produce portal hypertension and esophageal varices. The changes involving the pancreas and intestinal tract are manifested clinically as one form of the malabsorption syndrome. The increased loss of salt from the sweat glands results in poor tolerance to hot climates. Because of the tenacious mucus secretions in the paranasal sinuses, chronic sinusitis and nasal polyps are common complications.

Approximately 90% of children with this disease develop respiratory symptoms. The pulmonary manifestations may occur within the first few months of life but usually have their onset in later infancy. Any infant with recurrent bronchopneumonia or repeated attacks of bronchiolitis, croup, or asthma should be suspected of having cystic fibrosis, and appropriate laboratory tests should be performed.

Numerous pathologic changes are found in the lung, resulting primarily from infection secondary to bronchial obstruction produced by the tenacious viscid mucus. Abscess formation and bronchiectasis are common, but pleural effusion and empyema are rare. Respiratory failure is the primary cause of death in these children, while many others succumb to cor pulmonale or pulmonary hemorrhage.

Radiologically the earliest pulmonary manifestation is overinflation of the lungs or air trapping, such as is commonly seen in bronchiolitis or asthma (Fig. 5–52). Recurrent episodes of bronchopneumonia with varying degrees of confluence and atelectasis invariably occur (Fig. 5–53). Hilar and paratracheal lymphadenopathy are usually present. In the moderately or far advanced cases the radiographic features are characteristic, consisting of linear and patchy areas of infiltration, marked overinflation of the lungs, and small scattered rarefied areas representing either lung abscesses or bronchiectasis (Fig. 5–54). Mucoid impaction of bronchi may produce linear branching opacifications corresponding to bronchial segments, which contain viscid mucopurulent material (Fig. 5–55). Computerized tomography is helpful in cross-sectional imaging of the disease (Fig. 5–56). Magnetic resonance imaging is useful in differentiating the linear mucoid bronchial infections from pulmonary arteries (Fig. 5–57). The cardiac silhouette is small because of the tamponade effect of the emphysematous lungs, and the pulmonary arteries in the hilar areas may be increased in prominence because of the increased pulmonary resistance. Occasionally the areas of fibrosis and bleb formations may be localized (Fig. 5–58). Pneumothorax is an uncommon but serious complication, occurring in less than 3% of cases (Fig. 5–59).

If the major portion of the disease is localized to one segmental area, surgical resection may be of temporary benefit. Bronchography may be helpful in determining the degree of bronchiectasis if surgical resection is contemplated (Fig. 5–60). In cases of pulmonary hemorrhage selective bronchial artery embolization may be lifesaving (Fig. 5–61).

Pneumonia Complicating Congenital Heart Disease

Recurrent pneumonia is commonly encountered in infants and children with those forms of congenital heart disease associated with increased pulmonary blood

Text continued on page 198

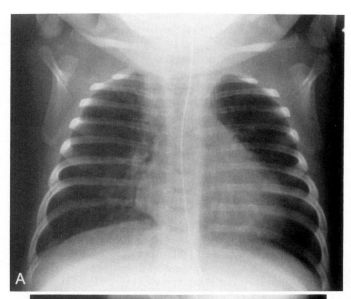

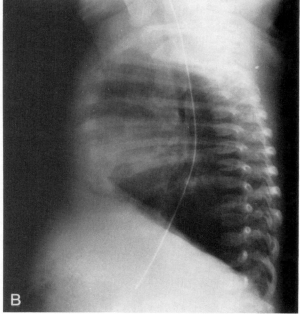

Figure 5–52. *Fibrocystic disease in a 2-month-old. A, The lungs are hyperinflated due to bilateral air trapping. There is no definite pneumonia, and the radiographic findings resemble those of bronchiolitis. B, The anteroposterior dimension of the chest is increased and flattened, similar to findings in cases of bronchiolitis in this age group.*

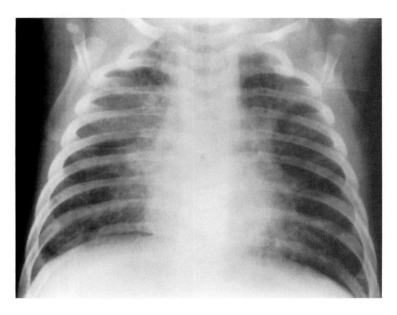

Figure 5–53. Pulmonary fibrocystic disease in a 2-month-old. There is bilateral air trapping and bronchopneumonia. Sweat testing showed the infant had cystic fibrosis.

A

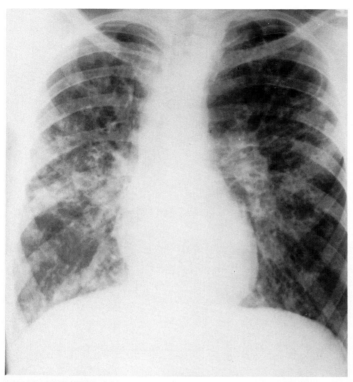

Figure 5–54. *Advanced pulmonary changes of fibrocystic disease in a 14-year-old. A, Frontal chest radiograph shows hyperinflation of the lungs, with diffuse pulmonary fibrosis and generalized interstitial pneumonia and bronchiectasis. B, Lateral view shows marked increase in the anteroposterior diameter of the chest.*

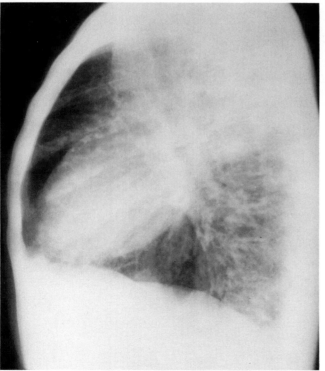

B

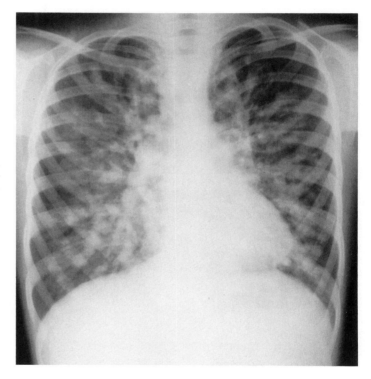

Figure 5–55. Fibrocystic disease in an 8-year-old child, showing multiple linear densities representing mucous plugs extending peripherally from the hilar areas.

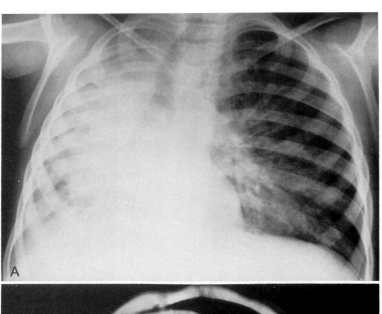

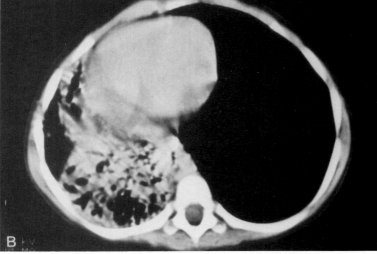

Figure 5–56. Fibrocystic disease. A, Chest radiograph shows bilateral pneumonia and loss of volume of the right lung. B, Computerized tomography emphasizes the severe bronchiectasis.

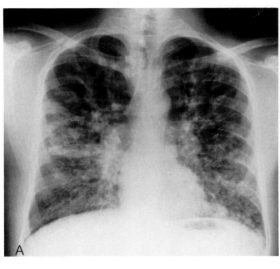

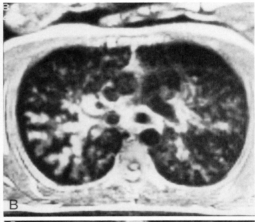

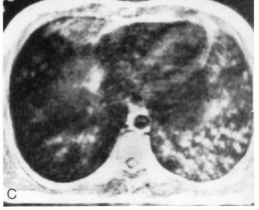

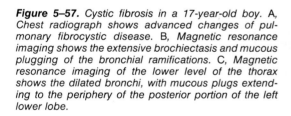

Figure 5–57. *Cystic fibrosis in a 17-year-old boy. A, Chest radiograph shows advanced changes of pulmonary fibrocystic disease. B, Magnetic resonance imaging shows the extensive brochiectasis and mucous plugging of the bronchial ramifications. C, Magnetic resonance imaging of the lower level of the thorax shows the dilated bronchi, with mucous plugs extending to the periphery of the posterior portion of the left lower lobe.*

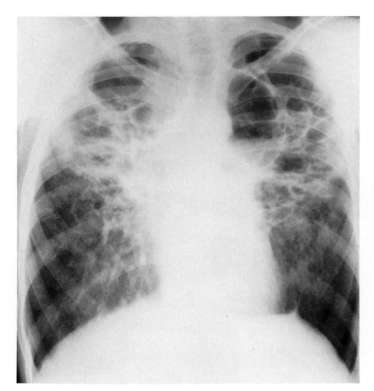

Figure 5–58. Fibrocystic disease in a 16-year-old boy showing hyperaeration of the lungs and localized areas of fibrosis and blebs in the perihilar and upper lobes bilaterally.

Figure 5–59. Pneumothorax complicating fibrocystic disease in a 14-year-old girl. The complete collapse of the left lung is unusual in patients with fibrocystic disease.

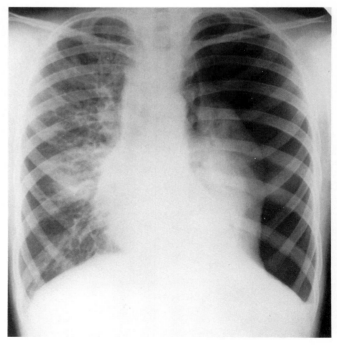

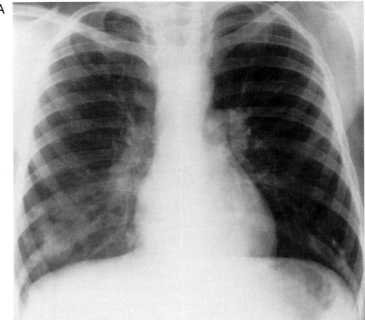

Figure 5–60. Fibrocystic disease in an 8-year-old child. A, Frontal view of the chest shows hyperaeration of the lungs, with infiltration localized primarily in the right and left lower lobes. B, Bronchogram of the right lower lobe shows localized bronchiectasis of the middle lobe.

Illustration continued on following page

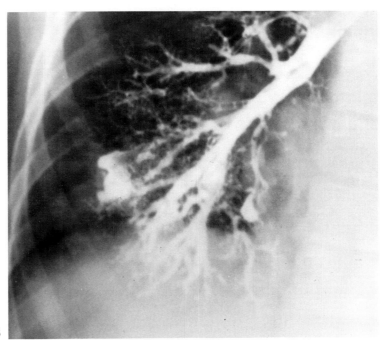

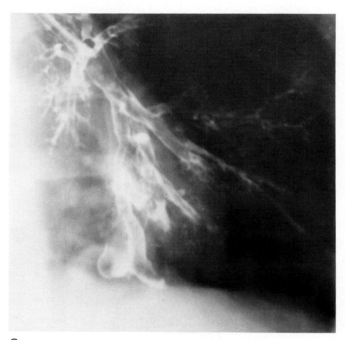

Figure 5–60. C, Bronchogram of the left lower lobe shows segmental bronchiectasis of the lower lobe. Segmental resection was accomplished, with resulting clinical improvement.

C

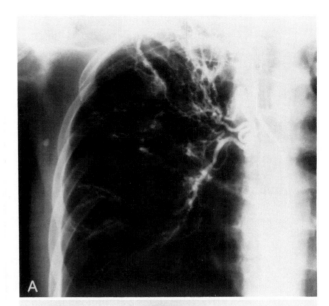

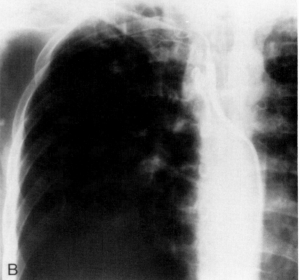

Figure 5–61. Cystic fibrosis in a 17-year-old boy with pulmonary hemorrhage. A, Selective catheterization of the bronchial artery shows increased vascularization of the right apex, representing the site of hemorrhage. B, Postembolization of this area shows obliteration of the bleeding vessel.

flow. The most common of these lesions are the ventricular and atrial shunts, patent ductus arteriosus, transposition of the great vessels, and true truncus arteriosus. Theoretically, patients with these defects are more susceptible to pneumonia because of the pressure on the bronchi by cardiac chamber enlargement, dilated pulmonary vessels, and inadequate lymphatic drainage. The severity and chronicity of the pneumonia seems to be related to the degree of congestive failure that many of these infants have. Young infants with congestive failure frequently aspirate during feeding, and as a consequence aspiration and atelectasis are often seen in their right upper lobe. Differentiation between pneumonia and the distended pulmonary veins and areas of pulmonary edema may be impossible by radiographic methods alone. Improvement in the degree of congestive failure is usually associated with resolution of the inflammatory process. Persistence of congestive failure is commonly associated with persistence of the pneumonia. Occasionally the pneumonia will not show resolution until surgical correction of the lesion. The radiographic pattern is commonly that of segmental atelectasis, with a mixed interstitial and alveolar distribution. Also, the degree of pulmonary hyperaeration, particularly in the young infant, is greater than that which would usually be seen with heart disease or lung disease alone (Fig. 5–62).

Aspiration Pneumonia

Aspiration pneumonia should be considered in any infant who has chronic pneumonia, particularly if it involves the right upper lobe and left perihilar areas (Fig. 5–63). These pulmonary segments are the most commonly involved areas in aspiration pneumonia because of their dependent positions. This is especially true in the right upper lobe, in which atelectasis commonly accompanies aspiration pneumonia. A number of etiologies should be considered, including esophageal atresia, tracheoesophageal fistula, pharyngeal incoordination, and vomiting due to gastroesophageal reflux, intestinal obstruction, or other causes. Esophageal atresia in the newborn infant is suspected when there is an excess amount of oral mucus and when a catheter cannot be passed into the stomach. Fluoroscopic examination of these infants should be done utilizing videotape and rapid spot films. Under fluoroscopic control, an end-hole catheter should be passed until it meets an obstruction. A small amount of contrast medium, no more than 1 ml, should be then injected into the upper esophageal pouch with the infant in a semiprone position to determine more accurately whether or not there is fistulous communication between the upper esophageal pouch and the trachea.

Evaluation of deglutition is mandatory in any infant suspected of having aspiration pneumonia. Pharyngeal incoordination with aspiration of contrast medium into the tracheobronchial tree occurs in a number of conditions, including weakness from prematurity, congenital dysautonomia, and brain damage. It also occurs occasionally in essentially normal term infants who, for some reason, have a temporary immaturity of the swallowing mechanism (Fig. 5–64) or who have fatigue aspiration. Gastroesophageal reflux is easily demonstrated by conventional fluoroscopy but may also be evaluated by radionuclide scintigraphy. In congenital dysautonomia there is pharyngeal incoordination, but apparently there is also abnormal activity of the cricopharyngeal muscle. If the aspiration pneumonia is secondary to obstruction, surgical correction is mandatory as soon as possible. Infants with severe pharyngeal incoordination and aspiration may require a gastrostomy. Chronic aspiration and pneumonia frequently result in bronchiectasis (Fig. 5–65). Iatrogenic perforation of the esophagus by a nasogastric or feeding tube may cause mediastinitis, pleural effusion, and pneumonia.

Massive aspiration may produce radiographic changes similar to those of pulmonary edema. The differentiation is made on the basis of the history and clinical information (Fig. 5–66).

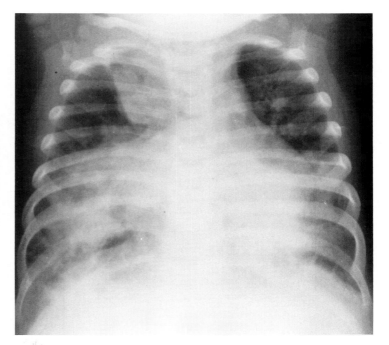

Figure 5–62. Pneumonia complicating congenital heart disease. Atrioventricular commune in an infant with Down's syndrome. The heart is enlarged and there is evidence of increased pulmonary flow and congestive heart failure. Extensive pneumonia is identified in both lower lobes. In addition, there are atelectasis and pneumonia involving the right upper lobe, possibly secondary to aspiration.

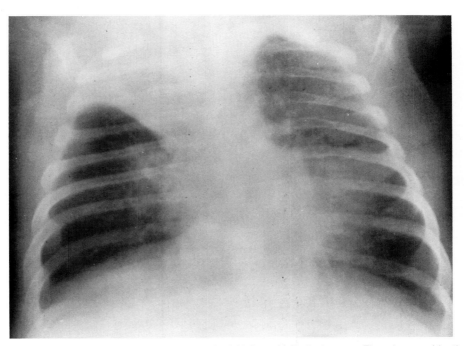

Figure 5–63. Aspiration pneumonia in a 1-month-old infant with brain damage. There is a combination of atelectasis and pneumonia in the right upper lobe and pneumonitis in the left perihilar area.

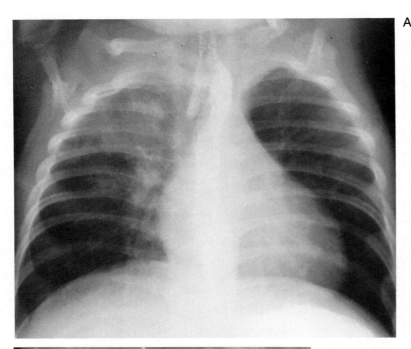

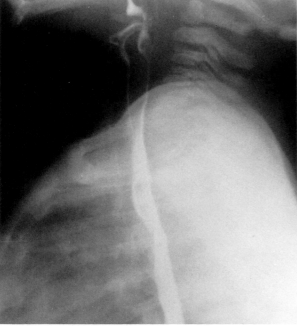

Figure 5–64. *Aspiration pneumonia in right upper lobe in infant with marked pharyngeal incoordination. A, Frontal chest radiograph shows pneumonia in the right upper lobe and barium in the esophagus and trachea. B, Lateral view shows ingested contrast medium in the trachea and the esophagus.*

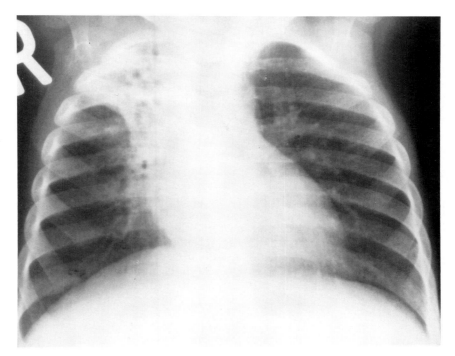

Figure 5–65. Chronic aspiration pneumonia with associated bronchiectasis in infant with brain damage.

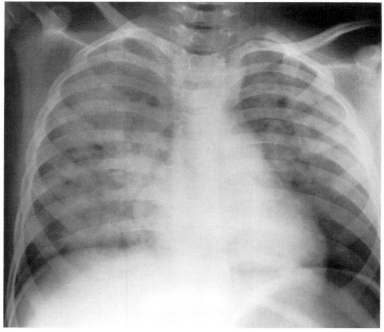

Figure 5–66. Massive aspiration of gastric contents in 8-year-old boy who was given a general anesthetic for reduction of a forearm fracture.

Aspiration of oily material may produce chronic pneumonitis, and should be a consideration in the differential diagnosis of chronic inflammatory disease in infants and children (Fig. 5–67). Oily material in any form is difficult for young infants to swallow without being aspirated, and consequently should not be given to those in this age group (Figs. 5–68 and 5–69). In addition, oily contrast material should not be used in the examination of the esophagus or upper gastrointestinal tract in infants because such substances are easily aspirated.

Aspiration in the ambulatory infant occurs usually in the right lower lobe, as in the adult.

Bronchiectasis

Bronchiectasis in the infant and young child is usually secondary to severe inflammatory changes of the small bronchial ramifications that may accompany a number of viral and bacterial infections, especially if incompletely treated. Necrotizing bronchiolitis represents a severe form of bronchiectasis in the young pediatric patient, and is usually a result of adenoviral infection. Bronchograms in these patients show extensive cylindric and saccular changes, which alter in size dramatically with inspiration and expiration (Fig. 5–70). Progression of this condition may produce bronchial pruning and bronchiolitis obliterans. If this complication is unilateral it is referred to as the Swyer-James syndrome. Congenital bronchiectasis is very rare. Tracheobronchiomegaly (Mounier-Kuhn syndrome) is also a rare congenital abnormality of the tracheobronchial tree. Immune deficiency diseases and the immotile cilia syndrome may also produce chronic respiratory disease. Bronchiectasis in this young age group may also be secondary to chronic aspiration or tracheoesophageal fistula, with resulting chronic infection and

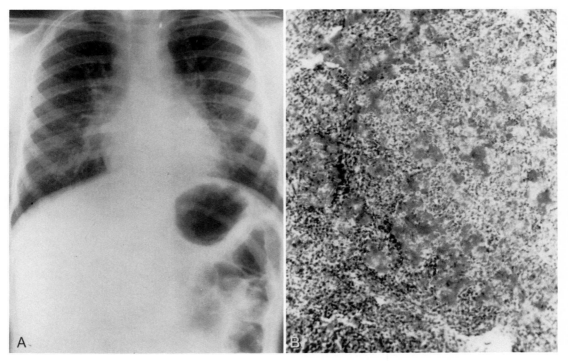

Figure 5–67. Aspiration of oil in bath water in a young infant. A, Chronic interstitial pneumonia was observed over a period of several weeks. B, Aspiration of a tracheobronchial tree shows many macrophages filled with oil.

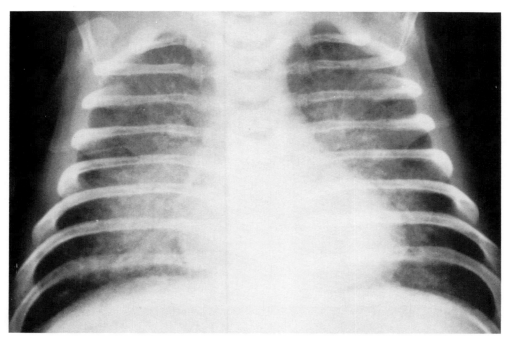

Figure 5–68. Olive oil aspiration in a 1-week-old infant who was given a tablespoon of olive oil.

Figure 5–69. Lipid pneumonia in child following prolonged use of petrolatum nose drops.

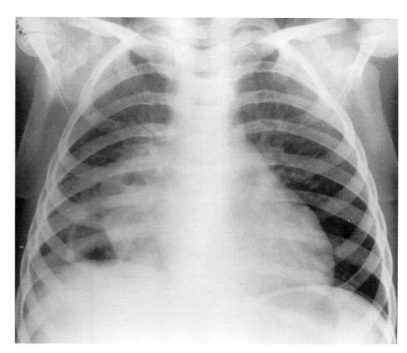

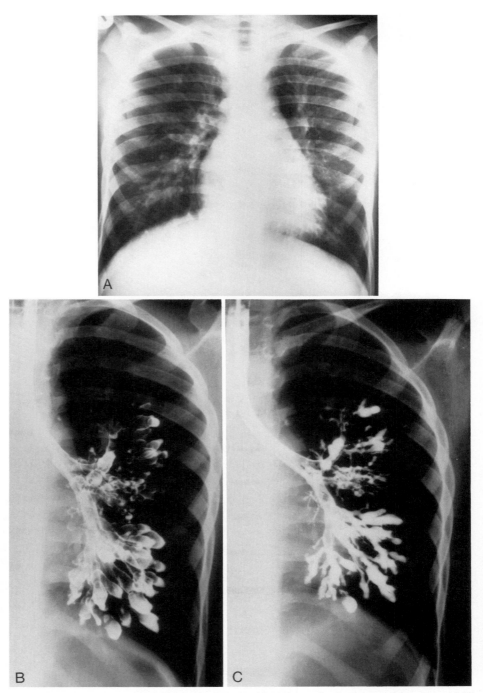

Figure 5–70. *Severe bronchiectasis in a 7-year-old patient who had necrotizing bronchiolitis associated with pertussis. A, Chest radiograph shows bilateral lower lobe infiltration. B and C, Bronchograms show marked cystic bronchiectasis, which changed dramatically in size during inspiration (B) and expiration (C).*

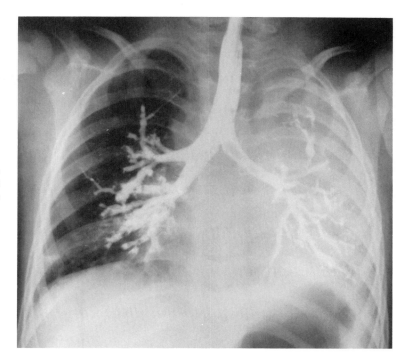

Figure 5–71. Bilateral cylindric bronchiectasis in a 2-year-old child who has a small tracheosophageal fistula.

atelectasis (Fig. 5–71). Chronic bronchiectasis in the child may also result from aspiration of infected material from suppurative tonsillitis (Fig. 5–72) or chronic sinusitis, from aspirated foreign bodies, and from incompletely treated pneumonia. In the ambulatory child, bronchiectasis is more common in the lower lobe segments, particularly the right lower and middle lobes. Other radiographic features consist of persistent areas of infiltration that may clear during antibiotic

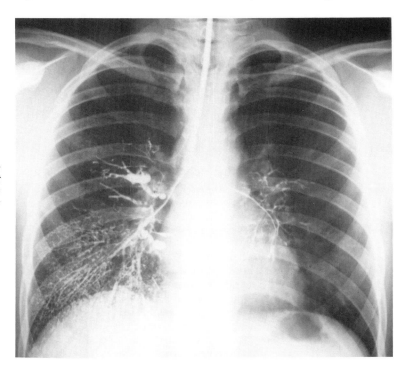

Figure 5–72. Chronic bronchiectasis of superior dorsal segment of right lower lobe in a 10-year-old boy with a long history of suppurative tonsillitis and recurrent pneumonia.

therapy but then recur in the same locations. In advanced cases small radiolucent areas representing the dilated involved bronchial segments can be identified. Occasionally, localized constriction of a bronchus proximal to the bronchiectasis is present, but whether this is an inflammatory bronchial stricture or a congenital disorder cannot be determined.

Bronchiectasis is also a feature of Kartagener's syndrome, which also includes sinusitis and situs inversus. Vessels arising from the aorta and leading to the bronchiectatic segments have been noted.

Bronchiectasis is invariably present in patients with advanced pulmonary fibrocystic disease.

Plain films of the chest are nearly always abnormal in bronchiectasis. Additional studies include technetium-99m perfusion and CT scans of the chest. If none of these are abnormal, it is very unlikely that bronchiectasis is present. Bronchograms define the extent of disease and the advisability of surgical resection. Bronchography in the pediatric patient should be regarded as a serious and hazardous procedure, and should be performed with the patient anesthetized with a general anesthetic administered by a competent pediatric anesthesiologist.

Pulmonary Sequestration

Pulmonary sequestration is a congenital malformation of the respiratory tract in which there is a small segment of lung that has no normal communication with the tracheobronchial tree and has a separate blood supply from systemic arteries. Pathologically there are two types, the more common intralobar sequestration, which lies within the normal visceral pleura, and the less common extralobar type, which is accessory lung tissue outside of the normal pleural boundaries. The exact embryologic defect is not definitely known, but it probably results from a small duplication of the lower anterior foregut, which differentiates into pulmonary tissue but retains its original blood supply from the aorta.

The sequestered segment never develops into normal respiratory tissue, and is usually airless. Partial aeration may occur, as well as aerated cystic areas, usually due to infection and fistulous communication with adjacent normal lung tissue (Fig. 5–73). The possibility of air entering the intralobar sequestration through the alveolar bronchiole communications (channels of Lambert) is another consideration. Sequestration (especially the intralobar type) occurs most often in the lower lobe areas. The extralobar type has been reported in nearly every portion of the thorax, and even in the upper abdomen (Fig. 5–74). The blood supply is usually from the thoracic or abdominal aorta, with the feeding artery varying in size. Venous drainage from the intralobar type is to the pulmonary circulation, while the extralobar variety drains to systemic veins. Although the lesion is congenital, clinical manifestations, usually consisting of repeated pulmonary infections, frequently do not occur until late childhood.

Radiographically, the chest x-ray will show an irregular oval or triangular density usually located in the medial and posterior portions of the lower lobe. Surrounding infiltration may be evident if there is secondary infection within the normal lung. If an abscess develops air-fluid levels may be present. There will be nonfilling of this segment bronchographically, with normal bronchi surrounding the lesion. Digital subtraction angiography is useful in evaluating the vascular supply and drainage of a sequestration. Aortography also provides a definitive diagnosis by demonstrating the anomalous blood supply, and it helps to differentiate the intralobar from the extralobar type by the difference in venous drainage.

Systemic blood supply to normal lungs with normal bronchial communication may rarely occur as a normal variant, or may be acquired in chronic inflammatory disease (pseudosequestration) (Fig. 5–75).

Surgical removal of the sequestration is the treatment of choice.

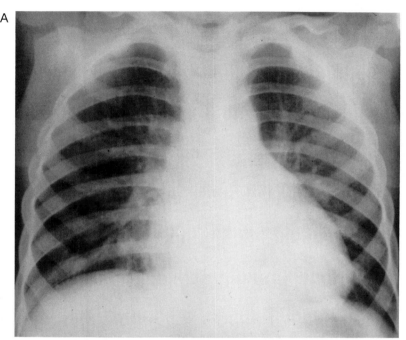

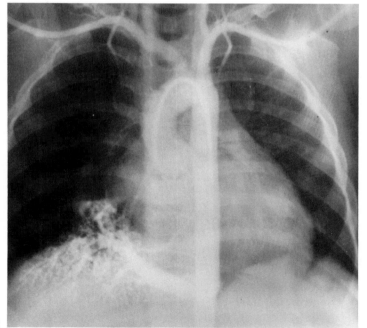

Figure 5–73. Intralobar pulmonary sequestrations. A, Chest radiograph shows abnormal density involving the right lower lobe. B, Aortogram shows anomalous blood supply from the aorta.

Illustration continued on following page

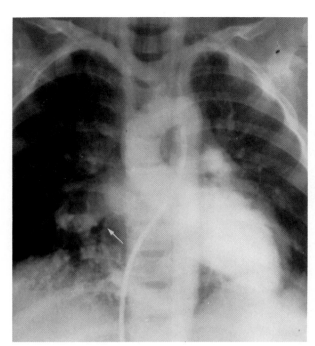

Figure 5–73. *C, Venous damage from the sequestrated segment is into the left atrium* (arrow).

C

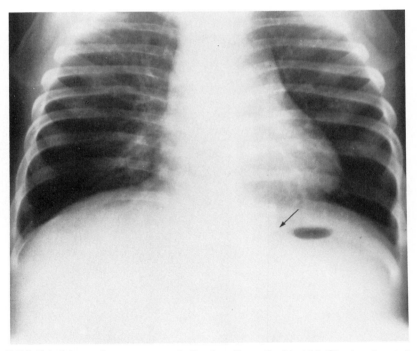

Figure 5–74. *Extralobar pulmonary sequestration in a 7-month-old child. Chest radiograph shows density in the left posterior mediastinum (arrow). At surgical exploration this was found to be accessory lung extending through a congenital defect in the left hemidiaphragm. The blood supply was from an anomalous bronchial artery, and it was considered to be an extralobar sequestration. Preoperative angiographic studies were not performed. (Courtesy of Dr. B. Felson, Cincinnati.)*

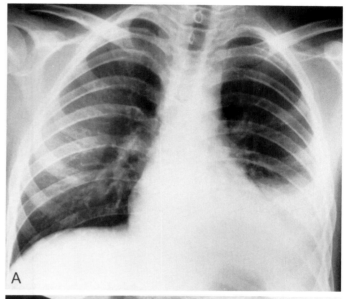

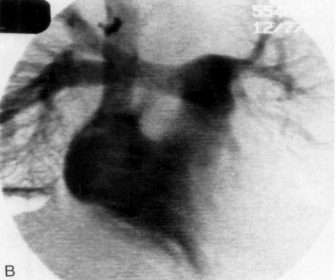

Figure 5–75. Chronic pneumonia (pseudo-sequestration) in a 14-year-old boy. A, Chest radiograph shows left lower lobe pneumonia, which had remained unchanged for several months. B, Digital subtraction study shows little appreciable blood flow through the pulmonary artery supplying the left lower lobe.

Illustration continued on following page

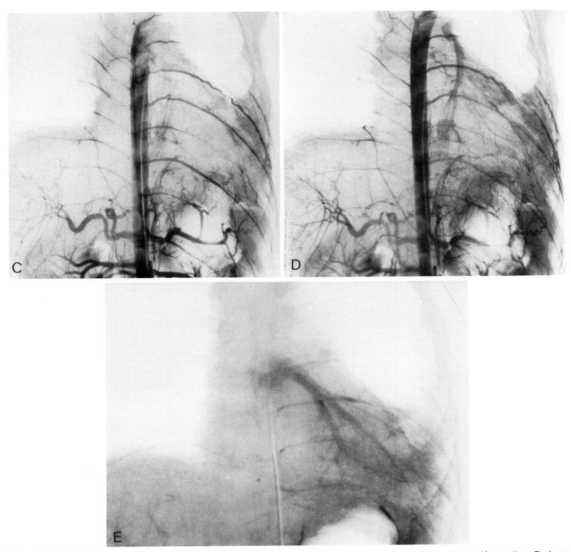

Figure 5–75. *C, Aortogram demonstrates several intercostal arteries supplying an arteriovenous malformation. D, Later phase of the aortogram shows the arteriovenous fistula, the network of intercostal vessels supplying the left lower lobe, and retrograde filling of the left pulmonary artery. E, Later phase shows pulmonary venous return into the left atrium.*

As described in Chapter 4, bronchopulmonary sequestration may be associated with cystic adenomatoid malformation.

Esophageal Bronchus

Esophageal bronchus is a rare type of foregut malformation that is usually classified with pulmonary sequestration (Fig. 5–76). The aberrant bronchi generally arise from the lower portion of the esophagus, and extend to the right lung. Chronic infection is commonly present, and the aberrant arterial blood supply to the area can usually be demonstrated by angiography. Frequently anomalous pulmonary venous return is also present.

Hypoimmune Diseases

The recognition of congenital and acquired deficiencies of the immunologic factors necessary for normal host resistance to disease and their radiographic manifestations has increased markedly during the past decade. The study and elucidation of the complexities involved in cellular and antibody reactions to pathogenic organisms, as well as to foreign tissue (including skin grafting and organ transplantation) currently represent an exciting and remarkable achievement in immunology.

It would be presumptuous to try to describe the extensive work done in this field. However, an understanding of certain fundamental aspects regarding the underlying process of the immunologic response is necessary. Basically, there are two distinct cell populations that presumably arise from the totipotential stem cell from which both the hematopoietic and lymphopoietic systems are derived (Fig. 5–77). The potential function of this cell type apparently depends on its location. If this cell circulates to the thymus it "nests" there, and developmental factors in that environment influence it to become a thymic (T) lymphocyte. If, on the other hand, it lodges and develops in an as yet undetermined site (perhaps the lymphoid area of the intestinal tract), it is influenced to develop along the plasma cell line and ultimately develops antibody functions. A deficiency in thymic stroma results in a lack of normal cellular immunity with resulting increased susceptibility, usually to viral, fungal, or protozoan disease.

There are many varieties of cellular and humoral deficiency. Acquired cellular immunity deficiency is seen in Hodgkin's disease as well as in other lymphomas, chronic lymphocytic leukemia, and sarcoidosis. Acquired humoral deficiency diseases are seen in thymomas and also in lymphomas. Acquired dysgammaglobulinemia is seen in multiple myeloma.

CONGENITAL IMMUNE DEFICIENCY

Our concern here is with congenital deficiency, particularly those situations in which lung disease occurs in infants. The best example of congenital cellular deficiency is the DiGeorge syndrome, in which there is a congenital absence of the thymus as well as of the parathyroid glands. The best example of the congenital form of humoral or antibody deficiency is Bruton's form of agammaglobulinemia.

In our experience the most common forms of congenital immune deficiency are seen in the combined cellular and humoral type, particularly in severe combined immune deficiency, or Swiss agammaglobulinemia. Ataxia telangiectasia, Nezelof's syndrome (Fig. 5–78), adenosine deaminase and nucleoside phosphorylase deficiency, and Wiskott-Aldrich syndrome are other less common forms of combined cellular and antibody deficiencies. The skeletal changes of costovertebral separation, flared anterior ribs, and squared-off scapulae and pneumonia should alert the radiologist to the probability of adenosine deaminase deficiency (Fig. 5–79). Short-limbed dwarfism with immunodeficiency and cartilage-hair hypoplasia are mainly forms of T-cell immunodeficiency, and pneumonia is a common complication.

Differentiation among most of these conditions is determined by clinical and laboratory methods. Only the more common forms of immune deficiency seen in the pediatric age group will be considered. The most common of these is severe combined immune deficiency disease. The radiographic findings occur early in infancy, and there is usually an associated absence of radiologically demonstrable lymphoid tissue. Recognition of the absence of the normal adenoid on lateral views of the nasopharynx may be helpful in suggesting that chronic or recurrent pneumonia is a result of immunologic deficiency (Fig. 5–80). However, it is important to know whether or not a previous adenoidectomy has been performed. It is equally important to realize that normal nasopharyngeal adenoid tissue is difficult to evaluate during the first year of life.

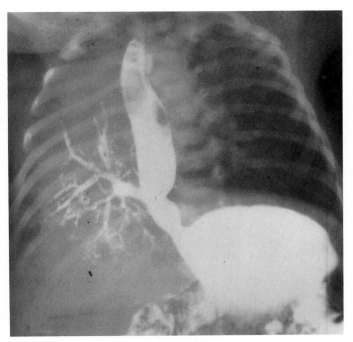

Figure 5–76. *Esophageal bronchus extending into the right lung, with resulting pneumonia.*

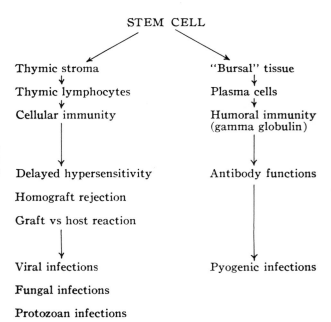

Figure 5–77. *Method of stem cell differentiation in the cellular and humoral immune functions. (From Presberg HJ, and Singleton EB: Combined immune deficiency disease. Radiology, 91:959, 1968.)*

STEM CELL

Thymic stroma

Thymic lymphocytes

Cellular immunity

Delayed hypersensitivity

Homograft rejection

Graft vs host reaction

Viral infections

Fungal infections

Protozoan infections

"Bursal" tissue

Plasma cells

Humoral immunity
(gamma globulin)

Antibody functions

Pyogenic infections

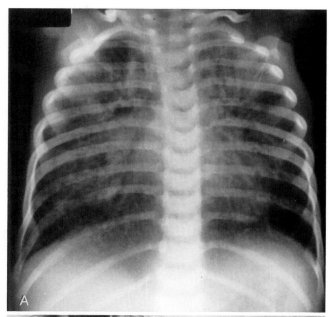

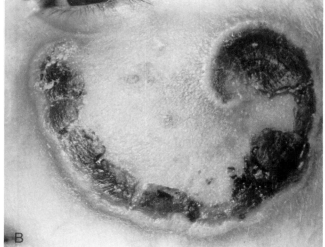

Figure 5–78. Nezelof's syndrome in a 1½-year-old who had received a smallpox vaccination. A, Chest radiography shows diffuse interstitial pneumonia. B, Skin lesion secondary to the patient's general vaccina.

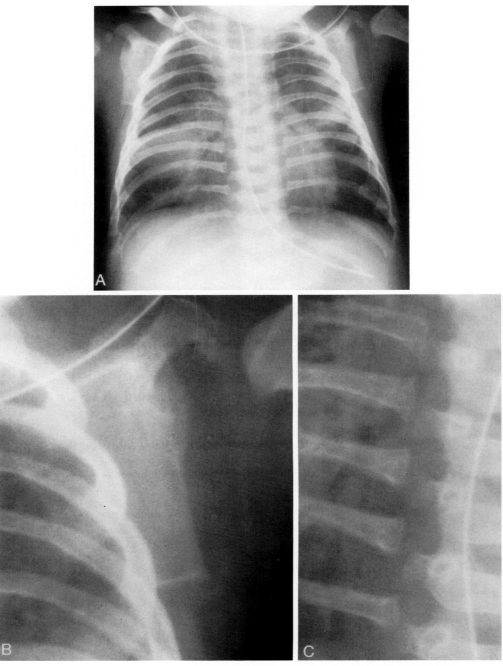

Figure 5–79. *Young infant with adenosine deaminase deficiency. A, Bilateral inflammatory infiltrates are present in both lungs. B, Radiograph of the scapulae shows the "cut-off" appearance of the scapular tip. C, Radiograph of the thoracic spine shows increased distance at the costovertebral junctions.*

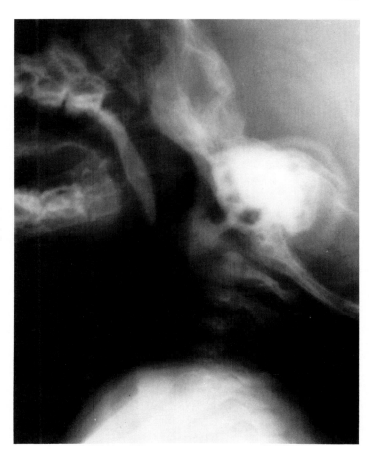

Figure 5–80. *Severe combined immune deficiency in a 7-month-old child with failure to thrive. Lateral view of the nasopharynx shows no radiographic evidence of adenoid tissue.*

The thymic shadow in immunologic deficiencies is abnormally small, giving the anterior mediastinum an "empty" appearance (Fig. 5–81). However, differentiation of secondary involution caused by chronic disease, steroid therapy, or cachexia and dysgenesis due to an immunologic defect is not always possible. In previous years, pneumomediastinography with carbon dioxide was used to evaluate the size of the thymus (Fig. 5–82), but computed tomography and magnetic imaging are now more informative. In the DiGeorge syndrome there is a congenital absence of the thymus and, because the thymus and parathyroid glands develop embryologically from the same branchial arch, hypocalcemia with resulting tetany is common. Aortic arch anomalies also occur frequently in this condition. A combination of these findings, as well as chronic recurrent infections, are important diagnostic features.

Most infants with immunologic deficiencies have chronic pulmonary diseases. In our experience, infants with combined immunologic deficiency have chronic lung disease due to pneumocystic pneumonitis.

Wiskott-Aldrich syndrome is a clinical entity characterized by dysgammaglobulinemia, recurrent otitis media, chronic lung disease, chronic eczema, and thrombocytopenia (Fig. 5–83). A lateral view of the nasopharynx may or may not show adenoidal hypoplasia.

ACQUIRED IMMUNE DEFICIENCY SYNDROME

Acquired immune deficiency syndrome (AIDS) may occur in infants as a result of transplacental, perinatal, or postnatal transmission. Pulmonary infections

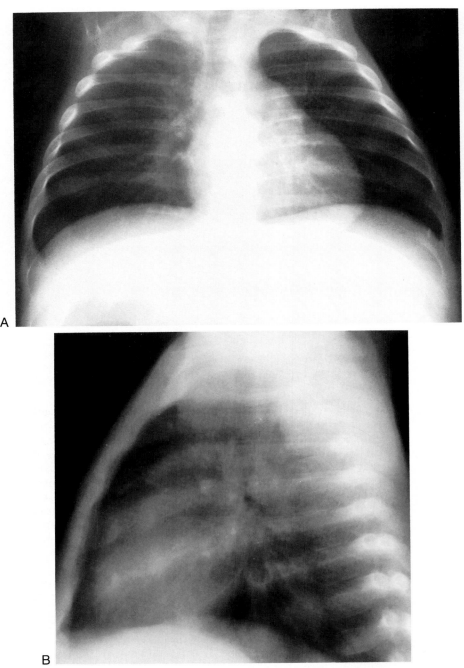

Figure 5–81. A, *Frontal chest radiograph shows absence of normal thymic tissue.* B, *Lateral view shows "empty" appearance of the anterior superior mediastinum.*

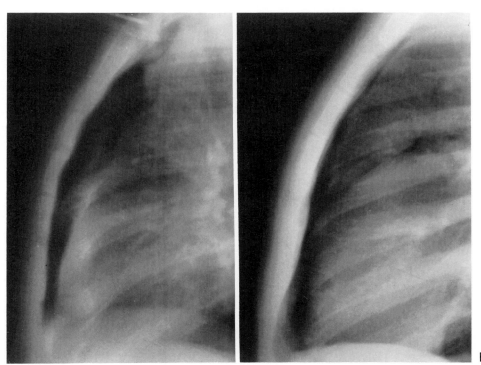

A   B

Figure 5–82. *Carbon dioxide insufflation of the anterior mediastinum. A, Lateral view of the chest following substernal injection of carbon dioxide shows an empty anterior superior mediastinum, with little appreciable thymic tissue being identified. B, Lateral view of the chest after carbon dioxide insufflation in infant with questionable hypoimmune syndrome shows normal thymic shadow. (From Presberg HJ, and Singleton EB: Combined immune deficiency disease. Radiology 91:959, 1968.)*

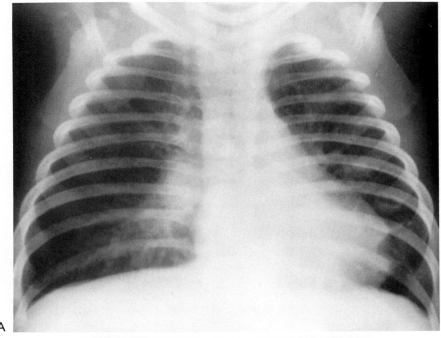

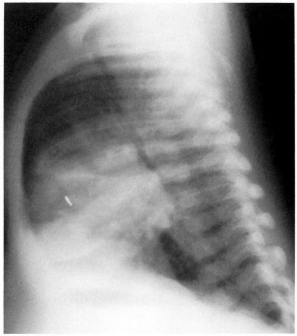

Figure 5–83. *Aldrich's syndrome in a 6-month-old child with chronic lung disease. A, Chest radiograph shows bronchopneumonia involving both lower lobes. B, Lateral view shows hyperinflation of the lungs as well as a clear anterior mediastinum. In this condition the thymus is not congenitally absent but has become atrophic because of chronic disease.*

are usually the result of the opportunistic organisms of Pneumocystis carinii, cytomegalovirus, or herpes simplex. The radiographic findings consist of perihilar infiltrates of varying degree of severity. Another type of pulmonary involvement that cannot be distinguished from that caused by opportunistic infections, but may be detected by lung biopsy or postmortem examination, consists of nodular peribronchiolar lymphoid hyperplasia. The focal aggregates of lymphoid tissue differentiate this condition from lymphoid interstitial pneumonitis. Clinically, patients with pulmonary lymphoid hyperplasia have a slower progressive course than those with only opportunistic infections. The radiographic features of pulmonary lymphoid hyperplasia consist of a nodular pattern distributed throughout the lung parenchyma, including its periphery. In the early stages the pattern may resemble miliary tuberculosis. With progression the nodules increase in size, and mediastinal adenopathy becomes more prominent (Fig. 5–84).

Chronic Granulomatous Disease of Childhood

This is a disease of infancy and childhood in which the basic defect is the inability of neutrophils and monocytes to destroy bacteria that they normally phagocytize. The disease commonly has its onset in early infancy, frequently within the first month of life, and is characterized by repeated infections, which often lead to early death. When first reported the disease was thought to be X-linked, occurring only in males, but it is now known to be autosomal recessive as well, and may affect both sexes.

Clinically, the disease is characterized by recurrent febrile illnesses in which many organs are involved. There may be eczematoid skin lesions, adenitis with suppuration, and varying forms of pleuropulmonary pathology. Intra-abdominal adenitis and hepatic abscesses with subsequent calcification may occur, and hepatosplenomegaly is often present. Osteomyelitis may also occur, but sequestration is rare. There may also be thickening and narrowing of the antrum of the stomach. Catalase-positive bacteria are the usual causes of the inflammatory lesions.

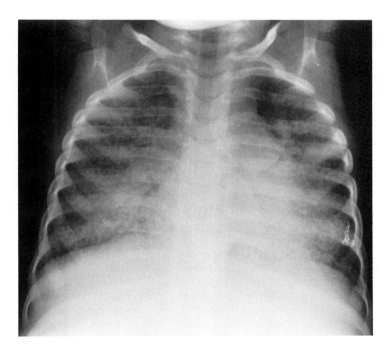

Figure 5–84. Pulmonary lymphoid hyperplasia as a result of AIDS in a 3-year-old boy whose mother was a prostitute. Small nodular densities occupy both lungs, with some confluence of the densities in the perihilar areas.

The pulmonary roentgenographic manifestations are variable, but most patients will demonstrate some form of pneumonia. Hilar and mediastinal adenopathy as well as pleural effusion commonly occur. Empyema and lung abscess are also common complications. If subphrenic abscess formation is present the diaphragm may be elevated, with a hazy margin. An interesting feature of the disease is the formation of spotty calcifications of varying size within the liver and spleen, secondary to healed granulomas. The radiographic combination of recurrent pneumonias and hepatic calcification should alert the radiologist to the possibility of chronic granulomatous disease of childhood (Fig. 5–85).

Hyper IgE syndrome (Buckley syndrome) is clinically similar to chronic granulomatous disease of childhood, but affects males and females. Staphylococcal infections are common, including recurrent and chronic pneumonias and frequent pneumatocele formation (Fig. 5–86). IgE levels are elevated, and polymorphonuclear leukocyte function is normal.

Agranulocytic pneumonia may be a complication of leukemia and aplastic anemia. Any pathogenic bacteria or virus may be the etiologic agent. Most leukemic children with agranulocytic pneumonia have Pseudomonas aeruginosa or staphylococcal infections. This pulmonary complication is usually a terminal condition. Radiographically there may be segmental involvement, but the usual radiographic appearance is that of a diffuse interstitial or mixed infiltration involving both lungs (Fig. 5–87).

Pneumocystis Carinii Pneumonia

This disease was first reported in Europe as interstitial plasma cell pneumonia in premature and debilitated infants. However, the lesion is more commonly an opportunistic infection in those suffering from chronic illnesses such as hematopoietic malignancies or congenital immune deficiency disorders, or in those receiving corticosteroids or cytotoxic drugs. It has also been seen endemically in foundling nurseries and within members of the same family.

Other organisms, such as varying types of bacteria, fungi, and cytomegalovirus, may be found concomitantly with the Pneumocystis protozoan.

Clinically, there may be a low-grade fever associated with respiratory distress and varying degrees of cyanosis. The physical findings in the chest are amazingly few compared to the radiographic findings. Laboratory studies are generally of little help.

There are several roentgenographic patterns, but the usual appearance is that of a fine, diffuse, granular, bilateral infiltration that begins in the hilar areas and spreads peripherally (Fig. 5–88). Interstitial emphysema, pneumothorax, or pneumomediastinum, either individually or in any combination, may develop, and generally proves fatal. If the disease progresses the peripheral lung fields become opacified by the infiltrate, and the lungs become virtually airless. There is usually no pleural reaction or hilar adenopathy. Rarely, the pulmonary involvement may be of a miliary form, and calcification may develop (Fig. 5–89).

The diagnosis is established by direct visualization of the organisms, either in tracheobronchial secretions or, more likely, by lung biopsy. The mortality rate is quite high, ranging between 20 and 50% of cases. Gallium-67 scans have been shown to be a sensitive test in doubtful cases.

Cytomegalic Inclusion Disease Pneumonia

Cytomegalic inclusion disease is caused by the cytomegalovirus and may occur in two forms, congenital or acquired. The congenital form may occur under two circumstances. In one form, the most virulent, the mother acquires the

Text continued on page 227

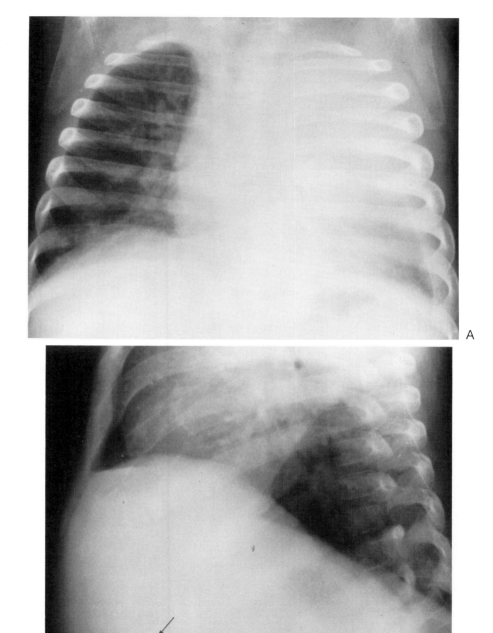

Figure 5–85. Chronic granulomatous disease of childhood in a 1-year-old child with chronic pneumonia. A, Chest radiograph shows left pleural effusion and consolidation of the left upper lobe. B, Lateral view shows calcification of the liver (arrow).

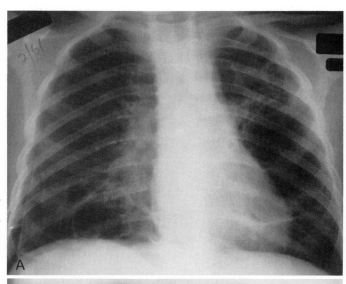

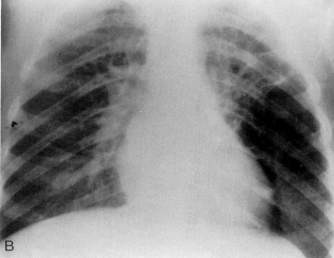

Figure 5–86. *Hyper IgE syndrome in a 4-year-old boy. A, Multiple small pneumatoceles are identified throughout both lungs. Right pneumothorax is also present. B, Repeat radiograph 3 months later shows additional pneumatocele formation, as well as upper lobe infiltrates.*

Illustration continued on opposite page

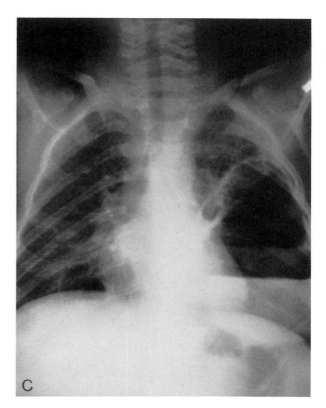

Figure 5–86. C, Repeat chest examination 1 year later shows large air-filled pneumatoceles in the left lung.

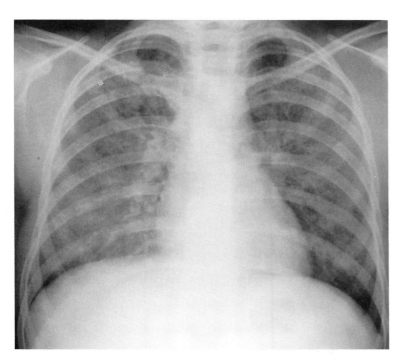

Figure 5–87. Agranulocytic pneumonia in child with terminal leukemia. Chest radiograph shows diffuse interstitial pneumonia involving both lungs.

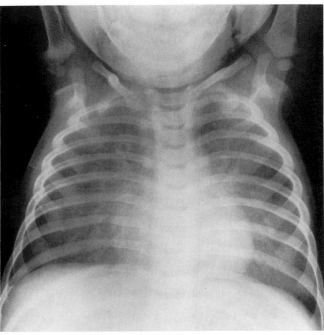

A

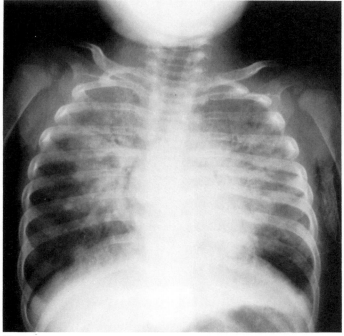

B

Figure 5–88. Pneumocystis pneumonia in two infants with severe combined immune deficiency disease. A, Chest radiograph of six-month-old shows diffuse interstitial pneumonitis involving primarily the perihilar areas. B, Chest radiograph of a 10-month-old shows similar radiating densities extending out from each hilus, with associated hyperaeration of the lungs.

Illustration continued on opposite page

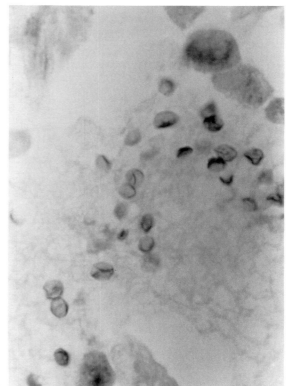

Figure 5–88. C, Photomicrograph of pneumocystic organisms (120 ×).

C

A

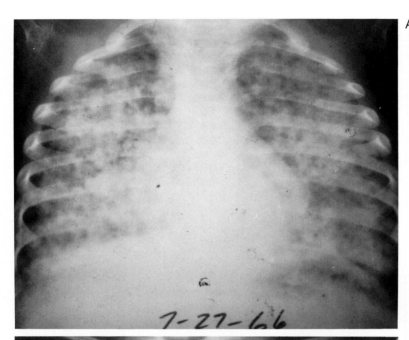

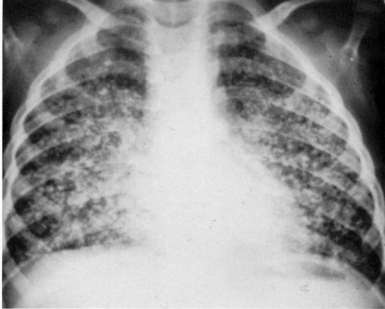

B

Figure 5–89. Chest radiograph of infant with hypoimmune syndrome and pneumocystis pneumonia. A, Disseminated nodular densities can be seen scattered throughout both lungs. B, Repeat chest radiograph several weeks later shows calcification of the nodules. (Courtesy of Dr. Guido Currarino, Dallas.)

cytomegalovirus during pregnancy, with subsequent infection of the fetus. This type may produce serious generalized disease, including severe pneumonia. Other clinical features include hepatosplenomegaly, skin rashes (occasionally petechial), hepatitis, and hemolytic anemia. A high percentage will develop central nervous system complications, including encephalitis, microcephaly (intracranial calcifications), optic and possibly auditory nerve involvement, and impaired intellectual and motor development. In another form of congenital infection the mother may have previously contracted cytomegalovirus disease and, during pregnancy, the virus is reactivated, with subsequent delivery of an infected child. The clinical findings in this form are usually not as severe as in the more serious type. In both forms the infant mortality rate is quite high.

In acquired cytomegalovirus disease babies may contract the organism from an infected cervix or from infected breast milk. These infants may develop mild pneumonia. Acquired disease may also be found in seronegative premature babies who have received seropositive blood. These infants may develop serious complications, including severe pneumonia. Cytomegalovirus pneumonia may also be found in children who are immunosuppressed for any reason, such as those receiving chemotherapy for malignancy, and those who have received an organ or bone marrow transplant. These patients may develop pneumonia by direct acquisition of the virus or by reactivation of the disease.

The most accurate method of establishing a diagnosis is isolation of the virus from the urine or throat. Typical cells containing intranuclear inclusions may be found in the urine, and the ELISA (enzyme-linked immunosorbent assay) is utilized for antibody studies.

Radiographic manifestations of cytomegalovirus pneumonia are variable. The disease may be found in one or more lobes, and may have a linear or patchy pattern of distribution. Occasionally the infiltrate may be rather symmetric bilaterally and, if severe enough, may simulate early pulmonary edema (Fig. 5–90). A rare complication is that of bronchiectasis (Fig. 5–91). Bone changes similar to those of rubella may be present. The differential diagnosis of a persistent interstitial pneumonia in a child with leukemia should include cytomegalic inclusion disease (Fig. 5–92), pneumocystic pneumonitis, agranulocytic pneumonia, and other viral pneumonias. The radiographic changes in each situation are frequently indistinguishable.

Childhood Tuberculosis

Most cases of childhood tuberculosis occur in older infants or young children, and are almost exclusively the result of contact with a parent, relative, or other caretaker who has active cavitary disease. Occasionally the source of infection is unknown, but all possible contacts should be investigated radiographically and given the tuberculin test. Fortunately, childhood tuberculosis as well as tuberculosis in the adult is becoming an uncommon illness and, when encountered, can be treated successfully. The importance of chemotherapy both in radiographically demonstrable tuberculosis and in children with positive skin tests is now clearly established, and is responsible for the success in controlling what was once one of the most common causes of death in children.

The pathogenesis of primary tuberculosis has been fully appreciated for many years. Tuberculosis bacilli, after reaching the alveoli, form an inflammatory exudate that spreads through the regional lymphatics to the mediastinal lymph nodes, producing the primary tuberculous complex. Pleural involvement is also common in primary infections (Fig. 5–93). Occasionally bronchial obstruction caused by enlarged peribronchial lymph nodes produces atelectasis, which was formerly known as epituberculosis (Fig. 5–94). Although any area of the lungs may be involved in primary tuberculosis, the important radiographic features

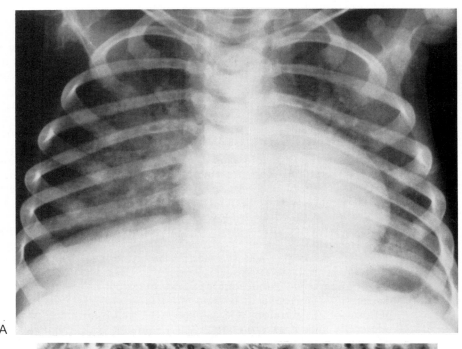

A

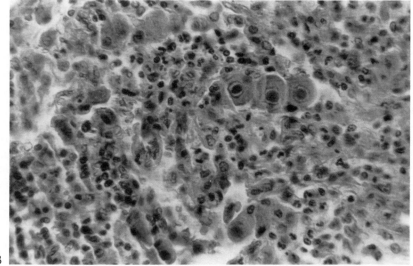

B

Figure 5–90. A, Congenital cytomegaloviral pneumonia in a 18-month-old child who had chronic lung disease from birth, with associated hepatosplenomegaly. Cytomegalic inclusion bodies had been recovered repeatedly from the urine. Chest radiograph shows diffuse bilateral interstitital pneumonia. Diagnosis was confirmed by lung biopsy and again by autopsy findings. B, Photomicrograph of intranuclear cytomegalic inclusion virus, producing a typical "bull's eye" appearance (45 ×).

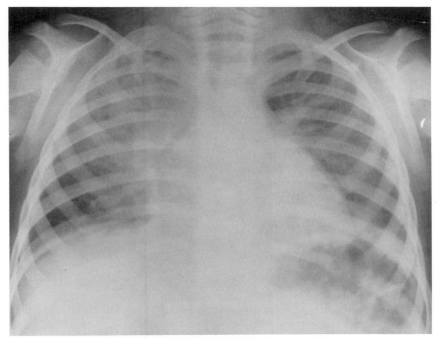

A

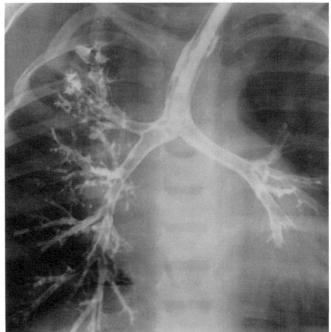

B

Figure 5–91. *Acquired chronic cytomegaloviral pneumonia in a 4-year-old child. A, Chest radiograph shows chronic bilateral bronchopneumonia involving predominantly the right upper lobe. B, Bronchogram shows bronchiectasis of right upper lobe segment. Resected specimen showed chronic infection secondary to cytomegalic inclusion disease.*

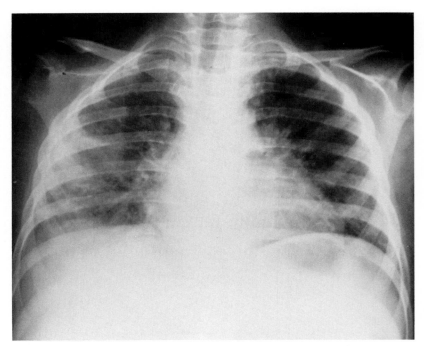

Figure 5–92. *Cytomegalic inclusion disease in a young child with leukemia. Chest radiograph shows chronic bilateral interstitial pneumonia.*

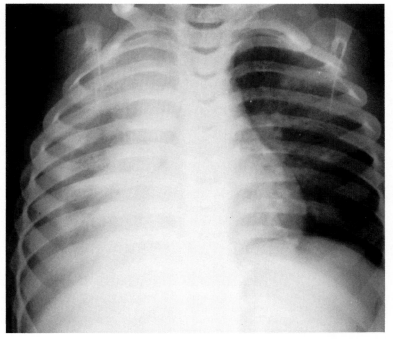

Figure 5–93. *Tuberculous pleural effusion and pneumonia in an 18-month-old boy whose only contact was the Sunday school teacher.*

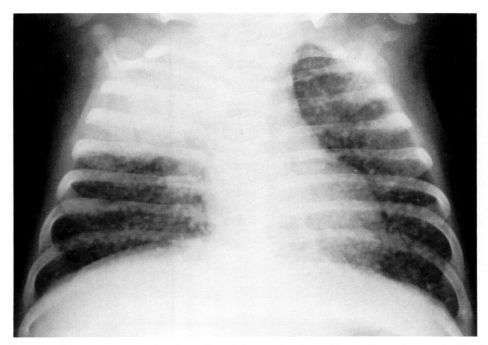

Figure 5–94. *Miliary tuberculosis in 5-month-old whose father had active cavitary tuberculosis. Chest radiograph shows disseminated miliary lesions throughout both lungs as well as large area of consolidation, which in part are probably due to atelectasis secondary to compression by mediastinal lymph nodes.*

consist of a chronic inflammatory infiltrate, usually with associated paratracheal adenopathy. A positive tuberculin test, even in the face of negative bacteriologic confirmation, should provide presumptive evidence that the pulmonary disease is the result of tuberculosis. Occasionally the accompanying adenitis will predominate, and the pulmonary changes will be minimal (Fig. 5–95). Mediastinal tuberculomas may be difficult to differentiate from lymph node enlargement secondary to other causes.

Miliary tuberculosis in the infant and child has the same pattern as that seen in the adult, and consists of disseminated small densities scattered throughout both lungs. The younger the infant the more rapid the inflammatory process develops and, late in the course of the disease, the once miliary lesions may have attained considerably larger size, simulating metastatic neoplasms. Negative tuberculin testing in fulminating tuberculosis should not detract from the importance of tuberculosis in the differential diagnosis.

Secondary or reinfection tuberculosis may be seen in the older child and, as in the adult, is usually apical in location and may be cavitary.

Pulmonary Mycoses

Mycotic infections of the lungs are uncommon in infants but should be considered in any child who has chronic, usually localized, pneumonia. Mycotic infections include histoplasmosis, coccidioidomycosis, actinomycosis, blastomycosis, geotrichosis, cryptococcosis, sporotrichosis, aspergillosis, nocardiosis, and mucormycosis. The radiographic differentiation of these conditions is impossible, with each producing areas of chronic pneumonitis with or without cavitation or calcification. Differentiation is dependent on appropriate laboratory tests.

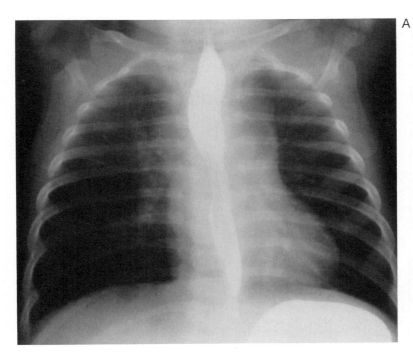

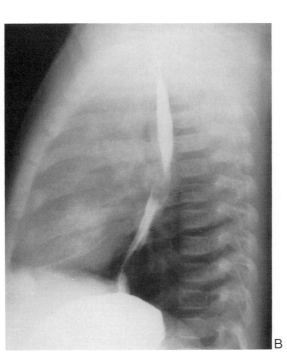

Figure 5–95. Subcarculoma in a 6-month-old infant whose grandfather had active tuberculosis. A, Frontal chest radiograph shows external compression on the esophagus by a mass in the subcarinal area. There is a minimal pulmonary infiltration in the right perihilar area. B, Lateral chest radiograph shows minimal compression on the midportion of the esophagus by the enlarged subcarinal lymph nodes.

Histoplasmosis is the most common chronic fungal infection of the lungs in children, and is certainly the most common lesion responsible for pulmonary and mediastinal lymph node calcification in children and adults. The radiographic findings are similar to those of other forms of chronic pneumonia, and differentiation is made by appropriate laboratory tests (Fig. 5–96). The lesions may be disseminated or localized. In our experience disseminated lesions are more common in younger patients. Pulmonary cavitation and pleural reaction are rare in the pediatric age group.

Pulmonary coccidioidomycosis is not common but follows histoplasmosis in relative degree of frequency of mycosis in infants and children. The radiographic changes are frequently similar, but cavitary disease as well as multiple disseminated lesions are more common in this condition (Fig. 5–97). Large pleural effusions have been reported. A history of exposure to a bird sanctuary or pigeon loft, or cave exploration, followed by clinical and radiographic findings of lung infection, should arouse suspicion of exposure either to coccidioidomycosis or histoplasmosis. As in other examples of unknown pulmonary infections, skin testing, appropriate agglutination tests, and even lung biopsies may be helpful in establishing the true diagnosis.

Pulmonary aspergillosis is caused by various species of the Aspergillus fungus and may occur in three clinical forms: allergic, invasive, or intracavitary. Allergic aspergillosis is usually a complication of chronic asthma and is presumably the result of inhalation of spores with resulting sensitization of the asthmatic patient. The radiologic changes usually consist of bronchiectasis of the upper lobes and sparing of the peripheral bronchi. Mucoid aspergillosis impactions may be seen on routine chest radiographs, appearing as nodular elongated areas of increased density (Fig. 5–98). In our experience aspergillosis is most commonly seen as a complication in patients with pulmonary fibrocystic disease. The radiographic identification of the aspergillosis lesion is virtually impossible because of the severe bronchiectasis and fibrosis that occur in patients with cystic fibrosis. The invasive form of aspergillosis is usually fatal, and more often appears as a secondary infection in patients with chronic immunologic deficiencies, such as leukemia and

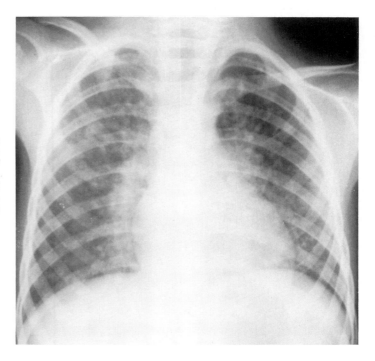

Figure 5–96. Pulmonary histoplasmosis in a 3-year-old child. Front chest radiograph shows disseminated ill-defined areas of density scattered throughout both lungs. Histoplasmin skin test was positive, and gradual clearing of the parenchymal disease occurred over a period of several months.

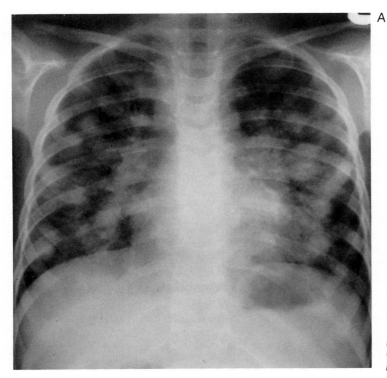

A

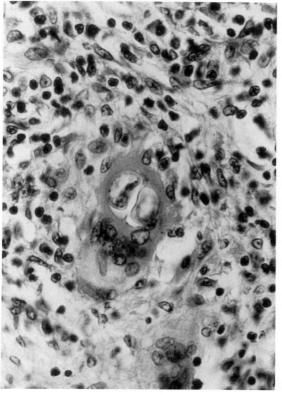

B

Figure 5–97. Coccidioidomycosis in a 6-year-old boy who became ill after exploring a cave. This patient, as well as several other children and the adults and family dog in the exploration trip, developed pulmonary coccidioidomycosis. A, Chest radiograph of the patient shows disseminated nodular lesions throughout both lungs. B, Photomicrograph showing the spirals of coccidioidomycosis (45 ×).

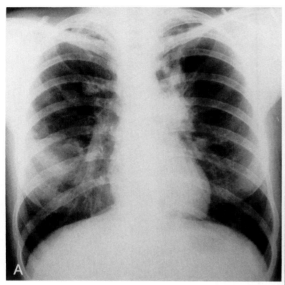
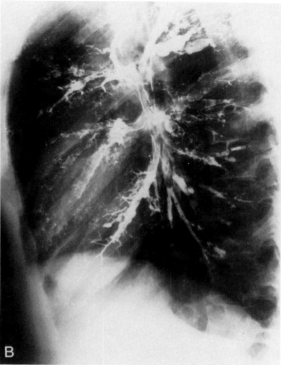

Figure 5–98. *Aspergillosis in a 17-year-old girl with a history of asthma. A, There is an area of consolidation in the right lower lobe, as well as patchy areas of density in both lungs and left hilar adenopathy. B, Bronchography shows bronchiectasis of the posterior segment of the right upper lobe, the right middle lobe, and the superior dorsal segment of the right upper lobe. Aspergilli fungi were obtained prior to bronchoscopy.*

lymphoma, and in patients who are on chemotherapy, including corticosteroids. It is much more commonly seen in the adult patient than in a patient in the pediatric age group. Pulmonary consolidation, central bronchiectasis, mucoid impaction, and "fungus ball" are characteristic radiographic findings.

The radiographic findings in mucormycosis are nonspecific, and are usually characterized by progressive diffuse and homogeneous consolidation of the lungs. It is an often fatal complication that occurs in the compromised patient with diabetes, leukemia, or lymphoma. Mucormycosis should be suspected in any diabetic child with chronic lung disease (Fig. 5–99).

Nocardiosis is a rare form of pulmonary mycotic infection that should also be considered in chronic, usually localized, pneumonia (Fig. 5–100).

Candida is a genus of yeastlike fungi that may be seen clinically as thrush in normal infants or as an opportunistic and serious infection in immune deficient patients (Fig. 5–101).

Sarcoidosis

Although sarcoidosis is rare in those in the pediatric age group, it should be considered in the differential diagnosis of mediastinal adenopathy and in unexplained pulmonary parenchymal disease. Although the disease in adults is more common in blacks, in our experience most cases occur in white children in the middle and late childhood age group.

The etiology has not been definitively determined. Whether it is a form of non-necrotic tuberculosis or a separate disease is unknown.

Pulmonary symptoms are usually mild and consist mainly of cough with some element of dyspnea, depending on the degree of lymphadenopathy and pulmonary

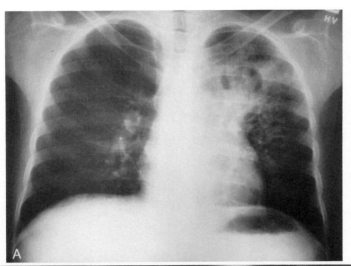

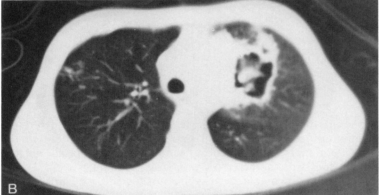

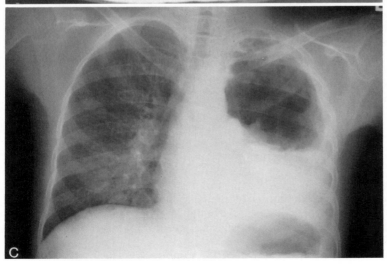

Figure 5–99. Mucormycosis in a 14-year-old diabetic girl. A, Chest radiograph shows the cavitary lesion in the left upper lobe. B, Computerized tomography shows the cavitary lesion, within which is a fungus ball. C, Repeat chest radiograph 3 months later shows increase in the size of the cavitary lesion.

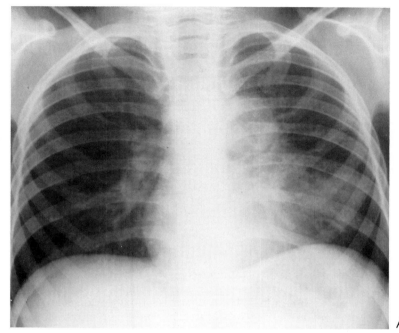

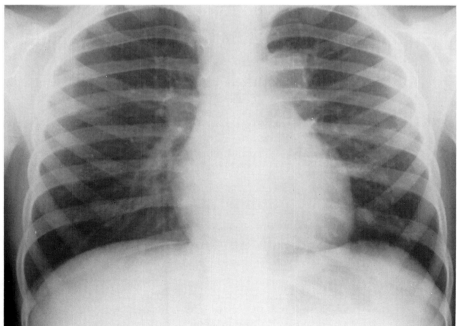

Figure 5–100. Nocardiosis in a 6-year-old boy. A, Chest radiographs show inflammatory infiltrate in the left lingula, with associated left hilar enlargement. B, Repeat chest radiograph after 5 months of sulfadiazine therapy. The parenchymal lesion has cleared, but the residual lymph node enlargement persists.

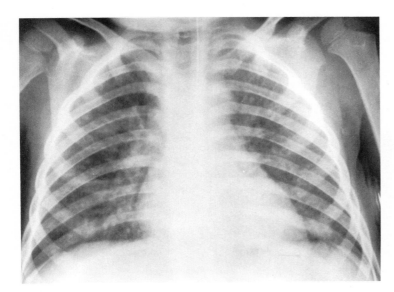

Figure 5–101. *Candidal pneumonia in 4-year-old boy with Burkitt's syndrome.*

parenchymal involvement. Negative tuberculin and fungal skin tests and abnormal pulmonary function studies are helpful in the diagnosis.

Radiographically the changes within the lungs are variable. The most common pattern is that of bilateral hilar and right paratracheal lymphadenopathy, with relatively clear lungs (Fig. 5–102). Other roentgenographic manifestations may be varying degrees of linear densities, diffuse patchy infiltrations, or miliary nodular patterns (Fig. 5–103). Pulmonary fibrosis and emphysema, although seen in adults with advanced disease, has not been definitely established as a complication in children. Lymphadenopathy is not always associated with the variable forms of pulmonary involvement. Pleural effusion and pneumothorax are rare complications in both adults and children. The prognosis in children, as in adults, is good. The bone lesions of sarcoidosis, which consist of small punched-out lesions with a lacelike trabecular pattern in the phalanges of the hands, are extremely uncommon in childhood sarcoidosis.

The diagnosis may be made by lymph node biopsy, which shows noncaseating granulomata and by excluding other granulomatous diseases.

Parasitosis

Parasitosis is not a common medical problem in this country, but it is widespread in the tropics as well as in many underdeveloped countries. Pulmonary complications may occur with many parasites, but only a few present severe problems.

Amebiasis. This is caused by Entamoeba histolytica. It most commonly affects the gastrointestinal tract, and may spread to the liver by the portal circulation. It has been estimated that 5 to 20% of such patients with intestinal involvement have liver disease. Pulmonary complications most frequently arise by direct spread from the involved liver or from a subphrenic abscess (Fig 5–104). Rarely, pulmonary involvement may occur by invasion of the inferior vena cava, with subsequent embolization, or through lymphatic spread to the thoracic duct and from there to the superior vena cava and lungs.

The symptomatic signs of pulmonary involvement are nonspecific and consist of cough, fever, chest pains, dyspnea, and hemoptysis.

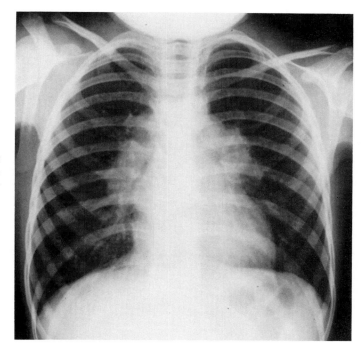

Figure 5–102. Sarcoidosis in a 5-year-old boy. There is bilateral hilar and right paratracheal adenopathy. (Courtesy of Dr. V. Condon, Salt Lake City.)

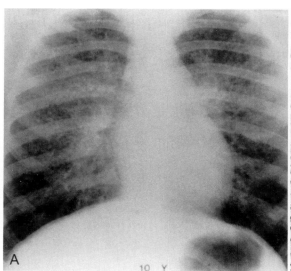

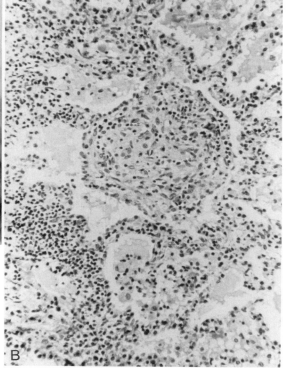

Figure 5–103. Sarcoidosis in a 10-year-old boy. A, Bilateral hilar adenopathy is present, as well as verticular nodular infiltrates throughout both lungs. B, Photomicrograph of lung biopsy shows noncaseous granuloma (40×).

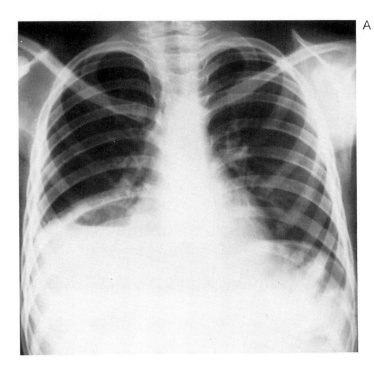

A

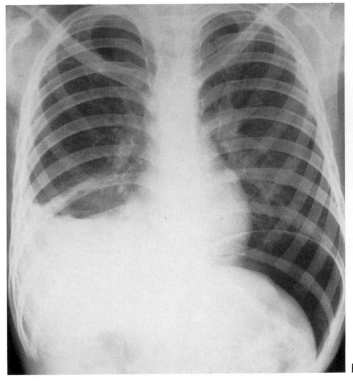

B

Figure 5–104. *Twelve-year-old boy with amebic abscess and right basilar pneumonitis. There was a history of fever, chest pain, and coughing up of "chocolate-type" pus. A, Posteroanterior chest film shows air-fluid level in the right lung base, which subsequently proved to be within the liver. The right hemidiaphragm is elevated and poorly defined. B, Posteroanterior chest film 4 days later following diagnostic pneumoperitoneum shows normal left hemidiaphragm. The right leaf of the diaphragm and liver do not separate because of the inflammatory reaction. (Courtesy of Unidad De Pediatria, Del Hospital General De Mexico, S. S. A.)*

The radiographic features are variable. Frequently there is elevation, paralysis, and partial obliteration of the right leaf of the diaphragm. Pleural reaction may be the only manifestation early in the disease but this in itself is not too common and, more frequently, there is segmental pneumonitis of the middle or right lower lobes. The left lung may also be affected, however. Pulmonary abscess formation and empyema may be seen and, on occasion, hepatobronchial fistulae complicate the clinical course. The latter is best demonstrated by bronchography.

The diagnosis is confirmed by demonstration of amebas in clinical specimens (i.e., stool), by culture, and by serologic studies.

Hydatid Disease. This is caused by the tapeworm Echinococcus granulosus. It presents virtually no problem in this country except for those who have migrated to the United States from an endemic area. The disease is passed to humans by contact with the contaminated feces of infected animals. The cyst that is produced has three layers: the outer layer, or pericyst, is a reaction by the host to the organism; the central layer, or ectocyst, is a protective covering; and the endocyst is the active germinal layer. The central portion of the cyst contains fluid of varying chemical composition, along with bits of the organism and other debris.

Symptomatology depends on the size of the cyst as well as on any complications that may arise from either infection or perforation of the cyst. As the cyst grows symptoms are caused by obstruction of surrounding normal structures, while infection may produce sputum and even hemoptysis. If the cyst ruptures and fluid is excreted slowly, there is persistent cough and expectoration. Sudden and massive rupture may cause severe respiratory distress and even death.

Radiographically the most common feature of hydatid disease is the presence of one or more rounded, well-defined, homogeneous radiodensities (Fig. 5–105). During deep inspiration the cyst may change its shape to an oval contour (Escudero-Nemerow sign). Air-fluid levels are seen if the cyst ruptures. When cyst tissue collapses on the fluid irregularity of the fluid layer may be seen; this has been described as the "water lily" sign. Similarly, growth of the cyst or rupture may allow some air to dissect between the layers of the cyst wall,

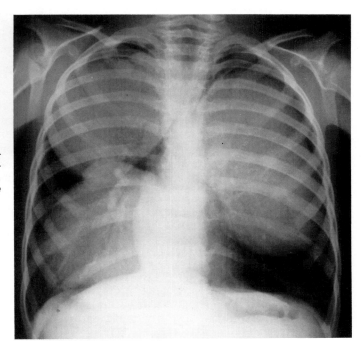

Figure 5–105. Hydatid cyst. Chest examination showed three large cysts, which at exploration were found to be hydatid cysts. (Courtesy of Rumel Chest Clinic, Salt Lake City.)

producing the so-called "crescent sign," typical of hydatid cyst formation. The cysts vary in size from small cysts of several centimeters to massive cysts that may occupy nearly the entire hemithorax. On occasion the position of the lesion may be such as to mimic mediastinal lesions or even diaphragmatic masses. Abscess formation may be closely mimicked if the cyst is partially evacuated. Calcifications of pulmonary hydatid cysts, pneumothorax, and pleural effusion are uncommon. Formation of daughter cysts, although seen infrequently, tends to produce a lobular appearance of the cyst. Surgical removal is the treatment of choice.

Pulmonary Dirofilariasis. This infection is caused by the organism Dirofilaria immitis, which is the common heartworm in dogs. It is rare in humans, but when it occurs it may produce one or more pulmonary nodules. The nodules do not generally calcify. Pathologically the nodule occurs as a result of occlusion of a pulmonary arteriole by the organism, with subsequent infarction. A small patch of pneumonitis may thus be the initial radiographic feature. The diagnosis is confirmed by microscopic examination of the affected tissue.

Pulmonary Paragonimiasis. This disease is found mainly in Asia, especially in Korea and the Pacific Islands. The pulmonary lesions cannot be differentiated radiographically from those of other chronic forms of pneumonitis. Occasionally intracranial involvement with calcification may be an associated complication, which is of diagnostic value. However, in this country the disease has been confined to those military personnel who have served in Asia. There are several specific forms of chronic interstitial pneumonias with no known etiology. Lung biopsy is necessary for a diagnosis.

Other Interstitial Pneumonias

IDIOPATHIC OR USUAL INTERSTITIAL PNEUMONIA (UIP)

Idiopathic interstitial pneumonia in infants and young children is a chronic pulmonary parenchymal disease that can be diagnosed only by lung biopsy. In our experience the pathologic reports have referred to chronic interstitial fibrosis. The condition is generally progressive but, on rare occasions, it may undergo slow resolution and lead to ultimate recovery. This is the most common of the chronic interstitial pneumonias.

The patients we have seen with chronic interstitial pneumonia in whom lung biopsy was reported as idiopathic interstitial pneumonia or as idiopathic interstitial fibrosis have usually shown a chronic course with persistent parenchymal disease over a period of many months or years (Fig. 5-106). Rarely there will be resolution of the parenchymal disease, with ultimate recovery. Apparently there is initial damage to the alveolar epithelium, followed by a monocytic infiltrate of the interstitial structures and fibroblastic infiltration. The etiology in all these cases is unknown but, in some instances, there may be prior viral infection, drug exposure (e.g., Cytoxan, hexamethonium, nitrofurantoin) or collagen vascular disease. A small percentage may be familial. Pulmonary parenchymal breakdown, pleural effusion, and pneumothoraces have not been encountered in our cases.

DESQUAMATIVE INTERSTITIAL PNEUMONIA (DIP)

This rare chronic interstitial pneumonia is of unknown etiology. Histologically the most striking feature is filling of the alveoli by large cells that resemble type II pneumocytes but are now considered to be macrophages. These and other histologic findings, as well as the radiographic features and favorable response to steroid therapy, have prompted this disease to be identified as a new type of chronic pneumonia. It occurs mainly in adults, but children may be affected. The symptomatology is variable and ranges from mild respiratory distress to severe pulmonary insufficiency.

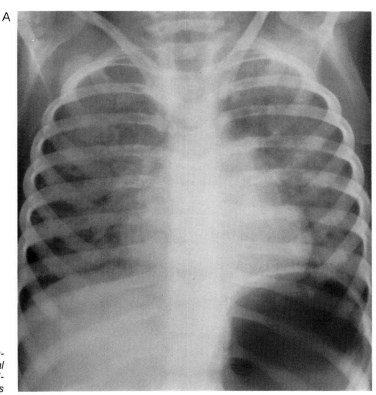

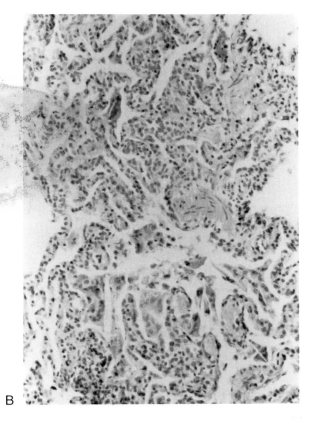

Figure 5–106. *Idiopathic interstitial pneumonia in a 3-year-old child.* A, *Frontal chest radiograph shows bilateral interstitial pneumonia, which was diagnosed as chronic interstitial fibrosis by lung biopsy.* B, *Photomicrograph of lung biopsy shows mononuclear cells infiltrating the interstitial structures of the lung, as well as fibroblastic activity (45 ×).*

Illustration continued on following page

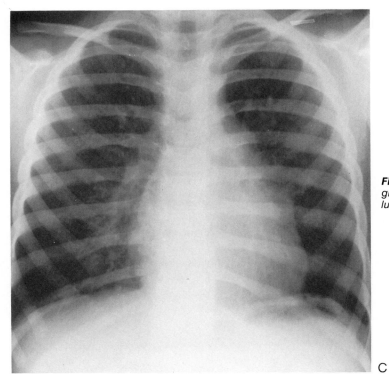

Figure 5–106. C, Follow-up chest radiograph 1 year later shows complete resolution.

C

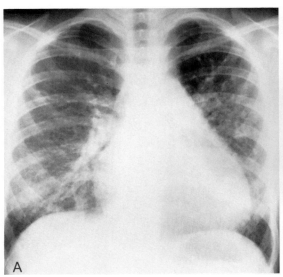

A

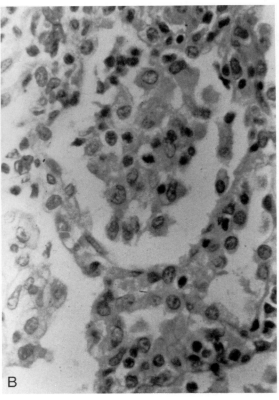

B

Figure 5–107. Desquamative interstitial pneumonia in a 15-year-old girl. A, Interstitial pattern involves both lungs. B, Photomicrograph of lung biopsy shows characteristic type cells that have been shed into the alveolus (45×).

Radiographically the pattern is surprisingly similar in many patients, consisting of hazy triangular opacities radiating from the hilus and usually involving the lower lobes that are closely associated with the fissures. The infiltrate generally spares the costophrenic angles. Infiltrates may be found elsewhere, and can be reticular or confluent (Fig. 5–107). The configuration is not characteristic, and diagnosis is usually made by lung biopsy. Atelectasis, pneumothorax, pleural effusion, and cor pulmonale are unusual complications. The response to steroid therapy has been reasonably good in most cases, and the prognosis appears to be favorable for long-term survival.

Lymphocytic Interstitial Pneumonia (LIP)

This is a very rare form of chronic interstitial pneumonia, with the peak incidence occurring in the fourth and fifth decades of life; however, the condition may occur in children. Symptomatology includes cough, dyspnea, fever, and weight loss. Enlargement of reticuloendothelial organs such as the lymph nodes or spleen is usually lacking.

The radiographic experience has been too limited to determine a typical x-ray pattern. Of the cases reported, the lesions are generally patchy and somewhat nodular, and seem to be located mainly in the lower lung fields (Fig. 5–108). In some cases, however, linear densities are observed. One of our cases showed severe hyperaeration of the lungs and radiographic changes resembling those of pulmonary fibrocystic diseases (Fig. 5–109). Lung biopsy is necessary for positive diagnosis.

Treatment is confined to steroids and other supportive measures.

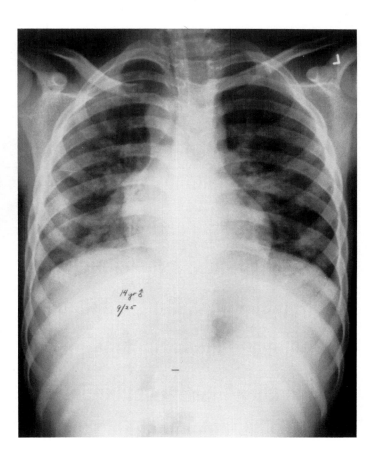

Figure 5–108. Lymphocytic interstitial pneumonia, in which nonspecific ill-defined interstitial infiltrates involve both lungs. This was proved by lung biopsy.

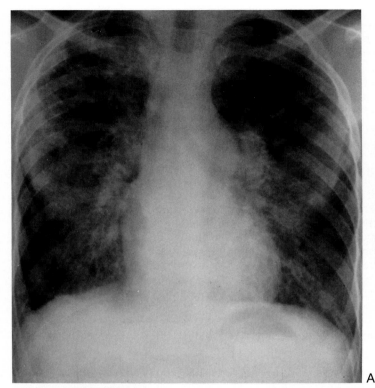

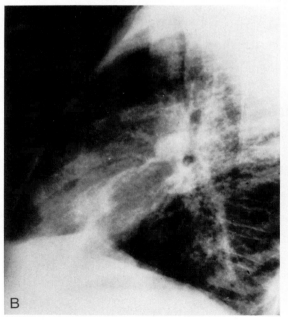

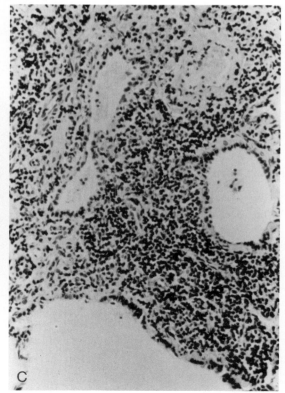

Figure 5–109. Lymphocytic interstitial pneumonia in a 14-year-old child. A, Chest radiographs show hyperinflation of the lungs, with linear densities scattered throughout both lungs and bilateral hilar adenopathy. B, Lateral view shows increase in anterioposterior dimension of the chest, with flattening of the diaphragm and interstitial pneumonia. C, Photomicrograph of lung biopsy shows lymphocytic infiltration into the interstitial structures of the lung (45×).

Lymphomatoid Granulomatosis

This rare condition in adults may occur in the pediatric patient. Although it is not a form of pneumonitis, it is placed in this section because of its radiologic similarity to various pneumonias. Fever, cough, malaise, and weight loss are the most frequent clinical symptoms. The pulmonary radiologic features are characterized by multiple nodules or masses, usually in the lower lungs, which may be unilateral or bilateral. Rapid change and cavitation occur. The radiologic features consist of diffuse nodular, or reticulonodular infiltration of the lungs similar to those seen in a number of conditions, such as multiple septic emboli, metastatic malignancies, acquired immune deficiency disease, and various fungal diseases (Fig. 5–110). Radiographically it is also indistinguishable from eosinophilic granuloma and Wegener's granulomatosis. Cavitation is common and hilar adenopathy is unusual. Histologically the condition apparently represents a lymphoproliferative granulomatous disease primarily involving the lungs, with associated vasculitis. In addition to pulmonary disease there is frequent involvement of the kidneys, central nervous system, skin, eyes, and heart. Untreated, the disease is usually fatal. A significant percentage of patients will progress to lymphoma. The angiopathic, destructive features of the lesions frequently result in vascular compromise and focal areas of infarction. However, because the disease is extremely rare in children, the complications found in the adult patient have not been observed in children.

Ectodermal Dysplasia

Two forms of this disease have been reported, the anhydrotic and hydrotic types. In both entities there is a deficiency of ectodermal derivatives. Clinical differentiation between the two is usually not too difficult, but a more important feature is the lack of sweating in the anhydrotic form. Both types usually show some alteration in the amount and texture of hair formation, along with varying skin changes.

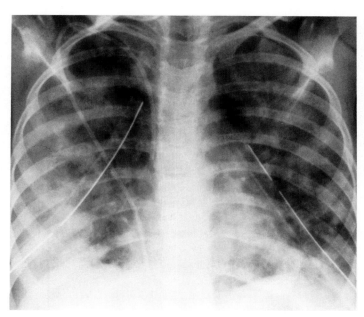

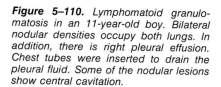

Figure 5–110. Lymphomatoid granulomatosis in an 11-year-old boy. Bilateral nodular densities occupy both lungs. In addition, there is right pleural effusion. Chest tubes were inserted to drain the pleural fluid. Some of the nodular lesions show central cavitation.

The anhydrotic form frequently presents with altered function of the sebaceous glands, along with partial or complete absence of teeth and frequently with a prominent "saddle nose" deformity. Abnormalities of entodermal derivatives may also be present, and frequently manifest themselves in the respiratory tract. Because these children have an absence of mucous glands, chronic sinusitis, bronchitis, and pneumonias may develop. Respiratory infections tend to be recurrent, and may be a result of the lack of the normal protective and cleansing functions of the mucus.

Radiographically the pulmonary infections are usually nonspecific. An important feature in the diagnosis is the sparsity or absence of tooth buds (Fig. 5–111).

Shwachman Syndrome

This syndrome is clinically similar in many respects to cystic fibrosis. Recurrent infections, particularly pneumonia, are common, as is malabsorption syndrome resulting from exocrine pancreatic insufficiency. There is associated growth retardation and leukopenia. The condition is probably autosomal recessive, and the lack of defense against infections is apparently due to defective neutrophil mobility.

The radiographic findings are limited to the chest and extremities. Recurrent pneumonia, which may be in the form of areas of consolidation or recurrent bronchopneumonia, is common (Fig. 5–112). The radiographic findings in the long bones, particularly in the lower extremities, consist of areas of rarefaction in the metaphysis, especially prominent in the distal femoral and proximal tibial metaphysis. Irregularity of the growth plate is common, as well as V-shaped deformity of the central portion of these growth plates.

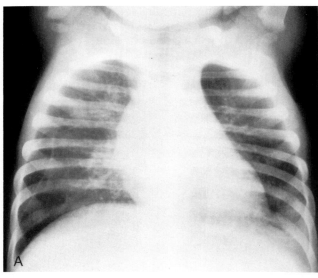

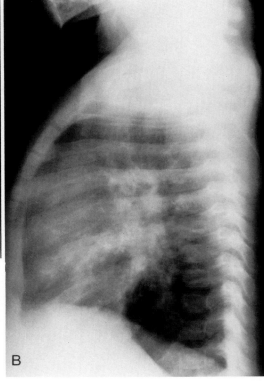

Figure 5–111. Anhydrotic ectodermal dysplasia in a young infant with chronic pneumonia. A, Chest radiograph shows bilateral pneumonia with pneumatoceles. B, Lateral chest radiograph shows pneumonia, hilar adenopathy, and deficiency of normal tooth buds.

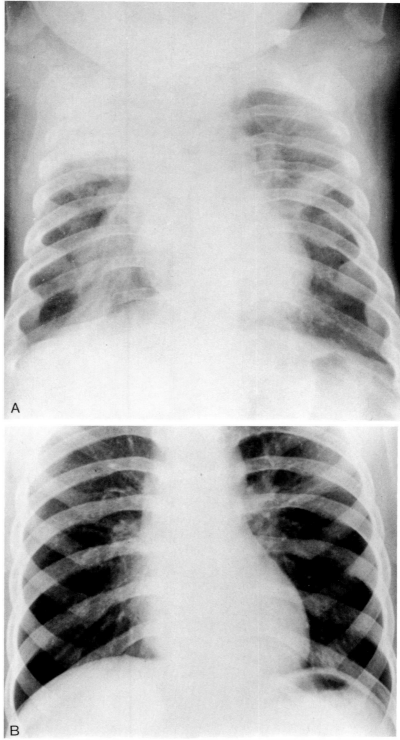

Figure 5–112. Shwachman syndrome. A, *At 6 months of age there is extensive pneumonia involving both lungs, with atelectasis of the right upper lobe. B, At 7 years of age there is moderate bilateral air trapping.*

Illustration continued on following page

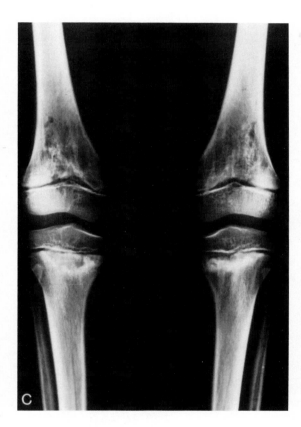

Figure 5–112. C, Metaphyseal defects of this condition are prominently demonstrated in the lower extremities.

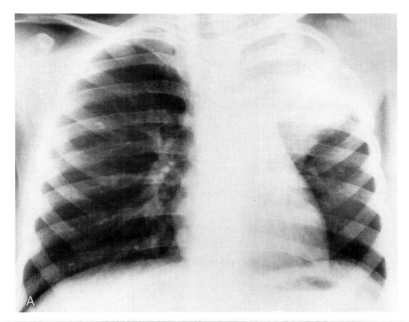

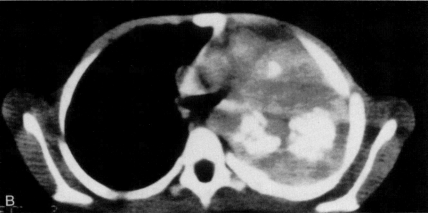

Figure 5–113. *Inflammatory pseudotumor in a 9-year-old boy. A, Chest radiograph shows consolidation of the left upper lobe, which was present for several months. B, Computerized tomography shows the large-mass lesion, with associated calcification.*

Inflammatory Pseudotumor

Inflammatory pseudotumor, or plasma cell granuloma of the lung, presents radiographically as a homogeneous area of consolidation resembling a neoplasm. The condition is considered to be a reparative process of an inflammatory lesion of unknown cause, with or without a history of a preceding respiratory illness. Many patients are asymptomatic. The lesion may be difficult to remove completely, and in some cases continues to grow after incomplete resection. Calcification may be identified within the lesion (Fig. 5–113).

SUGGESTED READINGS

NEONATAL PNEUMONIA

Group B Streptococcal Pneumonia

Ablow RC et al.: The radiographic features of early onset group B streptococcal neonatal sepsis. Radiology, 124:771, 1977.

Baker CJ, and Barrett FL: Transmission of group B streptococci among parturient women and their neonates. J Pediatr, 83:919, 1973.

Fraser RG, and Wortzman G: Acute pneumococcal lobar pneumonia: The significance of non-segmental lobar distribution. J Can Assoc Radiol, 10:37, 1959.

Kevy SV, and Lowe BA: Streptococcal pneumonia and empyema in childhood. N Engl J Med, 264:738, 1961.

Leonidas JC et al.: Radiologic findings in early onset neonatal group B streptococcal septicemia. Pediatrics, 59:1006, 1977.

McCracken GH: Group B streptococci: The new challenge in neonatal infections. J Pediatr, 82:703, 1973.

Weller MH, and Katzenstein AA: Radiologic findings in group B streptococcal sepsis. Radiology, 118:385, 1976.

Listeria Monocytogenes

Ahlfors CE et al.: Neonatal listeriosis. Am J Dis Child, 131:405, 1977.

Moore PH, and Brogdon BA: Granulomatosis infantiseptica. Radiology, 79:415, 1962.

Willich E: The radiological appearance of pulmonary listeriosis. Progr Pediatr Radiol, 1:160, 1967.

Chlamydia Pneumonia

Beem MO, and Saxon E: Pneumonia in infants infected with chlamydia trachomatis. Pediatr Res, 10:395, 1976.

Radkowski MA et al.: *Chlamydia* pneumonia in infants. Radiography in 125 cases. Am J Roentogenol, 137:703, 1981.

Stickney RN et al.: *Chlamydia trachomatis*: A cause of an infantile pneumonia syndrome. Am J Roentgenol, 131:914, 1978.

Tipple MA, Beem MD, and Saxon EM: Clinical characteristics of the afebrile pneumonia associated with *Chlamydia trachomatis* infections in infants less than 6 months of age. Pediatrics, 63:192, 1979.

TORCH

Feigin RD, and Cherry JD: Textbook of Pediatric Infectious Diseases. Philadelphia, WB Saunders, 1981.

McCracken GH Jr et al.: Congenital cytomegalic inclusion disease. A longitudinal study of 20 patients. Am J Dis Child, 117:522, 1969.

Phelan P, and Campbell P: Pulmonary complications of rubella embryopathy. J Pediatr, 75:202, 1969.

Whitley RJ et al.: Natural history of herpes simplex virus infections of mother and newborn. Pediatrics, 66:489, 1980.

Pneumonia Alba

Berdon WE: The neonate and the young infant (pneumonia). In Silverman FN (ed): Caffey's Pediatric X-Ray Diagnosis, 8th ed, pp 1782–1784. Chicago, Year Book Medical Publishers, 1985.

Cremin BJ, and Fisher RM: The lesions of congenital syphilis. Br J Radiol, 43:333, 1970.

Tuberculosis

Grady RC, and Zuelzer WW: Neonatal tuberculosis. Am J Dis Child, 90:381, 1955.
Hopkins R, Ermocilla R, and Cassady G: Congenital tuberculosis. So Med J, 69:1156, 1976.
Kendig EL Jr, and Rodgers WL: Tuberculosis in the neonatal period. Am Rev Tuberc, 77:418, 1958.
Polansky SM et al.: Congenital tuberculosis. Am J Roentgenol, 130:994, 1978.
Reisinger KS et al.: Congenital tuberculosis: Report of a case. Pediatrics, 54:74, 1974.

ACUTE DISORDERS

Bronchiolitis

Griscom NT, Wohl MEB, and Kirkpatrick JA Jr.: Lower respiratory infections: How infants differ from adults. Radiol Clin North Am, 16:367, 1978.
Gurwitz D, Mindorff C, and Levison H: Increased incidence of bronchial reactivity in children with a history of bronchiolitis. J Pediatr, 98:551, 1981.
Hall CB, Hall WJ, and Spurs DM: Clinical and physiological manifestations of bronchiolitis and pneumonia: Outcome of respiratory syncytial virus. Am J Dis Child, 133:798, 1979.
Henderson FW et al.: The etiologic and epidemiologic spectrum of bronchiolitis in pediatric practice. J Pediatr, 95:183, 1979.
Kirkpatrick JA, and Wagner ML: Roentgen manifestations of bronchiolitic inflammatory disease. Pediatr Clin North Am, 10:633, 1963.
Wright FH, and Beem NO: Diagnosis and treatment: Management of acute viral bronchiolitis in infancy. Pediatrics, 35:334, 1965.

Bronchitis

Turner JAP: Bronchitis. In Kendig EL Jr, and Chernick V (eds): Disorders of the Respiratory Tract in Children, 3rd ed, pp 361–366. Philadelphia, W.B. Saunders, 1977.

Pneumonia

Bacterial Pneumonia

Griscom NT, Wohl MEB, and Kirkpatrick JA Jr.: Lower respiratory infections: How infants differ from adults. Radiol Clin North Am, 16:367, 1978.
Kuhn JP: Bacterial pneumonias. In Silverman FN (ed): Caffey's Pediatric X-Ray Diagnosis, 8th ed, pp 1198–1200. Chicago, Year Book Medical Publishers, 1985.
Murphy TF et al.: Pneumonia: An eleven-year study in pediatric practice. Am J Epidemiol, 113:12, 1981.
Pearl M: Postinflammatory pseudotumor of the lung in children. Radiology, 105:391, 1972.
Rose RW, and Ward BH: Spherical pneumonias in children simulating pulmonary and mediastinal masses. Radiology, 106:179, 1973.
Smith MHD: Bacterial pneumonias: Gram-negative. In Kendig EL Jr, and Chernick V (eds): Disorders of the Respiratory Tract in Children, 3rd ed, pp 398–402. Philadelphia, W.B. Saunders, 1977.
Smith MHD: Bacterial pneumonias: Gram-positive. In Kendig EL Jr, and Chernick V (eds): Disorders of the Respiratory Tract in Children, 3rd ed, pp 378–397. Philadelphia, W.B. Saunders, 1977.

STAPHYLOCOCCAL PNEUMONIA

Ceruti E, Contreras J, and Neira M: Staphylococcal pneumonia in childhood. Long-term follow-up including pulmonary function studies. Am J Dis Child, 122:386, 1971.
Felman AH, and Shulman ST: Staphylococcal osteomyelitis, sepsis, and pulmonary disease. Observations of 10 patients with combined osseous and pulmonary infections. Radiology, 117:649, 1975.
Highman JH: Staphylococcal pneumonia and empyema in childhood. Am J Roentgenol, 106:103, 1969.
Huxtable KA, Tucher AS, and Wedgewood KRJ: Staphylococcal pneumonia in childhood. Long-term follow-up. Am J Dis Child, 108:262, 1964.
Mausbach TW, and Chao CT: Pneumonia and pleural effusion. Association with influenza A virus and *Staphylococcus aureus*. Am J Dis Child, 130:1005, 1976.

HAEMOPHILUS INFLUENZAE

Asmar BI et al.: *Haemophilus influenzae* type B pneumonia in 43 children. J Pediatr, 93:389, 1978.
Felson B: Chest Roentgenology, p 133. Philadelphia, W.B. Saunders, 1973.
Ginsberg CM, Howard JB, and Nelson JD: Report of 65 cases of *Haemophilus influenzae* and pneumonia. Pediatrics, 64:283, 1979.
Jacobs, NM, and Harris VJ: Acute hemophilus pneumonia in childhood. Am J Dis Child, 133:603, 1979.
Kaplan SL, and Feigan RD: Infections due to Hemophilus aphrophilus. In Behrman RE, and Vaughan VC (eds): Nelson Textbook of Pediatrics. Philadelphia, W. B. Saunders, 1983.

PERTUSSIS PNEUMONIA

Barnhard HJ, and Kniker WT: Roentgenologic findings in pertussis with particular emphasis on the "shaggy heart" sign. Am J Roentgenol, 84:445, 1960.

Bierling A: Childhood pneumonia, including pertussis pneumonia and bronchiectasis. A follow-up study of 151 patients. Acta Paediatr, 45:348, 1956.

Brooksaler F, and Nelson JD: Pertussis: A reappraisal and report of 190 confirmed cases. Am J Dis Child, 114:389, 1967.

Fawcitt J, and Parry HE: Lung changes in pertussis and measles in childhood. Br J Radiol, 30:76, 1957.

Radkowski MA, Kranzler JK et al.: Chlamydia pneumonia in infants. Radiography in 125 cases. Am J Roentgenol 137:703, 1981.

Viral Pneumonias

Denny FW: Viral pneumonia. In Kendig EL Jr, and Chernick V (eds): Disorders of the Respiratory Tract in Children, 3rd ed, pp 423–432. Philadelphia, W.B. Saunders, 1977.

Osborne D, Kirks DR, and Effman EL: Pneumonia in the child. In Putman CE (ed): Pulmonary Diagnosis: Imaging and Other Techniques, pp 230–232. New York, Appleton-Century-Crofts, 1981.

Osborne D: Radiologic appearance of viral diseases of the lower respiratory tract in infants and children. Am J Roentgenol, 130:29, 1978.

ADENOVIRAL PNEUMONIA

Becroft DMO: Histopathology of fatal adenovirus infection of the respiratory tract in children. J Clin Pathol, 20:561, 1967.

James AG et al.: Adenovirus type 21 bronchopneumonia in infants and young children. J Pediatr, 95:530, 1979.

Osborne, D, and White P: Radiology of epidemic adenovirus 21 infection of the lower respiratory tract in infants and young children. Am J Roentgenol, 133:379, 1979.

MEASLES PNEUMONIA (POSTMEASLES)

Fawcitt J, and Parry HE: Lung changes in pertussis and measles in childhood. A review of 1894 cases with a follow-up study of the pulmonary complications. Br J Radiol, 30:76, 1957.

Fulginiti VA et al.: Altered reactivity to measles virus. Atypical measles in children previously immunized with inactivated measles virus vaccine. JAMA, 202:1075, 1967.

Margolin FR, and Gandy TK: Pneumonia of atypical measles. Radiology, 131:653, 1979.

Mitnick J et al.: Nodular residua of atypical measles pneumonia. Am J Roentgenol, 134:257, 1980.

Wood BP, and Bernstein RM: Pulmonary nodules of "pneumonia" during the acute atypical measles illness. Ann Radiol (Paris), 21:193, 1978.

Young LW, Smith DI, and Glasgow LA: Pneumonia of atypical measles. Residual nodular lesions. Am J Roentgenol, 110:439, 1970.

GIANT CELL PNEUMONIA (MEASLES PNEUMONIA)

Hecht V: Die Riesenzellenpneumonia in Kindsalter, eine historische-experimentelle Studie. Beitr Pathol, 48:263, 1910.

McCarthy K et al.: Isolation of virus of measles from three fatal cases of giant cell pneumonia. Am J Dis Child, 96:500, 1958.

VARICELLA PNEUMONIA

Dahlstrom G et al.: Pulmonary calcifications following varicella and their effects on respiratory function. Scand J Respir Dis, 48:249, 1969.

Eisenklam EJ: Primary varicella pneumonia in a 3-year-old girl. J Pediatr, 69:452, 1966.

Nemir RL: Varicella pneumonia. In Kendig EL Jr, and Chernick V (eds): Disorders of the Respiratory Tract in Children, 3rd ed, p 955. Philadelphia, W.B. Saunders, 1977.

Sargent EN, Carson MJ, and Reilly ED: Varicella pneumonia. A report of 20 cases, with postmortem examination in six. Cal Med, 107:141, 1967.

Southward ME: Roentgen findings in chicken pox pneumonia. Review of the literature and a report of 5 cases. Am J Roentgenol, 76:733, 1956.

Primary Atypical Pneumonia (Mycoplasma Pneumonia)

Cameron DC, Borthwick RN, and Philip T: The radiographic pattern of acute mycoplasma pneumonitis. Clin Radiol, 28:173, 1977.

Denny F, Clyde WA Jr, and Gezen WP: Mycoplasm pneumonia disease: Clinical spectrum, pathophysiology, epidemiology, in control. J Infect Dis, 123:74, 1971.

Grix A, and Giammona ST: Pneumonitis with pleural effusion in children due to *Mycoplasma pneumoniae*. Am Rev Respir Dis, 109:665, 1974.

Kaufman JM, Cuvelier CA, and Van der Straeten M: Mycoplasma pneumonia with fulminant evolution into diffuse interstitial fibrosis. Thorax, 35:140, 1980.

Putman CE et al.: Mycoplasma pneumonia. Clinical and roentgenographic patterns. Am J Roentgenol, 124:417, 1975.

Hydrocarbon Pneumonia

Campbell JB: Pneumatocele formation following hydrocarbon ingestion. Am Rev Respir Dis, 101:414, 1970.

Daeschner CW Jr, Blattner RJ, and Collins VP: Hydrocarbon pneumonitis. Pediatr Clin North Am, 4:243, 1957.

Eade NR, Taussig LM, and Marks MI: Hydrocarbon pneumonitis. Pediatrics, 54:351, 1974.

Harris VJ, and Brown R: Pneumatoceles as a complication of chemical pneumonia after hydrocarbon ingestion. Am J Roentgenol, 125:531, 1975.

Wolfe BM, Brodeur AE, and Shields JB: The role of gastrointestinal absorption of kerosene in producing pneumonitis in dogs. J Pediatr, 76:867, 1970.

Wolfsdorf J, and Kundig H: Kerosene poisoning in primates. S Afr Med J, 46:617, 1972.

Near Drowning

Hunter TB, and Whitehouse WM: Freshwater near-drowning: Radiological aspects. Radiology, 112:51, 1974.

Modell JH: Drowning and near-drowning. In Kendig EL Jr, and Chernick V (eds): Disorders of the Respiratory Tract in Children, 3rd ed, p 498. Philadelphia, W.B. Saunders, 1977.

Peterson B: Morbidity of childhood near-drowning. Pediatrics, 59:364, 1977.

Putman CE et al.: Drowning: Another plunge. Am J Roentgenol, 125:543, 1975.

CHRONIC OR RECURRENT DISORDERS

Allergic Pneumonitis (Including Löffler's Pneumonia)

Chang CH, and Wittig HJ: Heiner's syndrome. Radiology, 92:507, 1969.

Epstein WL, and Kligman AM: Pathogenesis of eosinophilic pneumonitis (Löffler's syndrome). JAMA, 162:95, 1956.

Heiner DC, Sears JW, and Kniker WT: Multiple precipitants to cow's milk in chronic respiratory disease. A syndrome including poor growth, gastrointestinal symptoms, evidence of allergy, iron deficiency anemia and pulmonary hemosiderosis. Am J Dis Child, 103:634, 1962.

Howard WA: Loeffler's syndrome. In Kendig EL Jr, and Chernick V (eds): Disorders of the Respiratory Tract in Children, 3rd ed, pp 1023–1026. Philadelphia, W.B. Saunders, 1977.

Kuhn JP: Allergic reactions in the lungs. In Silverman FN (ed): Caffey's Pediatric X-Ray Diagnosis, 8th ed, p 1244. Chicago, Year Book Medical Publishers, 1985.

Löffler's syndrome (editorial). Br Med J, 3:569, 1968.

Roberts SR: Immunology of the lungs: An overview. Semin Roentgenol, 10:7, 1975.

Unger GF et al.: A radiologic approach to hypersensitivity pneumonias. Radiol Clin North Am, 11:339, 1973.

Reactive Airway Disease (Asthma)

Dees SC: Asthma. In Kendig EL Jr, and Chernick V: Disorders of the Respiratory Tract in Children, 3rd ed, p 620. Philadelphia, W.B. Saunders, 1977.

Eggleston PA et al.: Radiographic abnormalities and acute asthma in children. Pediatrics, 54:442, 1974.

Kirkpatrick JA Jr: The problem of chronic and recurrent pulmonary disease. Progr Pediatr Radiol, 1:294, 1967.

Kirsh MM, and Orvald TD: Mediastinal and subcutaneous emphysema complicating acute bronchial asthma. Chest, 57:580, 1970.

Rebuck AS: Radiologic aspects of severe asthma. Aust Radiol, 14:264, 1970.

Robinson AE, and Campbell JB: Bronchography in childhood asthma. Am J Roentgenol, 116:559, 1972.

Cystic Fibrosis

Anderson DH: Cystic fibrosis of the pancreas and its relation to celiac disease. A clinical and pathological study. Am J Dis Child, 56:344, 1938.

Brasfield D et al.: The chest roentgenogram in cystic fibrosis. A new scoring system. Pediatrics, 63:24, 1979.

Fellows KE et al.: Bronchial artery embolization in cystic fibrosis: Technique and long-term results. J Pediatr, 95:959, 1979.

Griscom NT et al.: Visible fatty liver. Radiology, 117:385, 1975.

Hodson CJ et al.: Pulmonary resection in cystic fibrosis: Results in 23 cases 1950–1970. Arch Dis Child, 47:499, 1972.

Holsclaw DS, Eckstein HB, and Mixon HH: Meconium ileus, a 20-year review of 109 cases. Am J Dis Child, 109:101, 1965.

L'Heureux PR et al.: Gallbladder disease in cystic fibrosis. Am J Roentgenol, 128:953, 1977.
Reilly BJ, Featherbee EA, and Weng TR: The correlation of radiological changes with pulmonary function in cystic fibrosis. Radiology, 98:281, 1971.
Shwachman H: Cystic fibrosis. In Kendig EL Jr, and Chernick V (eds): Disorders of the Respiratory Tract in Children, 3rd ed, p 760. Philadelphia, W.B. Saunders, 1977.
Shwachman H, and Kulczycki LL: Long-term study of 105 patients with cystic fibrosis. Am J Dis Child, 96:6, 1958.

Pneumonia Complicating Congenital Heart Disease

Kirkpatrick JA Jr: The problem of chronic and recurrent pulmonary disease. Progr Pediatr Radiol, 1:294, 1967.
Singleton EB: Pneumonias of early infancy. Tex State J Med, 52:901, 1962.

Aspiration Pneumonia

Bacsik RD: Meconium aspiration syndrome. Radiol Clin North Am, 24:463, 1977.
Bada HS, Alojipan LC, and Andrews BF: Premature rupture of membranes and its effect on the newborn. Pediatr Clin North Am, 24:441, 1977.
Bernstein J, and Wang J: Pathology of neonatal pneumonia. Am J Dis Child, 101:330, 1961.
Berquist WE et al.: Gastroesophageal reflux–associated recurrent pneumonia and chronic asthma in children. Pediatrics, 68:29, 1981.
Christie DL, O'Grady LR, and Mach DV: Incompetent lower esophageal sphincter and gastroesophageal reflux in recurrent acute pulmonary disease of infancy and childhood. J Pediatr, 93:23, 1978.
Cummings WA, and Reilly BJ: Fatigue aspiration: Cause of recurrent pneumonia in infants. Radiology, 105:387, 1972.
Darling DB, McCauley RGK, and Leonidas JC: Gastroesophageal reflux in infants and children: Correlation of radiologic severity and pulmonary pathology. Radiology, 127:735, 1978.
Euler AR et al.: Recurrent pulmonary disease in children: A complication of gastroesophageal reflux. Pediatrics, 63:47, 1979.
Gooding CA, and Gregory GA: Roentgenographic analysis of meconium aspiration of the newborn. Radiology, 100:131, 1971.
Heyman S, Kirkpatrick JA, and Winter HS: An improved radionuclide method for the diagnosis of gastroesophageal reflux and aspiration in children. Radiology, 131:479, 1979.
Hoffman RR Jr, Campbell RE, and Decker JP: Fetal aspiration syndrome. Clinical roentgenographic and pathologic features. Am J Roentgenol, 122:90, 1974.
McCauley RGK, et al.: Gastroesophageal reflux in infants and children: A useful classification and reliable radiologic technique for its demonstration. Am J Roentgenol, 130:47, 1978.
Naidich DP et al.: Computed tomography of bronchiectasis. J Comput Assist Tomogr, 6:437, 1982.
Sherman MP et al.: Tracheal aspiration and its clinical correlates in the diagnosis of congenital pneumonia. J Pediatr, 65:258, 1980.
Sondheimer JH, and Morris BA: Gastroesophageal reflux among severely retarded children. J Pediatr, 94:710, 1979.
Stahlman MT: Infections of the lung. In Kendig EL Jr, and Chernick V (eds): Disorders of the Respiratory Tract in Children, 3rd ed, p 292. Philadelphia, W.B. Saunders, 1977.

Bronchiectasis

Becroft DMO: Bronchiolitis obliterans. Bronchiectasis and other sequelae of adenovirus type 21 infection in young children. J Clin Pathol, 24:72, 1971.
Field CE: Bronchiectasis. Third report on a follow-up study of medical and surgical cases from childhood. Arch Dis Child, 44:551, 1969.
Glauser EM, Cook CD, and Harris GBC: Bronchiectasis: A review of 187 cases in children with follow-up pulmonary function studies in 58. Acta Paediatr Scand (Suppl), 165:1, 1966.
Gold R et al.: Adenoviral pneumonia and its complications in infancy and childhood. J Can Assoc Radiol, 20:218, 1969.
Macpherson RI, Comming GR, and Chernick V: Unilateral hyperlucent lung: A complication of viral pneumonia. J Can Assoc Radiol, 20:225, 1969.
Naidich DP et al.: Computed tomography of bronchiectasis. J Comput Assist Tomogr, 6:437, 1982.
Osborne D, and White P: Radiology of epidemic adenovirus 21 infection of the lower respiratory tract in infants and young children. Am J Roentgenol, 133:397, 1979.
Robinson AE, and Campbell JB: Bronchography in childhood asthma. Am J Roentgenol, 116:559, 1972.
Turner JAP et al.: Clinical expressions of immotile cilia syndrome. Pediatrics, 67:805, 1981.
Vandevivere J et al.: Bronchiectasis in childhood. Comparison of chest roentgenograms, bronchograms and lung scintigraphy. Pediatr Radiol, 9:193, 1980.

Pulmonary Sequestration and Esophageal Bronchus

Felson B: The many faces of pulmonary sequestration. Semin Roentgenol, 7:3, 1972.

Gerle RD et al.: Congenital bronchopulmonary-foregut malformation. Pulmonary sequestration communicating with the gastrointestinal tract. N Engl J Med, 278:1413, 1968.

Heithoff KB et al.: Bronchopulmonary foregut malformations. A unifying etiological concept. Am J Roentgenol, 126:46, 1976.

Kirks DR et al.: Systemic arterial supply to normal basilar segments of the left lower lobe. Am J Roentgenol, 126:817, 1976.

Skully RE, Mark EJ, and McNeely BU: Case records of the Massachusetts General Hospital. N Engl J Med, 309:1374, 1983.

Wagner ML, Singleton EB, and Egan ME: Digital subtraction angiography in children. Am J Radiol, 140:127, 1983.

Diseases Produced by Deficient Immunity and AIDS

Aldrich RA et al.: Pedigree demonstrating sex-linked recessive condition characterized by draining ears, eczematoid dermatitis and bloody diarrhea. Pediatrics, 13:133,1954.

Brown LR et al.: Ataxia-telangiectasia (Louis Bar syndrome) Semin Roentgenol, 11:67, 1976.

Bruton OC: Agammaglobulinemia. Pediatrics, 9:722, 1952.

Capitanio MA, and Kirkpatrick JA Jr: Nasopharyngeal lymphoid tissue. Roentgen observations in 257 children two years of age or less. Radiology, 96:389, 1970.

Cohen BA, Pomeranz S, and Rabinowitz JC: Pulmonary complications of AIDS. Radiologic features. Am J Roentgenol, 143:115, 1984.

DiGeorge AM: Discussions on new concepts of cellular basis of immunity. J Pediatr, 67:907, 1965.

Kirkpatrick JA Jr, and DiGeorge AM: Congenital absence of the thymus. Am J Roentgenol, 103:32, 1968.

Presberg HJ, and Singleton EB: Combined immune deficiency disease. Its radiographic expression. Radiology, 91:959, 1968.

Rubinstein A et al.: Pulmonary disease in children with acquired immune deficiency syndrome and AIDS-related complex. J Pediatr, 108:498, 1986.

Scott GB et al.: Acquired immunodeficiency syndrome in infants. N Engl J Med, 310:76, 1984.

Stiehm ER, and Fulginiti VA: Immunologic Disorders in Infants and Children, 2nd ed, pp 297–303. Philadelphia, W.B. Saunders, 1980.

Thomas PA et al.: Unexplained immune deficiency in children: A surveillance report. JAMA, 252:639, 1984.

Chronic Granulomatous Disease of Childhood

Berendes H, Bridges RA, and Good RA: A fatal granulomatosis of childhood. Minn Med, 40:309, 1957.

Bowen A, and Gibson MD: Chronic granulomatous disease with gastric antral narrowing. Pediatr Radiol, 10:119, 1980.

Buckley RH et al.: Extreme hyperimmunoglobulinemia E and undue susceptibility to infections. Pediatrics, 49:59, 1972.

Griscom NT et al.: Gastric antral narrowing in chronic granulomatous disease of childhood. Pediatrics, 54:456, 1974.

Merten DF, Buckley RH, and Pratt PC: Hyperimmunoglobulinemia E syndrome: Radiologic observations. Radiology, 132:71, 1979.

Wolfson J et al.: Roentgenologic manifestations in children with a genetic defect of polymorphonuclear leukocyte function. Radiology, 91:37, 1968.

Pneumocystis Carinii Pneumonia

Barron TF et al.: Pneumocystis carinii pneumonia studies by gallium-67 scanning. Radiology, 154:791, 1985.

Bazaz GR et al.: Pneumocystis carinii pneumonia in three full-term siblings. J Pediatr, 76:767, 1970.

Capitanio MA, and Kirkpatrick JA Jr: Pneumocystis carinii pneumonia. Am J Roentgenol, 97:174, 1966.

Green R: Opportunistic pneumonias. Semin Roentgenol, 15:50, 1980.

Hughes WT: Pneumocystis carinii pneumonitis. In Kendig EL Jr, and Chernick V (eds): Disorder of the Respiratory Tract in Children, 3rd ed, pp 403–411. Philadelphia, W.B. Saunders, 1977.

Stagno S et al.: *Pneumocystis carinii* pneumonitis in young immunocompetent infants. Pediatrics, 66:56, 1980.

Cytomegalic Inclusion Disease Pneumonia

Hanshaw JB: Congenital and acquired *Cytomegalovirus* infection. Pediatr Clin North Am, 13:279, 1966.

Howard WA: Cytomegalic inclusion disease. In Kendig EL Jr, and Chernick V (eds): Disorders of the Respiratory Tract in Children, 3rd ed, p 936. Philadelphia, W.B. Saunders, 1977.

Merten DF, and Gooding CA: Skeletal manifestations of cytomegalic inclusion disease. Radiology, 95:333, 1970.

Spector SA et al.: Cytomegaloviruria in older infants in intensive care nurseries. J Pediatr, 95:444, 1979.

Stagno S et al.: Infant pneumonitis associated with cytomegalovirus, Chlamydia, Pneumocystis, and Ureaplasma: A prospective study. Pediatrics, 68:322, 1981.

Whitley RJ et al.: Protracted pneumonitis in young infants associated with perinatally acquired cytomegaloviral infection. J Pediatr, 89:16, 1976.

Childhood Tuberculosis

Giammona ST et al.: Massive lymphadenopathy in primary pulmonary tuberculosis in children. Am Rev Respir Dis, 100:480, 1969.

Kendig EL Jr: Tuberculosis. In Kendig EL Jr, and Chernick V (eds): Disorders of the Respiratory Tract in Children, 3rd ed, pp 787–843. Philadelphia, W.B. Saunders, 1977.

Lincoln EM, and Sewell EM: Tuberculosis in Children, p 81. New York, McGraw-Hill, 1963.

Woodring JH et al.: Update: The radiographic features of pulmonary tuberculosis. Am J Roentgenol, 146:497, 1986.

Pulmonary Mycosis

Christie A: Histoplasmosis. In Kendig EL Jr, and Chernick V (eds): Disorders of the Respiratory Tract in Children, 3rd ed, pp 865–878. Philadelphia, W.B. Saunders, 1977.

Greendyke WH, Resnick DL, and Harvey WG: The varied roentgen manifestations of primary coccidioidomycosis. Am J Roentgenol, 109:491, 1970.

Klein DL, and Gamsu G: Thoracic manifestations of aspergillosis. Am J Roentgenol, 134:543, 1980.

Kuhn JP: Pulmonary mycoses. In Silverman FN (ed): Caffey's Pediatric X-Ray Diagnosis, 8th ed, pp 1228–1233. Chicago, Year Book Medical Publishers, 1985.

Mintzer RA et al.: The spectrum of radiologic findings in allergic bronchopulmonary aspergillosis. Radiology, 127:301, 1978.

Pinckney L, and Parker BR: Primary coccidioidomycosis in children presenting with massive pleural effusion. Am J Roentgenol, 130:247, 1978.

Richardson HD Jr, Anderson JA, and McCay BN: Acute pulmonary coccidioidomycosis in children. J Pediatr, 70:376, 1967.

Schwarz J: Histoplasmosis. New York, Praeger, 1981.

Schwarz J, and Baum GL: Fungus diseases of the lung. Semin Roentgenol, 5:1, 1970.

Seabury JH: Candidiasis. In Kendig EL Jr, and Chernick V (eds): Disorders of the Respiratory Tract in Children, 3rd ed, pp 921–923. Philadelphia, W.B. Saunders, 1977.

Seabury JH: The mycoses (excluding histoplasmosis). In Kendig EL Jr, and Chernick V (eds): Disorders of the Respiratory Tract in Children, 3rd ed, pp 879–935. Philadelphia, W.B. Saunders, 1977.

Stites DT, and Glezen WP: Pulmonary nocardiosis in childhood. A case report. Am J Dis Child, 114:101, 1967.

Sarcoidosis

Kendig EL Jr: The clinical picture of sarcoidosis in children. Pediatrics, 54:289, 1971.

Kendig EL Jr: Sarcoidosis. In Kendig EL Jr, and Chernick V (eds): Disorders of the Respiratory Tract in Children, 3rd ed, pp 852–864. Philadelphia, W.B. Saunders, 1977.

Kirks DR, McCormick VD, and Greenspan RH: Pulmonary sarcoidosis. Roentgenologic analysis of 150 patients. Am J Roentgenol, 177:777, 1973.

Merten DF, Kirks DR, and Grossman H: Pulmonary sarcoidosis in childhood. Am J Roentgenol, 135:673, 1980.

Parasitosis

Burton K et al.: Pulmonary paragonimiasis in Laotian refugee children. Pediatrics, 70:246, 1982.

Deskin CA, Colvin SH Jr, and Beaver PC: Pulmonary dirofilariasis: Cause of pulmonary nodular disease. JAMA, 198:665, 1966.

Grunebaum M: Radiologic manifestations of lung echinococcus in children. Pediatr Radiol, 3:65, 1975.

Herrera-Lilerandi R: Thoracic repercussions of amoebiasis. J Thorac Cardiovasc Surg, 52:361, 1966.

McPhil JL, and Arora EA: Intrathoracic hydatid disease. Dis Chest, 52:772, 1967.

Tauzon RA, Firestone EF, and Blaustein AE: Human pulmonary dirofilariasis manifesting as a "coin" lesion. A case report. JAMA, 199:45, 1967.

Wall MA, and McGhee G: Paragonimiasis. Am J Dis Child, 136:828, 1982.

Interstitial Pneumonia

Idiopathic or Usual Interstitial Pneumonia (UIP)

Gaensler EA, Carrington CB, and Coutu RE: Chronic interstitial pneumonias. Clin Notes Respir Dis, 10:3, 1972.

Liebow AA: Definition and classifications of interstitial pneumonias in human pathology. Progr Respir Res, 8:1, 1975.

Liebow AA: New concepts and entities in pulmonary disease. In Liebow AA, and Smith DE (eds): The Lung, pp 332–336. Baltimore, Williams & Wilkins, 1967.

Thurlbeck WM: Cryptogenic or idiopathic fibrosing alveolitis. In Kendig EL Jr, and Chernick V (eds): Disorders of the Respiratory Tract in Children, 3rd ed, pp 518–522. Philadelphia, W.B. Saunders, 1977.

Desquamative Interstitial Pneumonia (DIP)

Feigin DS, and Friedman PJ: Chest radiography in desquamative interstitial pneumonitis: Review of 37 patients. Am J Roentgenol, 134:491, 1980.

Fromm GB, Dunn JD, and Harris JD: Desquamative interstitial pneumonitis. Chest, 77:4, 552, 1980.

Gaensler EA, Carrington CB, and Coutu RE: Chronic interstitial pneumonias. Clin Notes Respir Dis, 10:3, 1972.

Gaensler EA, Goff AN, and Prowse CN: Desquamative interstitial pneumonia. N Engl J Med, 274:113, 1966.

Howatt WF et al.: Desquamative interstitial pneumonia: Case report of an infant unresponsive to treatment. Am J Dis Child, 126:346, 1973.

Liebow AA, Steer RA, and Billingsley JG: Desquamative interstitial pneumonia. Am J Med, 39:369, 1965.

Rosennow EC, O'Connell EJ, and Harrison EG: Desquamative interstitial pneumonias in children. Am J Dis Child, 120:344, 1970.

Lymphocytic Interstitial Pneumonia (LIP)

Carrington CB, and Liebow AA: Lymphocytic interstitial pneumonia. Presented at the Scientific Proceedings of the American Association of Pathologists and Bacteriologists, Cleveland, March 4, 1966.

Glickstein M et al.: Nonlymphomatous lymphoid disorders of the lung. Am J Roentgenol, 147:227, 1986.

Halprin GM, Famirez-R J, and Pratt PC: Lymphoid interstitial pneumonia. Chest, 62:418, 1972.

Liebow AA, and Carrington CB: Diffuse pulmonary lymphoreticular infiltrations associated with dysproteinemia. Med Clin North Am, 57:809, 1973.

Lymphomatoid Granulomatosis

Bassani F et al.: Chronic granulomatous disease. Pediatr Radiol, 11:105, 1981.

Bridges RA et al.: A fatal granulomatous disease of childhood: The clinical, pathological and laboratory features of a new syndrome. Am J Dis Child, 97:387, 1959.

Glickstein M et al.: Non-lymphomatous lymphoid disorders of the lungs. Am J Roentgenol, 147:227, 1986.

Gold RH, et al.: Roentgenographic features of the neutrophil dysfunction syndromes. Radiology, 92:1045, 1969.

Katzenstein AA, Carrington CB, and Liebow AA: Lymphomatoid granulomatosis: A clinical pathologic study of 152 cases. Cancer, 43:360, 1979.

Liebow AA, Carrington CR, and Friedman PJ: Lymphomatoid granulomatosis. Hum Pathol, 3:457, 1972.

Sutcliffe J et al.: Chronic granulomatous disease. Br J Radiol, 43:110, 1970.

Ectodermal Dysplasia

Capitanio MA et al.: Congenital anhydrotic ectodermal dysplasia. Am J Roentgenol, 103:168, 1968.

DeJager J: Respiratory tract lesions in so-called congenital ectodermal dysplasia. J Pathol Bacteriol, 96:502, 1968.

Shwachman Syndrome

Danks DM et al.: Metaphyseal chondrodysplasia, neutropenia, and pancreatic insufficiency presenting with respiratory distress in the neonatal period. Arch Dis Child, 51:697, 1976.

Shwachman H et al: The syndrome of pancreatic insufficiency and bone marrow dysfunction. J Pediatr, 65:645, 1964.

Stanley P, and Sutcliffe J: Metaphyseal chondrodysplasia with dwarfism, pancreatic insufficiency and neutropenia. Pediatr Radiol, 1:119, 1973.

Taybi H, Mitchell AD, and Friedman GD: Metaphyseal dysostosis and the associated syndrome of pancreatic insufficiency and blood disorders. Radiology, 93:563, 1969.

Inflammatory Pseudotumor

Bahadori M, and Liebow AA: Plasma cell granulomas of the lung. Cancer, 31:191, 1973.

Glickstein M, et al.: Nonlymphomatous lymphoid disorders of the lungs. Am J Roentgenol, 147:227, 1986.

McCall I, and Woo-Ming M: Radiological appearances of plasma cell granuloma of the lung. Clin Radiol, 29:145, 1978.

Monzon CM et al.: Plasma cell granuloma of the lung in children. Pediatrics, 70:168, 1982.

Schwartz EE, Katz SM, and Mandell GA: Post-inflammatory pseudotumors of the lung: Fibrous histiocytoma and related lesions. Radiology, 136:609, 1980.

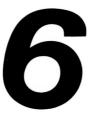

TUMORS

Computerized tomography (CT) provides a valuable cross-sectional image of intrathoracic neoplasms. Any patient with an intrathoracic mass should have the advantage of computerized tomographic evaluation, not only for a more accurate diagnosis but also to facilitate surgical resection. In addition, small lesions, especially pleural neoplasms, frequently can be identified only by CT. Especially important is the use of CT for post-treatment follow-up studies and for the detection of metastases.

BENIGN PULMONARY NEOPLASMS

Benign neoplasms of the lungs are extremely uncommon in the pediatric patient. Various conditions have been reported, including mesodermal tumors, leiomyomas, neurogenic tumors, hamartomas, and bronchial adenomas. The latter two conditions are relatively more common than the others.

Bronchial Adenomas

These should be considered in the differential diagnosis of a child with chronic cough, recurrent pneumonia, or clinical findings similar to those seen with aspiration of a foreign object. The pathologic varieties are the same as in the adult—that is, carcinoid, cylindroma, and mucoepidermoid adenoma. The carcinoid tumor is the most common, and accounts for 90% of bronchial adenomas.

Clinical features depend on the location of the tumor, which in the pediatric age group is usually endobronchial and centrally located. They consist of cough, wheezing and, frequently, hemoptysis.

The usual radiographic finding in the pediatric patient is that of recurrent pneumonia, with or without atelectasis. If a major bronchus is involved air trapping may develop, producing fluoroscopic and radiographic features similar to those seen with an aspirated foreign body. Peripheral bronchial adenomas may present as coin lesions, and may even contain stippled areas of calcification. If the lesion is large and arises from a bronchus in the hilar area, it may present as a hilar mass.

Bronchograms may delineate the filling defect if it is located in one of the larger bronchial segments, seen radiographically as a smooth, round, intraluminal

261

mass (Fig. 6–1). The diagnosis is confirmed by bronchoscopy or resection of the lesion and by histologic examination.

Hamartomas

These benign tumors presumably represent embryologic remnants of pulmonary tissue, and are composed mainly of cartilaginous overgrowth. These lesions rarely produce symptoms and are discovered during routine chest radiography.

Radiographically the lesion is usually sharply circumscribed, and may contain calcium. Consequently, radiographic differentiation from a granuloma is virtually impossible. The lesion may be variable in size but apparently, in the young patient, may be relatively larger than that seen in the adult. Hamartomas may gradually enlarge and undergo cystic changes.

Juvenile Papilloma of the Larynx

This is the most common tumor that occurs in the respiratory tree of infants and children (see Fig. 4–20). The etiology is unknown, but viral infections have been suggested. An unusual occurrence is the distal spread of the neoplasm into the bronchi and lungs. Although malignant change has occurred, it has only been reported in those cases that were previously irradiated. The mode of spread to the distal bronchi and lungs is unclear, but presumably is the result of aspiration of papillomatous material. Pulmonary changes in those cases that have peripheral papillomatosis show nodular densities, and radiolucent areas representing cystic bronchiectasis may develop in the later stages of the disease (see Fig. 4–20). The similarity of the extreme cystic bronchiectasis to that seen in necrotizing bronchiolitis is striking.

PULMONARY AND BRONCHIAL CYSTS

Cystic adenomatoid malformation of the lung is a congenital cystic disease, described in Chapter 4. Air trapping within the cyst results in respiratory distress, usually in the neonatal period. Milder forms may not be identified until infancy or childhood (Fig. 6–2). Congenital bronchogenic cysts are difficult to evaluate radiographically because of their similarity to postinflammatory cysts. However, many cases of congenital bronchogenic cysts have been reported. Apparently they arise from abnormal budding of the primitive trachea or from abnormal branching of the tracheobronchial tree.

Most bronchogenic cysts do not communicate with the major tracheobronchial passages, and are filled with secretions.

The patient is usually asymptomatic, although hemoptysis, cough, chest pain, and pulmonary infection may be presenting features that require radiographic investigation. Although the cysts may occur in the periphery of the lungs, congenital cysts, in our experience, are more common in an area contiguous to the mediastinum. Mediastinal bronchogenic cysts in infants may cause severe respiratory distress as a result of bronchial compression.

If the cyst communicates with the bronchial tree and is filled with air, the radiographic findings may be very similar to those of a pneumatocele (Fig. 6–3). The cysts are usually sharply defined and variable in size. If infected, or if secretions are trapped within the area, they form an air-fluid level (Fig. 6–4). If completely filled with fluid, the lesion appears as a solid mass (Fig. 6–5). The mediastinal bronchogenic cyst is usually homogeneous in density and less likely to communicate with the tracheobronchial tree. The typical location of such cysts

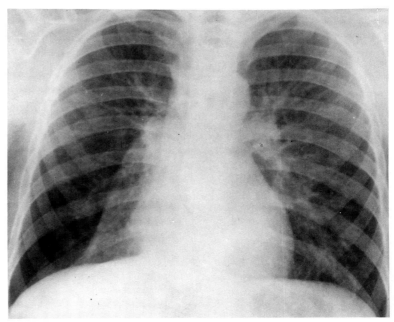

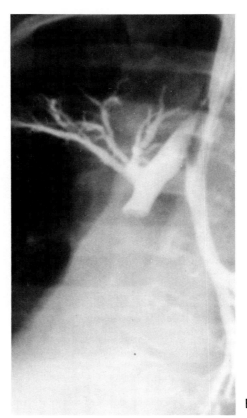

Figure 6–1. Bronchial adenoma in 9-year-old boy. A, Frontal chest radiograph shows atelectasis of the right lower lobe. B, Bronchogram shows smooth-filling defect involving the bronchus intermedius. Histologically the lesion was a cylindroma.

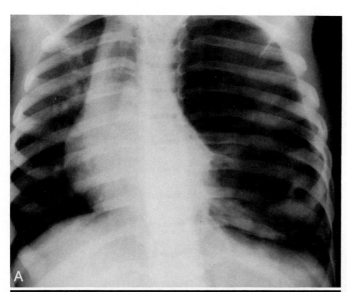

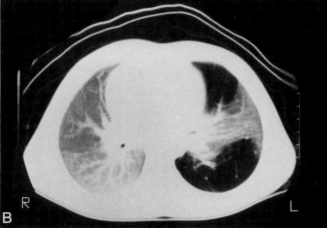

Figure 6–2. *Cystic adenomatoid malformation of the lung in a 2-year-old child. A, Chest radiograph shows air trapping of the left lung, with displacement of mediastinal structures to the right. B, Computerized tomography shows the area of air trapping, as well as a band of compressed tissue within the hyperinflated lobe.*

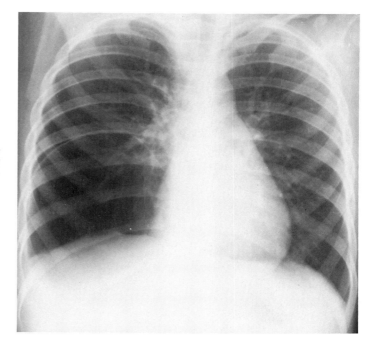

Figure 6–3. Pulmonary cyst. This is a large thin-walled cyst in the right base of a young child. The histologic diagnosis after resection was bronchial cyst.

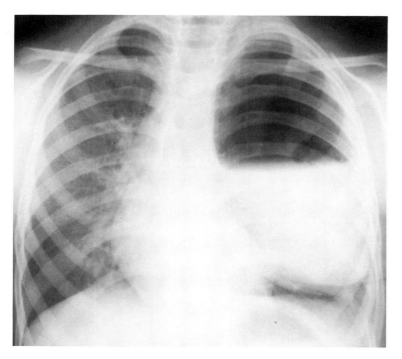

Figure 6–4. Large air-fluid-filled cyst of the left lung in a 7-year-old child. The histologic diagnosis was bronchial cyst.

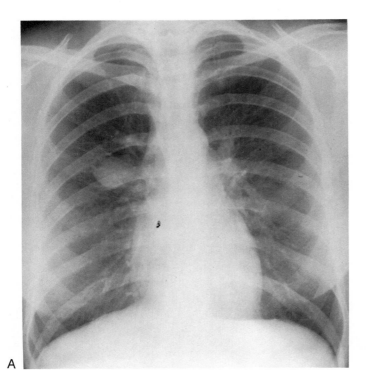

A

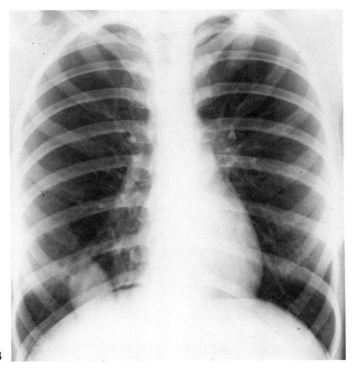

B

Figure 6–5. Solitary fluid-filled congenital bronchogenic cyst. A, Fifteen-year-old asymptomatic girl with a round density lateral to the right hilus. The histologic diagnosis was congenital bronchogenic cyst. B, Fourteen-year-old asymptomatic girl with oval-shaped density in the right lower lobe. The histologic diagnosis was congenital bronchogenic cyst.

is in the subcarinal area, and the parenchymal ones are usually in the lower lung fields. Computerized tomography is helpful for accurate anatomic localization (Figs. 6–6, 6–7, and 6–8). Bronchial cysts may occasionally be found posteriorly, and mimic neurogenic tumors (Fig. 6–9). Fluid-filled cysts in the young patient may be mistaken for hamartomas, granulomas, or hematomas (Fig. 6–10). Mucoid impaction distal to an atretic bronchus or bronchiole may produce a density similar to a benign tumor or granuloma. Radiographic differentiation of air-filled bronchial cysts from pneumatoceles may be extremely difficult, but pneumatoceles have a history of antecedent pneumonia, have an extremely thin wall, and over a period of many weeks or months show gradual reduction and then disappear.

Histologically, the differentiation between a congenital bronchial cyst and an acquired cyst may be impossible. The presence of smooth muscle or cartilage in the wall of the cyst suggests its congenital origin, but an acquired cyst may, as a result of its expansion and the compression of surrounding lung tissue, show similar histologic findings (Fig. 6–11). Consequently, any cystic pulmonary lesion found in an asymptomatic child should be treated conservatively. Pneumatoceles will show gradual regression and disappear over a period of weeks or months, whereas the true bronchogenic cyst will remain unchanged. However, we have seen one postinflammatory cyst that remained unchanged for 2 years (Fig. 6–12).

Text continued on page 272

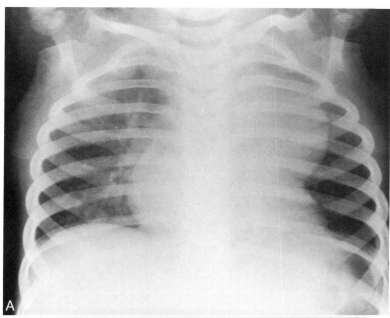

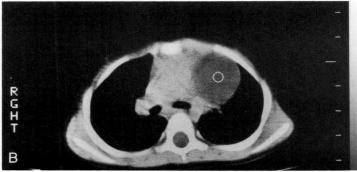

Figure 6–6. Bronchial cyst in a 2-year-old girl. A, Chest radiograph shows a sharply demarcated mass in the left superior mediastinum. B, Computerized tomography shows the mediastinal location of the mass, as well as the low attenuation density.

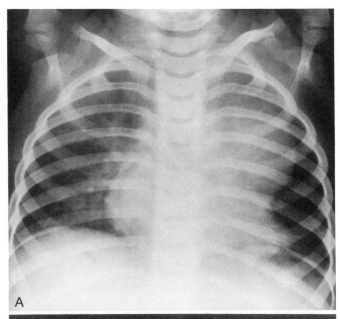

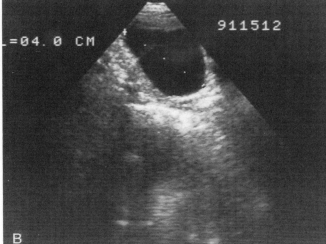

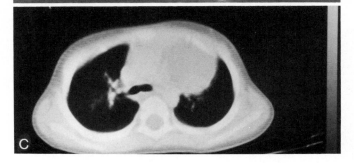

Figure 6–7. *Bronchial cyst in a 2-year-old girl. A, Chest radiograph shows sharply demarcated mass lesions similar to that seen in the previous case. B, Ultrasound examination demonstrates the echo-free cystic lesion. C, Computerized tomography reveals the mediastinal location of the cyst.*

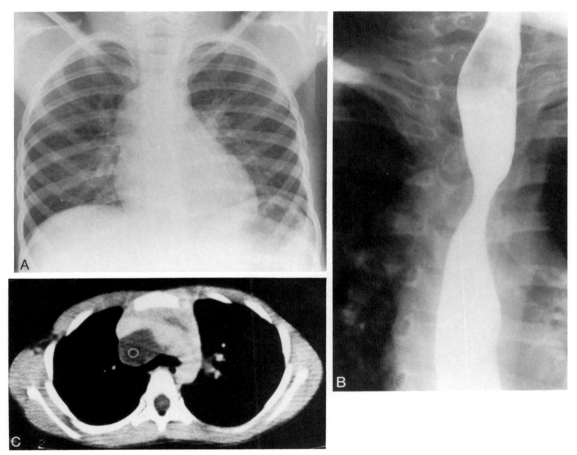

Figure 6–8. Bronchial cyst in a 4-year-old girl. A, Chest radiograph shows a mass in the right superior mediastinum. B, Esophagram demonstrates indentation by the mass on the right side of the esophagus. C, Computerized tomography shows the low attenuation of the mass, which after surgical resection was found to be a bronchial cyst.

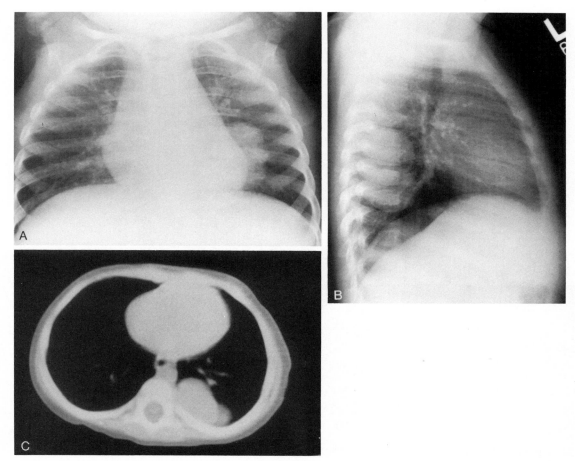

Figure 6–9. Bronchial cyst in a 1-year-old girl. A, Chest radiograph shows lobulated, sharply demarcated mass in the left retrocardiac area. B, Lateral view shows the posterior location of the lesion. C, Computerized tomography emphasizes the posterior location adjacent to the costovertebral angle, suggesting neoplasm of neurogenic origin. After surgical resection the lesion was found to be a bronchial cyst.

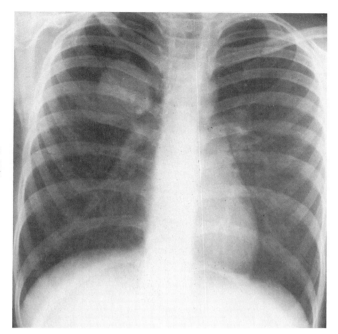

Figure 6–10. *Traumatic hematoma of the lung in a 4-year-old child. The frontal projection shows a round sharply demarcated density in the right upper lobe.*

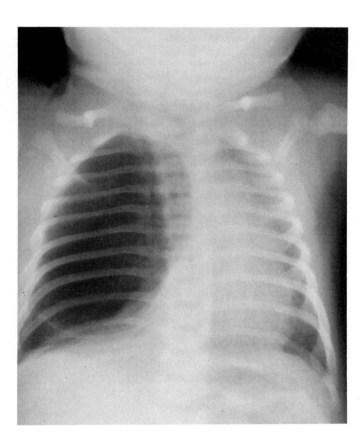

Figure 6–11. *Thin-walled cyst in the right lung of a 3-month-old. The histologic diagnosis was bronchogenic cyst. Although the histology of these cases suggests its congenital origin, each may be a postinflammatory acquired cyst. (Courtesy of Dr. V. Condon.)*

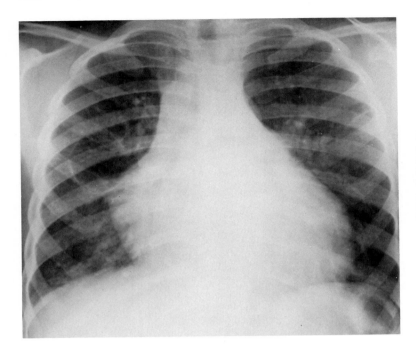

Figure 6–12. Postinflammatory cyst of the right lung in a 6-year-old child with sickle cell anemia. Chest radiograph 2 years after staphylococcal pneumonia shows no change in the appearance of the cyst, which has been present since the initial infection.

MEDIASTINAL TUMORS

These are more common than primary lung tumors in the pediatric patient. The major compartments of the mediastinum consist of the anterior, middle, and posterior segments; each has its own normal anatomic structures from which various neoplasms arise. The anterior mediastinum is the area between the sternum and the anterior portion of the pericardium, and contains the thymus and lymph nodes. The middle mediastinum is composed of the heart, pericardial sac, trachea and major bronchi, and associated lymph nodes. The posterior mediastinum, which is located between the posterior pericardial reflection and the posterior chest wall, contains the esophagus, descending thoracic aorta, intercostal nerves, and sympathetic and parasympathetic nerve trunks. Masses arising from these structures may encroach on adjacent areas of the mediastinum, and may even extend into the adjacent thoracic space and lungs. However, by determining the location of the major portion of the mass in one of the mediastinal compartments, the differential considerations are reduced in number.

Benign Masses

An anterior mediastinal mass in an infant is usually a large thymus, which is a normal variant, but at times may be difficult to differentiate from a significant mediastinal mass. Fluoroscopy is helpful by showing a change in the size of the thymus with inspiration and expiration and, by turning the child to oblique positions, by identifying the characteristic inferior corner of the thymus and the indentations of the costal cartilages. An anterior mediastinal mass, regardless of size in an asymptomatic infant, should be considered to be the thymus (see Fig. 2–8). CT and MRI may also be helpful in differentiating the thymus from other anterior mediastinal structures. Benign neoplasms arising in the anterior mediastinum include teratomas and dermoids (Fig. 6–13) and, rarely, lipomas (Fig. 6–14), hemangiomas, and cystic hygromas.

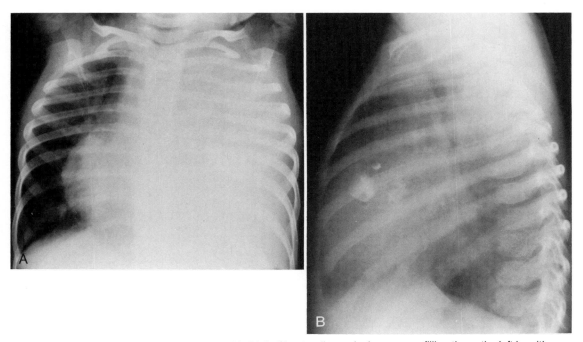

Figure 6–13. Mediastinal teratoma in a 2-year-old girl. A, Chest radiograph shows mass filling the entire left hemithorax. B, Lateral radiograph shows the areas of calcification within the mass to better advantage in the frontal projection. The histologic diagnosis was benign teratoma.

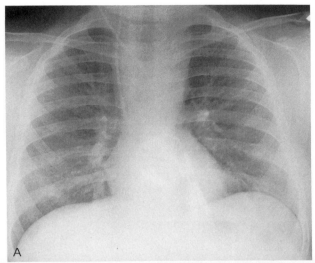

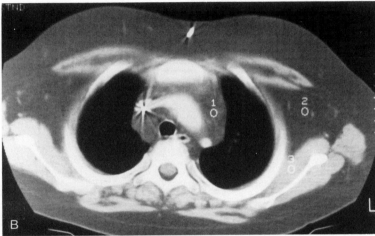

Figure 6–14. Mediastinal lipomatosis in a 9-year-old boy with leukemia who had been treated for 4 months with corticosteroids. A, Chest radiograph shows widening of the superior mediastinum without tracheal compression. B, Computerized tomography shows the superior mediastinal mass to be of fat density. (From Shukla LW, Katz JA, and Wagner ML: Mediastinal lipomatosis: A complication of high dose steroid therapy in children. Pediatr Radiol, in press.)

Benign masses arising in the middle mediastinum include bronchial cysts, pericardial cysts, pericardial defects (Fig. 6–15), and cystic hygromas (lymphangiomas), which are usually peritracheal in location (Fig. 6–16). Bizarre lymphangiomas may develop in any portion of the mediastinum (Fig. 6–17). Inflammatory lesions of the lymph nodes may also produce enlargement of the hilar lymph nodes. Benign neoplasms arising in the posterior mediastinum include neuromas, usually arising from the intercostal nerves, ganglioneuromas (Fig. 6–18), and neurenteric cysts (esophageal duplications) (Fig. 6–19).

Malignant Masses

Malignancies of the mediastinum usually arise from those anatomic structures normally found in the different mediastinal compartments, except for malignant teratomas, which develop in the anterior mediastinum (Fig. 6–20). Lymphosarcomas, T-cell lymphomas, and leukemic infiltration of the thymus develop in the anterior mediastinum (Fig. 6–21). CT is extremely helpful, not only in identifying the location and extent of the lesion, but also in evaluating the response to

Text continued on page 282

Figure 6–15. *Herniation of left atrium through pericardial defect in a 10-year-old girl. A, Chest radiograph shows an abnormal convex left cardiac border. B, Computerized tomography indicates cross-sectional anatomy of the abnormal density extending to the left and anteriorly. Angiocardiography demonstrated contrast medium within the herniated left atrial appendage.*

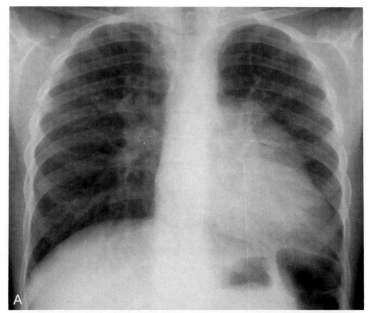

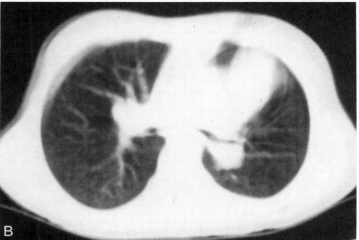

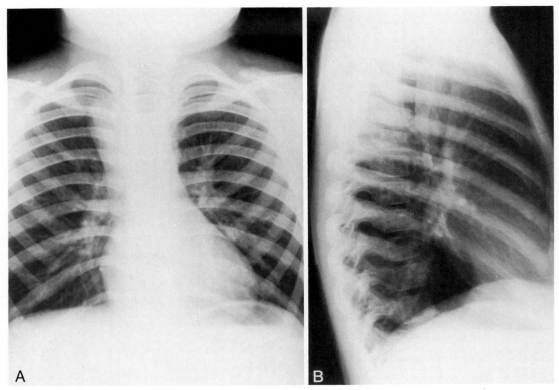

Figure 6–16. Cystic hygroma in a 7-year-old boy. A, Chest radiograph shows mediastinal mass in the right superior mediastinum. B, Lateral view identifies the mass in a paratracheal location. The histologic diagnosis was cystic hygroma (lymphangioma).

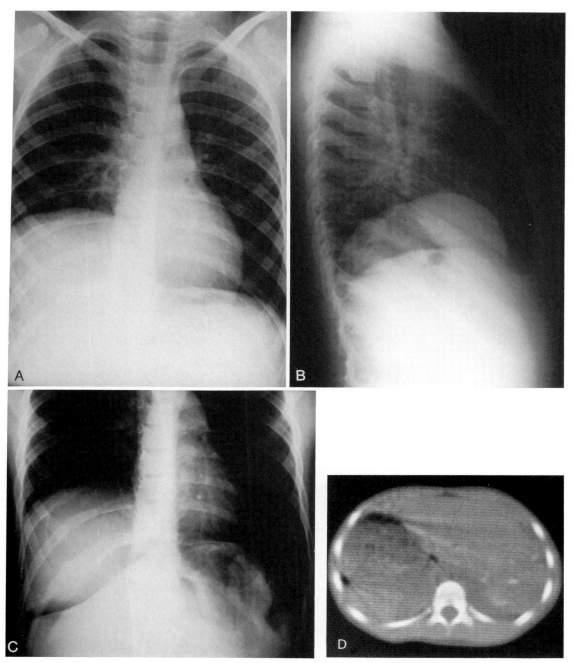

Figure 6–17. Intrathoracic lymphangioma. A, Convex mass simulating elevated right hemidiaphragm is seen in the right lower hemithorax. B, Lateral view shows the mass mimicking either eventration or paralysis of the right hemidiaphragm. Thoracotomy demonstrated the mediastinal origin. C, Diagnostic pneumoperitoneum reveals calcification within the mass, which depresses the right hemidiaphragm. D, Computerized tomography shows the large calcium-containing mass in cross-section. The histologic diagnosis after resection was a large lymphangioma.

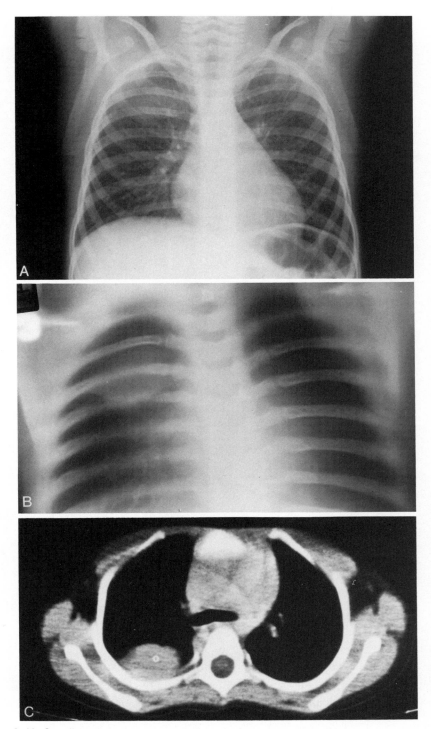

Figure 6–18. *Ganglioneuroma in a 7-year-old boy. A, Chest radiograph shows ill-defined density in the right upper lobe. B, Linear tomography demonstrates the lesion to be posterior and adjacent to the ribs. C, Computerized tomography shows the cross-sectional anatomy of the posterior thoracic mass. The histologic diagnosis was ganglioneuroma.*

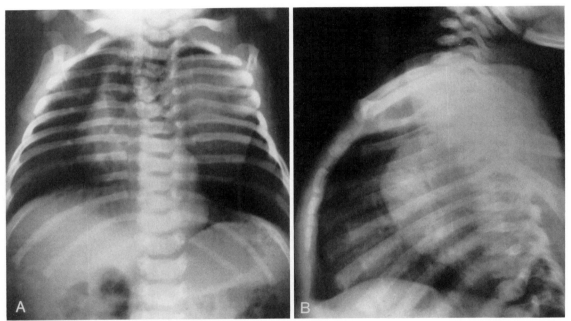

Figure 6–19. *Neurenteric cyst in a 1-month-old infant with respiratory difficulties. A, Chest radiograph shows mass in the left hemithorax, with associated vertebral anomalies. B, Lateral radiograph shows the posterior location of the mass. After surgical resection the mass was found to be a neurenteric cyst lined with gastric mucosa. (From Singleton EB, Wagner ML, and Dutton RV: Radiology of the Alimentary Tract in Infants and Children, 2nd ed. Philadelphia, W. B. Saunders, 1977.)*

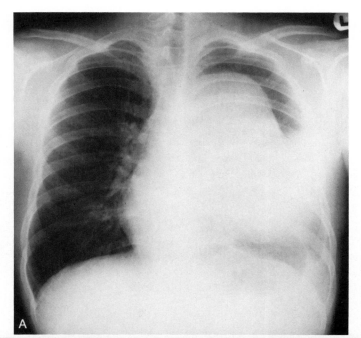

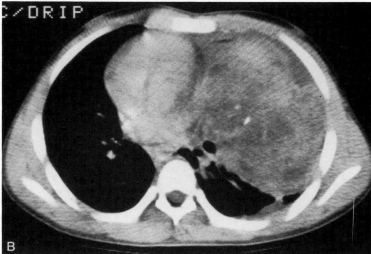

Figure 6–20. *Malignant teratoma in a 13-year-old boy. A, A large mediastinal mass obscures the left cardiac border. B, Computerized tomography shows the extent of the large mass as well as areas of calcification. The low-density areas represent necrosis.*

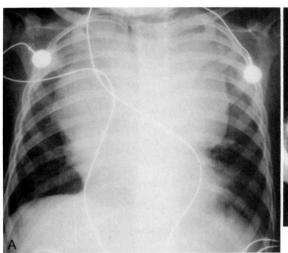
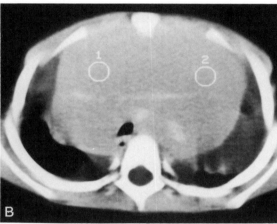
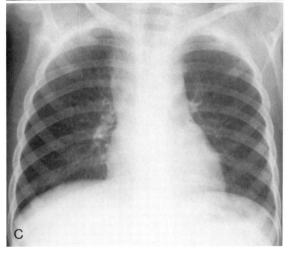

Figure 6–21. *T-cell lymphoma in the anterior mediastinum of a 3½-year-old boy. A, The large paramediastinal mass obscures detail of the superior mediastinal structures and displaces the trachea to the right. B, Computerized tomography reveals the anterior location of the mass. C, Repeat chest radiograph 1 week after chemotherapy shows marked regression in the size of the mass.*

treatment (Fig. 6–21). Rhabdomyosarcoma may rarely arise in the anterior mediastinum. Any of these conditions may produce pleural effusions as well as a disturbance of pulmonary aeration secondary to pressure on bronchial segments. The rapid regression in size of these masses, especially of the lymphomas, and the clinical improvement of the patient that occurs when chemotherapeutic drugs are used, frequently seems miraculous. Unfortunately, a recurrence usually occurs, commonly associated with systemic leukemia.

Hodgkin's disease and other lymphomas arise from lymph nodes in the anterior and midmediastinal area, and present in various radiographic patterns with and without pulmonary parenchymal involvement (Figs. 6–22, 6–23 and 6–24). The great majority of posterior mediastinal malignancies arise from the sympathetic and parasympathetic nerve trunks, and are ganglioneuroblastomas and neuroblastomas (Figs. 6–25 and 6–26). Rib erosion is commonly found adjacent to these neoplasms, and myelography may be essential to exclude

Text continued on page 287

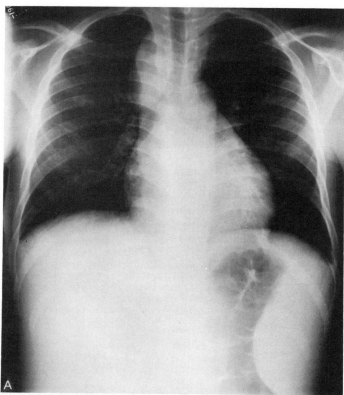

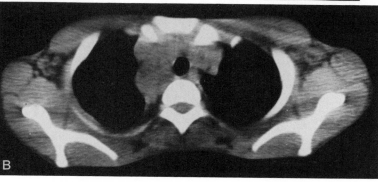

Figure 6–22. Hodgkin's disease in a 15-year-old boy. A, Chest radiograph shows the right superior mediastinal mass and enlargement of the spleen. B, Computerized tomography demonstrates cross-sectional anatomy of the right paratracheal mass.

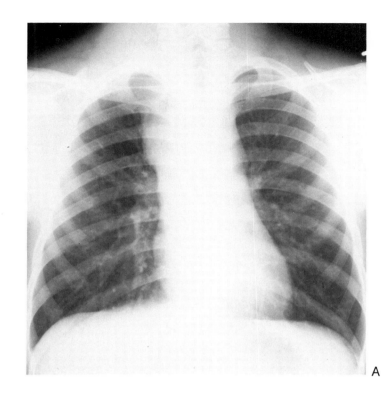

A

Figure 6–23. Hodgkin's disease in a 10-year-old boy. A, Initial chest radiograph shows localized para-tracheal lymphadenopathy and right supraclavicular adenopathy. B, Chest radiograph 2 years later shows parenchymal involvement consisting of patchy and linear densities. Pulmonary Hodgkin's disease was confirmed by autopsy.

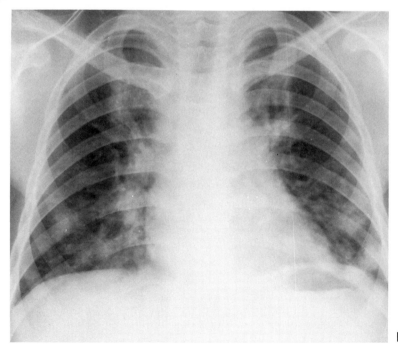

B

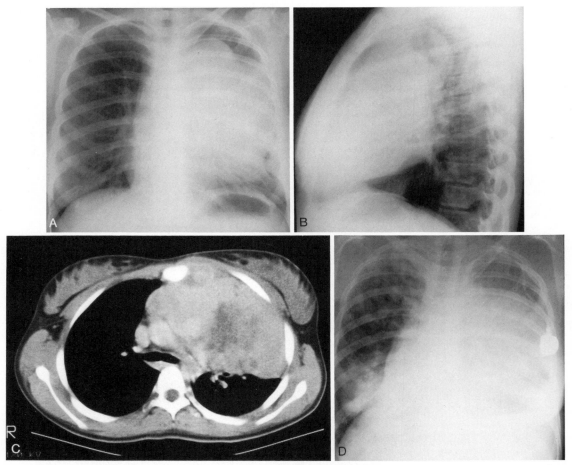

Figure 6–24. Hodgkin's disease in a 14-year-old girl. A, Chest radiographs show large mass in the left mediastinum, extending to the lateral portion of the chest wall. The histologic diagnosis was Hodgkin's disease. B, Lateral radiograph indicates the anterior location of the mass, with extension into the midportion of the mediastinum. C, Computerized tomography shows the necrotic mass involving the pericardium and anterior chest wall. D, Repeat chest radiograph 2 years later demonstrates increase in size of mass as well as nodular parenchymal involvement.

Illustration continued on opposite page

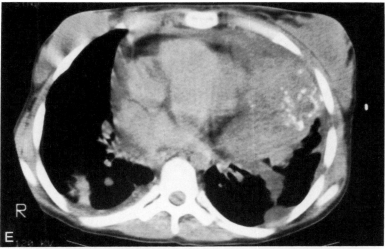

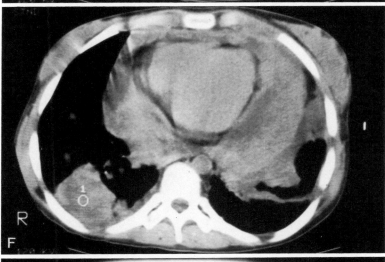

Figure 6–24. E, Computerized tomography shows the large mass occupying the anterior midmediastinum, with associated areas of calcification and pulmonary parenchymal involvement. F, Computerized tomography at a slightly lower level indicates the mass encircling the heart, as well as a large mass adjacent to the posterior right chest wall. G, Computerized tomography with pulmonary window settings shows the nodular involvement of the lung parenchyma.

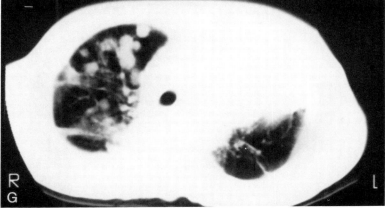

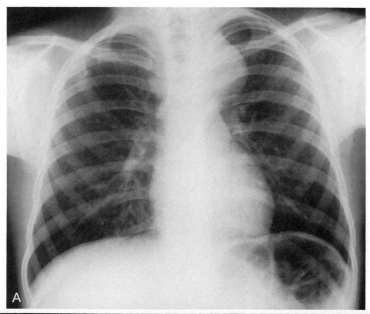

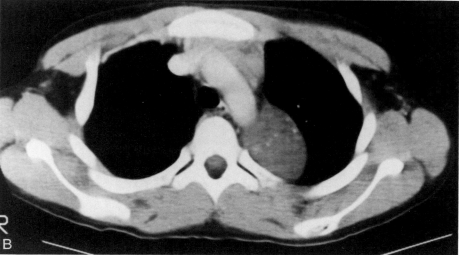

Figure 6–25. *Ganglioneuroblastoma of the posterior mediastinum in an 11-year-old boy. A, Chest radiograph shows the left posterior mediastinal mass. B, Computerized tomography reveals the mass adjacent to the costovertebral angle, and demonstrates calcification within the lesion not seen on routine radiographs. The histologic diagnosis was ganglioneuroblastoma.*

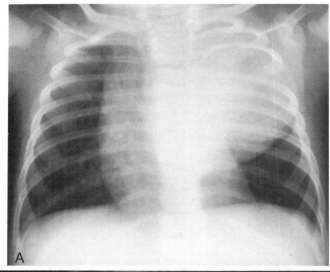

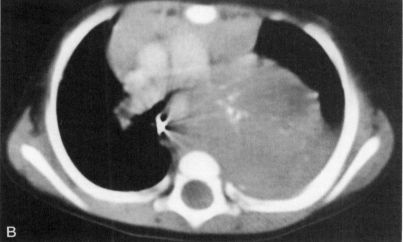

Figure 6–26. Neuroblastoma in a 5-month-old boy. A, Chest radiographs show large mass occupying the left upper hemithorax, with erosion and displacement of the posterior portions of the left third and fourth ribs. B, Computerized tomography demonstrates the large size of the mass as well as the calcific component. The histologic diagnosis was neuroblastoma.

intraspinal (extradural) extension of a paraspinal tumor. Germinoma is a rare mediastinal tumor that may develop in the posterior mediastinum and simulate neuroblastoma.

PRIMARY PULMONARY MALIGNANCIES

Primary malignancies of the lungs in infants and children are extremely rare, and primary sarcomas and carcinomas, although reported, are so uncommon as to be deleted from most differential considerations of abnormal lung densities in the pediatric patient. Bronchial carcinoma is extremely rare, and may have the same radiographic findings as a granuloma or some other parenchymal mass (Fig. 6–27).

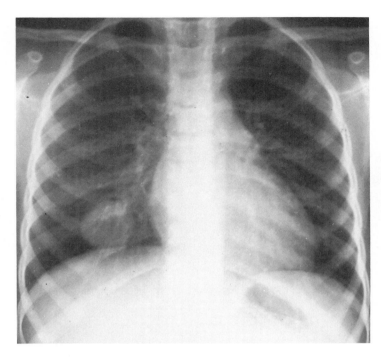

Figure 6–27. Discrete lesion in right lower lobe in a 6-year-old girl. The histologic diagnosis was primary adenocarcinoma. (Courtesy of W. Hall, United States Air Force Hospital, San Antonio, Texas.)

Pulmonary blastoma is a rare primary lung malignancy that also generally has a nodular or granulomatous configuration (Fig. 6–28).

Fibromatosis with visceral involvement involves the lungs, liver, and other viscera, as well as the skeleton and subcutaneous areas. The condition is usually fatal during infancy. The pulmonary lesions appear as discrete nodular densities (Fig. 6–29).

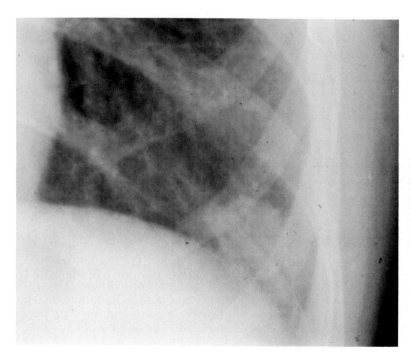

Figure 6–28. Primary lung malignancy. Nodular lesion in the left lower lobe of a 14-year-old child. The histologic diagnosis was pulmonary blastoma.

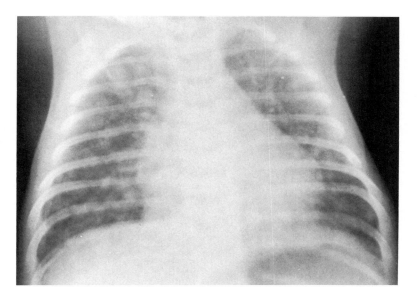

Figure 6–29. *Visceral fibromatosis in a young infant. Diffuse nodular densities are scattered throughout both lungs. Subcutaneous fibromas as well as additional visceral involvement were also present.*

The Askin tumor, a rare, malignant, small-cell tumor of the thoracopulmonary region, is found in children and young adults. It occurs predominately in females and must be differentiated from rhabdomyosarcoma, Ewing's sarcoma, neuroblastoma, and malignant lymphoma. The mass originates in the soft tissues of the chest wall or the periphery of the lung. The pleura is frequently involved, and there is often rib destruction (Fig. 6–30). On rare occasions, there is soft tissue calcification. The radiographic features, however, are nonspecific. Recurrence usually occurs locally, but occasional distant metastases, generally to bone, can be found. The prognosis is poor.

Mensenchymal tumors of the thorax may produce marked deformity of the thoracic cage, including rib destruction (Fig. 6–31).

METASTASES

Metastatic tumors are far more common than primary neoplasms, and may arise from various distant primary malignancies to involve the lungs and regional lymph nodes. Wilms' tumor is the most frequent malignancy that produces pulmonary metastases in children. The roentgenographic manifestations are those of pulmonary nodules, ranging in size from barely discernible densities to large, well-defined masses. Although solitary metastases are not uncommon, multiple bilateral deposits occur more frequently (Figs. 6–32 and 6–33). Pleural effusion is commonly associated with the metastases. Surgical resection of metastases should be performed when feasible. The combination of chemotherapy, radiation therapy, and radical surgery on the primary, as well as metastatic, lesions of Wilms' tumors has resulted in a much greater cure rate than was formerly achieved (Fig. 6–34).

From the radiographic standpoint, pulmonary metastases usually do not offer a clue as to the primary site of the malignancy, except in some cases of osteogenic sarcoma, in which bone may be produced within the pulmonary lesion (Fig. 6–35). Other metastases from osteogenic sarcoma may be indistinguishable from those of other metastatic lesions. Pneumothorax is inexplicably a complication of metastatic osteosarcoma.

Other soft tissue malignancies that might metastasize to the lungs include Ewing's sarcoma (Fig. 6–36), embryonal tumors of the testes or ovaries (Figs. 6–37 and 6–38), rhabdomyosarcomas, hepatic malignancies (Fig. 6–39), leiomyosar-

Text continued on page 299

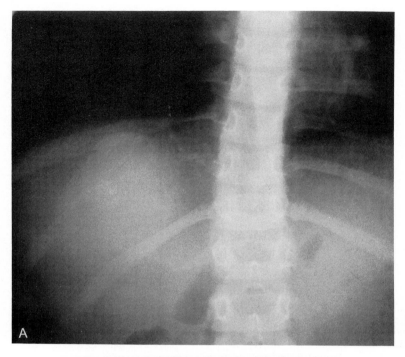

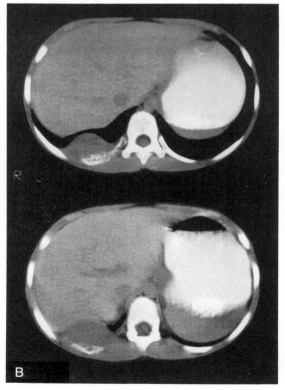

Figure 6–30. Askin tumor in a 6-year-old boy. A, *Soft tissue mass in the lower right hemothorax has produced destruction of the right eleventh rib.* B, *Computerized tomography shows the mass in the posterior pulmonary sulcus with destruction of the adjacent rib.*

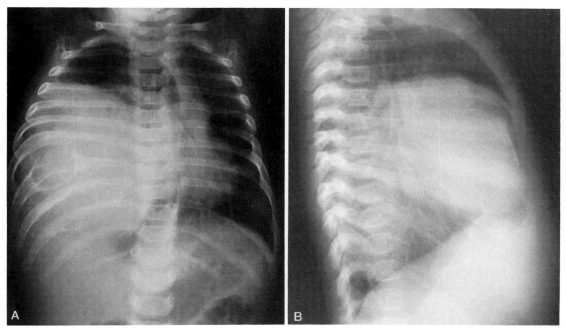

Figure 6–31. Mesenchymal tumor in a young child. A, Chest radiograph shows areas of rib involvement as well as a large mass occupying the thorax, with displacement of the mediastinal structures to the left. B, Lateral view demonstrates areas of calcification within the mass, as well as emphasizing its enormous size. (Courtesy of Dr. J. A. Kirkpatrick.)

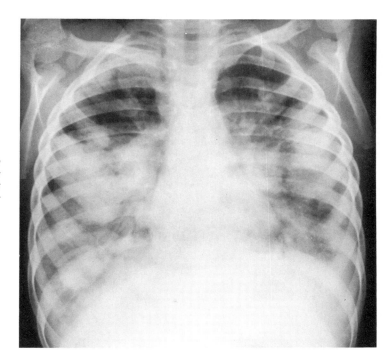

Figure 6–32. Metastatic Wilms' tumor in a 4-year-old boy. Chest radiographs show multiple pulmonary metastases with confluence of many of the metastatic nodules.

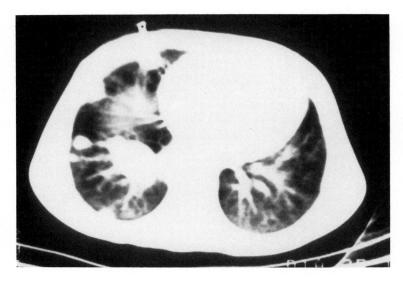

Figure 6–33. *Computerized tomography of the lungs in a child shows metastatic neoplasm from a Wilms' tumor.*

Figure 6–34. *Metastatic Wilms' tumor in a 7-year-old girl. A, Frontal chest radiograph shows large well-defined density in the right midlung field. A Wilms' tumor was previously removed and the patient has been on chemotherapy.*

Illustration continued on opposite page

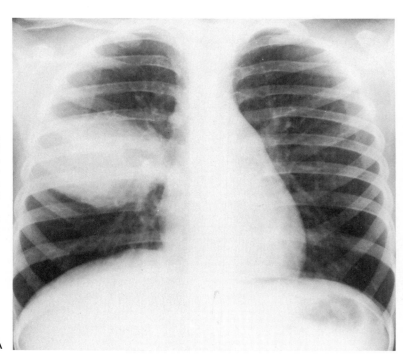

A

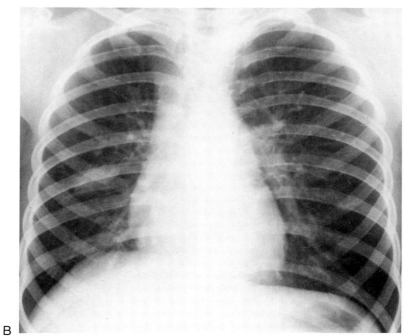

B

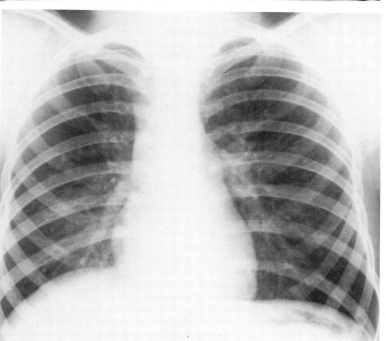

C

Figure 6–34. B, *Five months later there is marked regression of the solitary metastasis following chemotherapy and radiotherapy to the right chest.* C, *Five months later the chest is radiographically normal.*
Illustration continued on following page

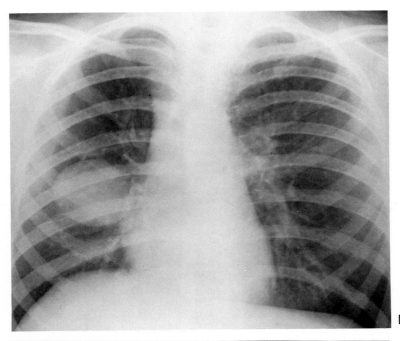

D

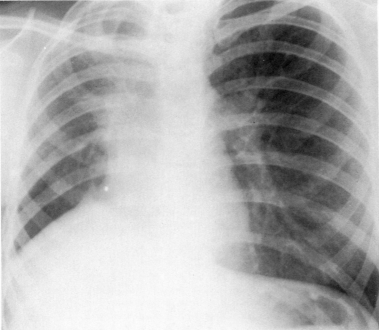

E

Figure 6–34. D, *Nine months later there is a recurrence of the solitary metastasis in the right chest. E, Frontal chest radiograph 1 year later. There has been surgical resection of the metastatic nodule. The mediastinum and heart are retracted to the right, and there is elevation of the right hemidiaphragm. No other metastatic lesions are identified.*

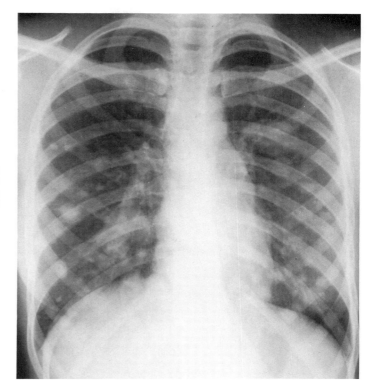

Figure 6–35. Pulmonary metastases in a 12-year-old girl who had an osteogenic sarcoma of the femur. The metastases are dense, and many of them contain small flecks of bone density.

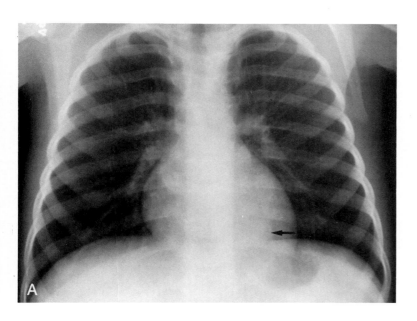

Figure 6–36. Metastatic Ewing's sarcoma in a 5-year-old boy. A, Chest radiograph shows solitary metastatic lesion (arrow).

Illustration continued on following page

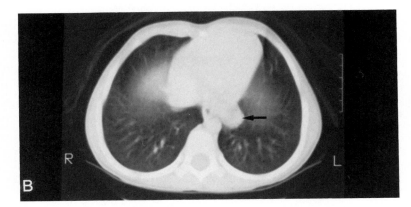

Figure 6–36. B, *Computerized tomography demonstrates cross-sectional location of the metastases.*

Figure 6–37. *One-year-old boy with metastatic embryonal carcinoma of the testes to the mediastinal lymph nodes and lungs.*

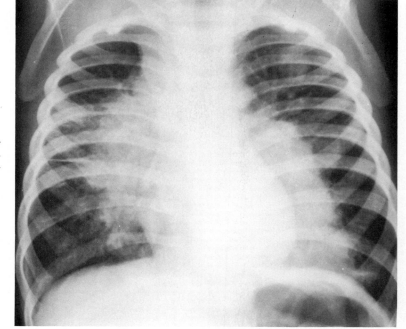

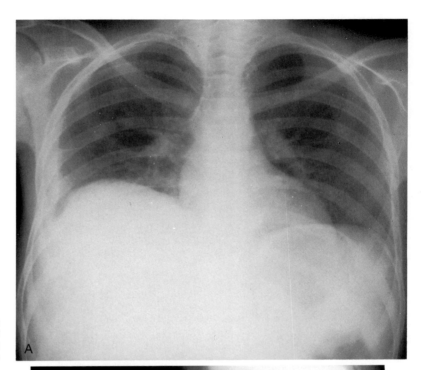

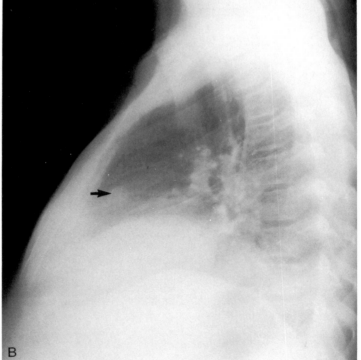

Figure 6–38. Metastatic ovarian germ cell tumor in a 13-year-old girl. A, Chest radiograph shows right pleural effusion and elevation of the right hemidiaphragm. B, Lateral radiograph indicates a solitary nodular metastasis in the substernal area (arrow).

Illustration continued on following page

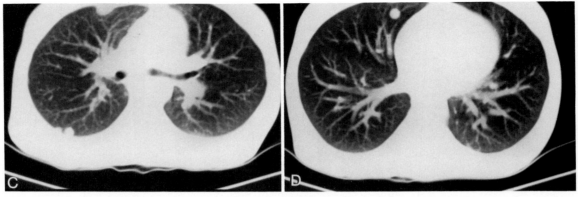

Figure 6–38. C, Computerized tomography demonstrates the pleural metastatic lesions adjacent to the pleural posteriorly, as well as a subpleural lesion anteriorly. D, Cross-sectional tomography at a lower level shows the solitary metastatic lesion behind the anterior chest wall, which was noted on the lateral chest radiograph.

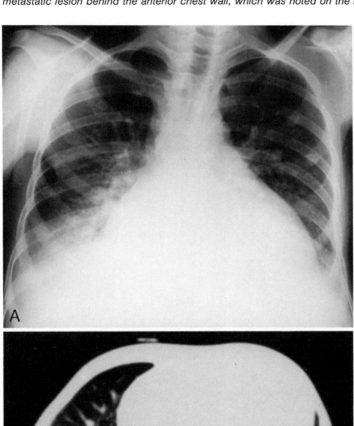

Figure 6–39. Metastatic adenocarcinoma involving the lungs in a child who in infancy had von Gierke's glycogen storage disease, which developed into adenocarcinoma of the liver. A, Chest radiographs show multiple nodular metastatic lesions scattered throughout both lungs. B, Computerized tomography shows the multiple pulmonary metastases to better advantage.

comas (Fig. 6–40), retinoblastomas, and thyroid malignancies. As in the adult, the occasional thyroid cancer may produce small multinodular densities that are several millimeters in diameter and tend to be more concentrated in the lower lung fields (Fig. 6–41). On very rare occasions neuroblastomas will metastasize to the lungs, but the overwhelming number spread to the thoracic cage, pleura, and mediastinal nodes (Figs. 6–42 and 6–43). Yolk sac (endodermal sinus) tumors may lead to extensive and bizarre mediastinal and pulmonary metastases (Fig. 6–44).

During the last decade, the superiority of chest CT over conventional radiography and linear tomography to detect pulmonary metastases has often been documented. Conversely, one must guard against the problem of overdiagnosis (pseudometastases) because of a diversity of benign lesions, including granulomas, round pneumonias, hamartomas, radiation fibrosis, cytotoxic chemotherapy (e.g., bleomycin), and atelectasis (simple or post-anesthetic).

It is of interest that pulmonary metastases usually do not produce atelectasis or obstructive emphysema as compared to endobronchial tumors, but cavitation and pneumothorax may occur.

RETICULOENDOTHELIOSES

The group of diseases known as the reticuloendothelioses consists of various conditions that show considerable clinical and pathologic overlap. In general, the conditions can be divided into the lipid forms, consisting primarily of Gaucher's disease and Niemann-Pick disease, and the nonlipid form, histiocytosis X, which includes eosinophilic granuloma, Hand-Schüller-Christian disease, and Letterer-Siwe disease. There are a number of hypotheses regarding the pathology and pathogenesis of the latter three conditions. The current popular opinion is that they represent disseminated forms of eosinophilic granuloma, with the differentiation being dependent on the severity of the disease and on the clinical findings. This relationship is based primarily on a histologic similarity between the condi-

Text continued on page 304

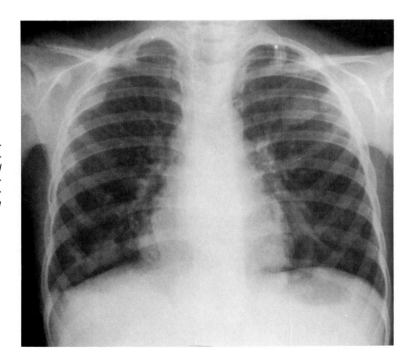

Figure 6–40. *Metastatic leiomyosarcoma in a 5-year-old boy whose primary malignancy was in the inguinal canal. Chest radiograph shows multiple metastatic nodules, with associated metastasis to the right clavicle and right third rib.*

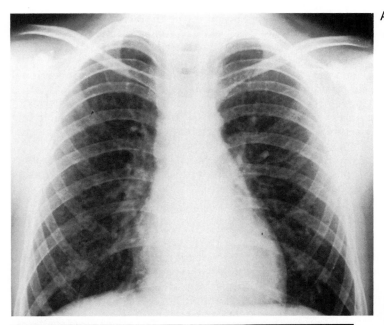

A

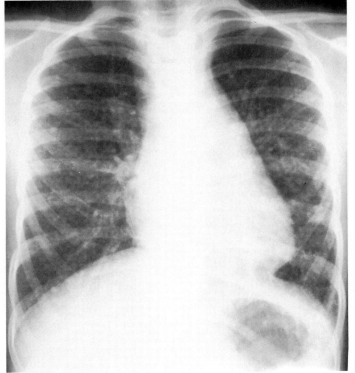

B

Figure 6–41. A, Metastatic thyroid carcinoma in a 13-year-old boy. Chest radiograph shows multiple small discrete metastatic lesions. B, Disseminated thyroid metastases in a 6-year-old girl. The miliarylike metastases have shown stabilization after treatment with radioactive iodine.

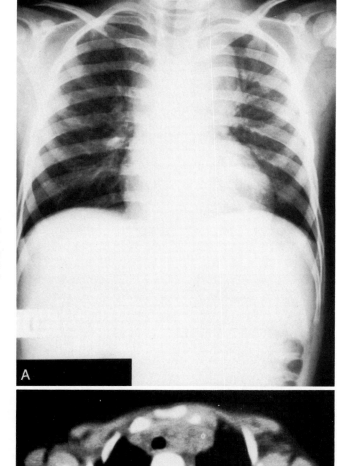

Figure 6–42. Metastatic neuroblastoma in a 3-year-old boy. A, Chest radiograph shows a superior mediastinal mass obscuring the left superior mediastinum. B, Computerized tomography reveals the left paratracheal location of the mass. The histologic diagnosis was metastatic neuroblastoma.

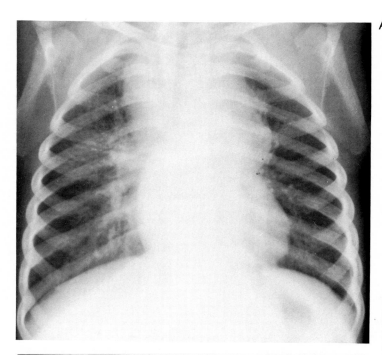

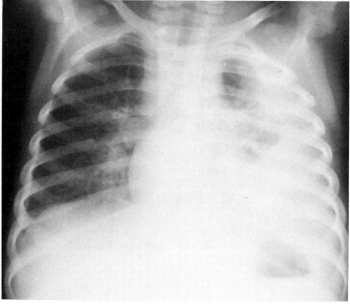

Figure 6–43. Metastatic neuroblastoma in a 4-year-old girl. A, Initial metastases were to the hilar and paratracheal lymph nodes. B, Repeat chest radiograph 4 months later after irradiation of mediastinal lymph nodes shows extensive left pleural effusion.

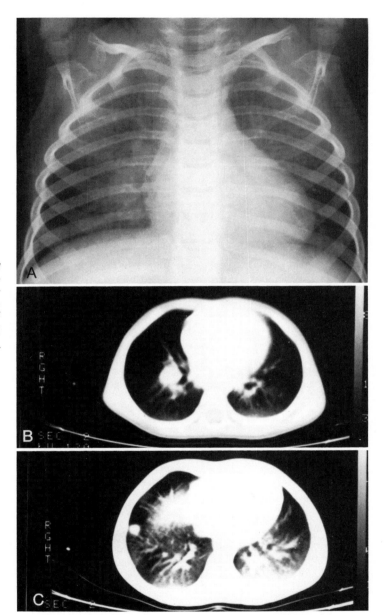

Figure 6–44. Metastatic endodermal sinus tumor (yolk sac tumor) in a 2-year-old boy. A, Chest radiograph shows ill-defined mass in the right hilar area. B, Computerized tomography demonstrates the right hilar mass to better advantage. C, Repeat computerized tomography 1 month later shows an increase in the number of metastatic lesions.

tions and also on the observation that eosinophilic granuloma occasionally progresses to Hand-Schüller-Christian disease, and even to Letterer-Siwe disease. There may also be an as yet unknown underlying immunologic deficiency involved in these conditions.

There are many diverse causes of histiocytic proliferation (histiocytosis). The collective term, histiocytosis X, representing three distinct clinical syndromes, is one of many causes. Histiocytosis X is histiologically unique and is characterized by a proliferative disorder of Langerhans' cells, in which Langerhans' or Bierbeck granules can be demonstrated in histiocytes by electron microscopy. It is generally acknowledged that these conditions are unrelated to the lipid forms of reticuloendotheliosis, namely Gaucher's disease and Niemann-Pick diseases. The basic abnormality in the latter disorders is an abnormal storage of lipid due to an error in lipid metabolism, whereas the cholesterol-containing foam cells, described in

A

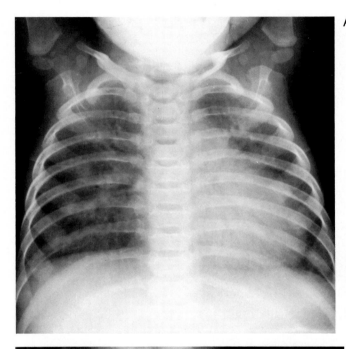

Figure 6–45. *Letterer-Siwe disease. A, Chest radiograph of a 7-month-old infant shows abnormal linear densities extending out into both lungs. There is a destructive lesion of the left clavicle. B, Chest radiograph of a 2-year-old child shows linear nodular densities involving both lungs.*

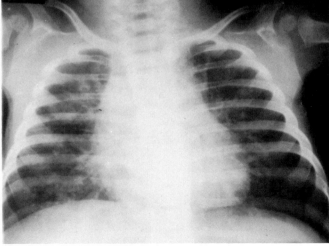

B

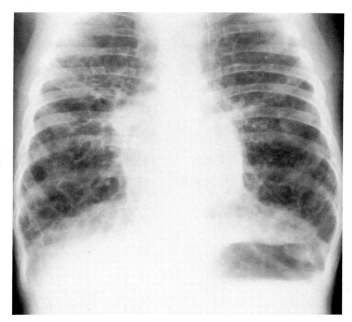

Figure 6–46. Hand-Schüller-Christian disease in a 5-year-old-child. Chest radiograph shows multiple cystic areas involving both lungs.

eosinophilic granuloma and its disseminated forms, are not a reflection of a disturbance of cholesterol metabolism but represent either increased intracellular cholesterol synthesis or the collection of cholesterol from neighboring necrotic tissue.

The primary differences between eosinophilic granuloma, Hand-Schüller-Christian disease, and Letterer-Siwe disease are the clinical manifestations. Eosinophilic granuloma of bone may be a solitary lesion in an asymptomatic individual but may also be disseminated, involving multiple bones as well as the skin, liver, spleen, lungs, and lymph nodes. The disseminated form is associated with clinical abnormalities such as diabetes insipidus, purpura, anemia, fever, and various other conditions. The fulminating form in infants is Letterer-Siwe disease. In older children the condition is more benign, has a more chronic course, and is generally classified as Hand-Schüller-Christian disease.

The radiographic findings in the lungs of both Hand-Schüller-Christian disease and Letterer-Siwe disease are variable, and may appear as linear nodular infiltrations (Fig. 6–45) or as marked honeycombing with multiple vacuoles (Fig. 6–46). Varying degrees of hilar lymphadenopathy may be present. In our experience, lymph node involvement in the hilar and mediastinal regions are less obvious as the peripheral pulmonary infiltrates progress. Although the reticular and honeycombed pattern, classically described in eosinophilic granuloma of the lung, is more common in the older child and in the adult, it may occur in the young infant. In these conditions multiple cystic lesions of varying size are scattered diffusely throughout the lungs, which appear considerably hyperinflated. Pneumothorax is an occasional complication. The pathogenesis of these cysts is debatable, but evidence suggests that they result from proliferation of nodular infiltrates with destruction of lung parenchyma and subsequent central necrosis, followed by cystic expansion in the necrotic areas and secondary entrapment of air.

The congenital form of reticuloendotheliosis is usually of the Letterer-Siwe type. Pulmonary manifestations are more often those of the linear nodular variety. Pleural involvement is uncommon in our experience, unless secondarily affected by overlying rib pathology.

Occasionally, the only intrathoracic manifestations are those of hilar and

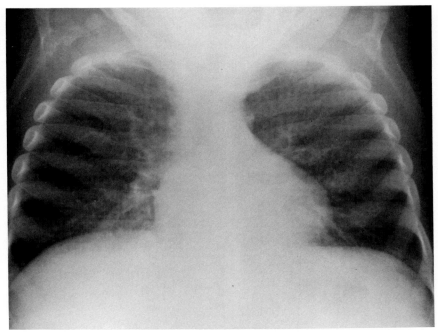

Figure 6–47. *Niemann-Pick disease. Chest radiograph shows disseminated small densities scattered throughout both lungs.*

mediastinal enlargement. In some cases the thymus may be diffusely infiltrated, producing considerable enlargement of this structure.

Pulmonary involvement may occur rarely in Gaucher's disease and Niemann-Pick disease (Fig. 6–47). The radiographic pattern in the cases we have seen consists of a reticular and finely nodular density involving both lungs, with little appreciable lymph node enlargement.

SUGGESTED READINGS

BENIGN PULMONARY NEOPLASMS

Bronchial Adenoma

Baldwin JN, and Grimes OF: Bronchial adenomas. Surg Gynecol Obstet, 124:813, 1967.

Condon VR, and Phillips EW: Bronchial adenoma in children. A review of the literature and report of three cases. Am J Roentgenol, 88:543, 1962.

Guistra PE, and Stassa G: The multiple presentations of bronchial adenomas. Radiology, 93:1013, 1969.

Heimburger IL, Kilman JW, and Battersby JS: Peripheral bronchial adenomas. J Thorac Cardiovasc Surg, 52:542, 1966.

Sane SM, and Girdany BR: Cysts and neoplasms in the infant lung. Semin Roentgenol, 7:122, 1972.

Verska JJ, and Connolly JE: Bronchial adenomas in children. J Thorac Cardiovasc Surg, 55:411, 1968.

Hamartoma

Blair TC, and McElvein RB: Hamartoma of the lung. A clinical study of 25 cases. Dis Chest, 44:296, 1963.

Doppman J, and Wilson G: Cystic pulmonary hamartoma. Br J Radiol, 38:629, 1965.

Olsen P: Hamartomas of the lung. Dan Med Bull, 15:117, 1968.

Sagel SS, and Ablow RC: Hamartoma: On occasion a rapidly growing tumor of the lung. Radiology, 91:971, 1968

Weisel W, Glicklich M, and Landis FB: Pulmonary hamartoma, an enlarging neoplasm. Arch Surg, 71:128, 1955.

Papillomatosis

Borkowsky W, Martin D, and Lawrence S: Juvenile laryngeal papillomatosis with pulmonary spread. Am J Dis Child, 138:667, 1984.

Cohen SR et al.: Papilloma of the larynx and tracheobronchial tree in children: A retrospective study. Ann Otol, 89:497, 1980.

Mendelson DS et al.: Bronchogenic cysts with high CT numbers. Am J Roentgenol, 140:463, 1983.

Nakata H et al.: Computed tomography of mediastinal bronchogenic cysts. J Comput Assist Tomogr, 6:733, 1982.

Rogers LF, and Osmer JC: Bronchogenic cysts—a review of 46 cases. Am J Roentgenol, 91:273, 1964.

Sullivan MA: Case of the day (Case 5: Mediastinal cyst). Am J Roentgenol, 138:1202, 1982.

Mediastinal Tumors

Bower RJ, and Kiesewetter WM: Mediastinal masses in infants and children. Arch Surg 112:1003, 1977.

Castellino RA et al.: Radiographic findings in previously untreated children with non-Hodgkin's lymphoma. Radiology, 117:657, 1975.

Cho CS, Blank N, and Castellino RA: Computerized tomography evaluation of chest wall involvement in lymphoma. Cancer, 55:1892, 1985.

Cohen MD et al.: The diagnostic dilemma of the posterior mediastinal thymus: CT manifestations. Radiology, 146:691, 1983.

Davis LA, and McCreadie SR: The enlarged thymus gland in leukemia in childhood. Am J Roentgenol, 88:924, 1962.

Felson B: The mediastinum. Semin Roentgenol, 4:41, 1969.

Felson B: The mediastinal compartments. In Chest Roentenology, pp 416–420. Philadelphia, W.B. Saunders, 1973.

Gaisie G, and Oh KS: Paraspinal interfaces in the lower thoracic area in children: Evaluation by CT. Radiology, 149:133, 1983.

Grossman H et al.: Roentgenographic changes in childhood Hodgkin's disease. Am J Roentgenol, 108:354, 1970.

Hope JW, Borns PF, and Koop CE: Radiologic diagnosis of mediastinal masses in infants and children. Radiol Clin North Am, 1:17, 1963.

Kirks DR et al.: Myelography in the evaluation of paravertebral mass lesions in infants and children. Radiology, 119:603, 1976.

Kirks DR et al.: Tracheal compression by mediastinal masses in children: CT evaluation. Am J Roentgenol, 141:647, 1983.

Kirks DR, and Korobkin M: Computed tomography of the chest in infants and children: Techniques and mediastinal evaluation. Radiol Clin North Am, 19:409, 1981.

Kirks DR, and Korobkin M: Computed tomography of the chest wall, pleura, and pulmonary parenchyma in infants and children. Radiol Clin North Am, 19:421, 1981.

Lee J, Sagel S, and Stanley R (eds): Computed Body Tomography, pp 55–131. New York, Raven Press, 1983.

Mainzer F, and Taybi H: Thymic enlargement and pleural effusion: An unusual roentgenographic complex in childhood leukemia. Am J Roentgenol, 112:35, 1971.

Muller NL, Webb WR, and Gamsu G: Subcarinal lymph node enlargement: Radiographic findings and CT correlation. Am J Roentgenol, 145:15, 1985.

O'Brien RT et al.: Superior vena cava syndrome in children. West J Med, 135:143, 1981.

Parker BE, Catellino RA, and Kaplan HS: Pediatric Hodgkin's disease. I. Radiographic evaluation. Cancer, 37:2430, 1976.

Press GA et al.: Thoracic wall involvement by Hodgkin's disease and non-Hodgkin lymphoma: CT evaluation. Radiology, 157:195, 1985.

Pugath RD et al.: CT diagnosis of benign mediastinal abnormalities. Am J Roentgenol, 134:685, 1980.

Putnam CE: Pulmonary Diagnosis—Imaging and Other Techniques, pp 277–284. New York, Appleton-Century-Crofts, 1981.

Sones PJ Jr et al.: Effectiveness of CT in evaluating intrathoracic masses. Am J Roentgenol, 139:469, 1982.

Webb WR: Advances in computed tomography of the thorax. Radiol Clin North Am, 21:723, 1983.

Weinberg B et al.: Posterior mediastinal teratoma (cystic dermoid): Diagnosis by computerized tomography. Chest, 77:694, 1980.

PRIMARY PULMONARY MALIGNANCIES

Askin FB, Rosai J et al.: Malignant small cell tumor of the thoracopulmonary region in childhood. Cancer, 43:2438, 1979.

Campbell AN, Wagget J, and Mott MG: Benign mesenchymoma of the chest wall in infancy. J Surg Oncol, 21:267, 1982.

Cangir A, and Haggard ME: Miscellaneous childhood tumors. In Sutow WW, Fernbach DJ, and Vietti TJ (eds): Clinical Pediatric Oncology, 3rd ed, pp 791–792. St. Louis, C.V. Mosby, 1984.

Cayley CK, Caez HJ, and Mersheimer W: Primary bronchogenic carcinoma of the lung in children. Review of the literature; Report of a case. Am J Dis Child, 82:49, 1951.

Condon VR, and Allen RP: Congenital generalized fibromatosis: Case report with roentgen manifestations. Radiology, 76:444, 1961.

Fink IJ, Kurtz DW et al.: Malignant thorocopulmonary small cell ("Askin") tumor. Am J Roentgenol, 145:517, 1985.

Grossman H et al.: Roentgenographic changes in childhood. Hodgkin's disease. Am J Roentgenol, 108:354, 1970.

Minken SL, Craver WL, and Adams JT: Pulmonary blastoma. Arch Pathol, 86:442, 1968.

Morettin LB, Mueller E, and Schreiber M: Generalized hamartomatosis. Am J Roentgenol, 114:722, 1972.

Ownby D, Lyon G, and Spock A: Primary leiomyosarcoma of the lung in childhood. Am J Dis Child, 130:1132, 1976.

Solomon A et al.: Pulmonary blastoma. Pediatr Radiol, 12:148, 1982.

Spencer H: Pulmonary blastomas. J Pathol, 82:161, 1961.

Sumner TE et al.: Pulmonary blastoma in a child. Am J Roentgenol, 133:147, 1979.

METASTASES

Cohen M et al.: Efficacy of whole lung tomography in diagnosing metastases from solid tumors in children. Radiology, 141:375, 1981.

Cohen M et al.: Pulmonary pseudometastases in children with malignant tumors. Radiology 141:371, 1981.

Cohen M et al.: Lung CT for detection of metastases: Solid tissue neoplasms in children. Am J Roentgenol, 139:895, 1982.

Coussement AM, and Gooding CA: Cavitating pulmonary metastatic disease in children. Am J Roentgenol, 117:833, 1973.

Damgaard-Pedersen K, and Qvist T: Pediatric pulmonary CT-scanning, anesthesia-induced changes. Pediatr Radiol, 9:145, 1980.

Glasier CM, and Siegel MJ: Multiple pulmonary nodules: Unusual manifestation of bleomycin toxicity. Am J Roentgenol, 137:155, 1981.

Hidalgo H et al.: The problem of benign pulmonary nodules in children receiving cytotoxic chemotherapy. Am J Roentgenol, 140:21, 1983.

Kassner EG, Goldman HS, and Elguezabal A: Cavitating lung nodules and pneumothorax in children with metastatic Wilms' tumor. Am J Roentgenol, 126:728, 1976.

Kirks DR, and Korobkin M: Computed tomography of the chest wall, pleura, and pulmonary parenchyma in infants and children. Radiol Clin North Am, 19:421, 1981.

Pagani JJ, and Libshitz HI: CT manifestations of radiation-induced change in chest tissue. J Comput Assist Tomogr, 6:243, 1982.

Schaner EG et al.: Comparison of computed and conventional whole lung tomography in detecting pulmonary nodules: A prospective radiologic-pathologic study. Am J Roentgenol, 131:51, 1978.

Singleton EB et al.: Sclerosing osteogenic sarcomatosis. Am J Roentgenol, 88:483, 1962.

Smoger BR et al.: The search for pulmonary metastases in pediatric patients: CT vs. conventional radiology. Ann Radiol, 25:47, 1982.

Spittle MR et al.: The association of spontaneous pneumothorax with pulmonary metastases in bone tumors of children. Clin Radiol 19:400, 1968.

Wedemeyer PD et al.: Resection of metastases in Wilms' tumor: A report of three cases cured of pulmonary and hepatic metastases. Pediatrics 41:446, 1968.

RETICULOENDOTHELIOSIS

Basset F et al.: Pulmonary histiocytosis X. Am Rev Respir Dis, 118:811, 1978.

Bekerman C et al.: Gallium-67 citrate imaging studies of the lung. Semin Nucl Med, 10:286, 1980.

Hertz CG, and Hambrick GW Jr: Congenital Letterer-Siwe disease. A case treated with vincristine and corticosteroids. Am J Dis Child, 116:553, 1968.

Kittredge RD, Geller A, and Finby N: The reticuloendothelioses in the lung. Am J Roentgenol, 100:588, 1967.

Lichtenstein L: Histiocytosis X. Integration of eosinophilic granuloma of bone, "Letterer-Siwe disease," and "Hand-Schüller-Christian disease" as related manifestations of a single nosological entity. Arch Pathol, 56:84, 1953.

Lucaya J: Histiocytosis X. Am J Dis Child, 121:289, 1971.

Miller DR: Familial reticuloendothelioses: Concurrence of disease in five siblings. Pediatrics, 38:986, 1966.

Roland AS, Merdinger WF, and Froeb HF: Recurrent spontaneous pneumothorax. A clue to the diagnosis of histiocytosis X. N Engl J Med, 270:73, 1964.

Siemsen JK, Grebe SF, and Waxman AD: Gallium studies of the lung. Semin Nucl Med 8:235, 1978.

Takahashi M, Martel W, and Overman HA: The variable roentgenographic appearance of idiopathic histiocytosis. Clin Radiol, 17:48, 1966.

Weber WN, Margolin FR, and Nielsen SL: Pulmonary histiocytosis X. A review of 18 patients with reports of 6 cases. Am J Roentgenol, 107:280, 1969.

Winzelberg GG et al.: Combined gated cardiac blood pool scintigraphy and Ga-citrate scintigraphy for detection of cardiac lymphproliferative disorders. Radiology, 141:191, 1981.

7 PULMONARY VASCULAR DISEASES

CONGENITAL PULMONARY	PULMONARY
VASCULAR ABNORMALITIES	LYMPHANGIOMYOMATOSIS
PULMONARY LYMPHANGIECTASIA	VASCULITIS
	PULMONARY HEMOSIDEROSIS

Arteriography is usually necessary for accurate anatomic demonstration of pulmonary vascular anomalies. One of the more recently developed imaging modalities used in the diagnosis of pulmonary vascular abnormalities is digital subtraction angiography. Initial experiences in young infants using hand injections of moderate amounts of contrast medium into a peripheral vein has produced diagnostic images of pulmonary artery and pulmonary vascular anomalies. However, improvement in the quality of the images is achieved by more central venous injection via catheter, utilizing smaller quantities of contrast material. In addition, motion artifacts are diminished and the contrast and spatial resolution are improved. Improvement in imaging has also been enhanced by the improvement in digital subtraction equipment that provides automatic masking and greater digital acquisition and storage capabilities. Most current angiographic units include digital subtraction capabilities.

Sedation is imperative in any successful angiographic imaging in the pediatric patient. The medications utilized have been described in Chapter 1.

Enhanced computerized tomography (CT) is helpful in imaging many vascular abnormalities of the lungs. Magnetic resonance imaging may also be used, but in our experience it is less reliable than arteriography.

CONGENITAL PULMONARY VASCULAR ABNORMALITIES

Pulmonary arteriovenous communications may be single or multiple lesions, and frequently have associated hemangiomas or telangiectasias in other portions of the body. Clinical manifestations include cyanosis of varying degree, polycythemia, clubbing of the fingers, and occasionally an auscultatory murmur over the lesion.

Radiographic examination shows, in the larger lesions, a homogeneous density of variable size and shape that is frequently in continuity with the hilar vascular shadows. Laminographic studies are useful in showing afferent and efferent vessels extending to the lesions (Fig. 7–1). Digital subtraction angiography or angiocardiography are the most useful diagnostic procedures (Fig. 7–2).

If there are multiple minute fistulae associated with cutaneous or mucosal telangiectasias and a hereditary history, the pulmonary lesions may be described as part of Osler-Weber-Rendu disease, or hereditary hemorrhagic telangiectasia. In this condition chest radiographs may appear normal but pulmonary arteriograms

A

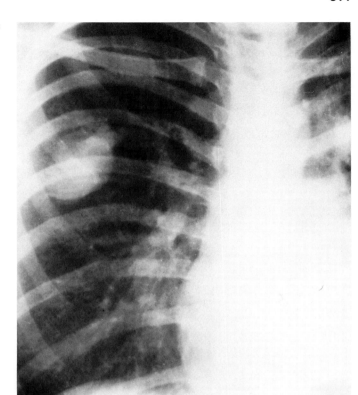

Figure 7–1. Pulmonary arteriovenous fistula in a 10-year-old child. A, Chest radiograph shows right upper lobe lesion. B, Lamino-grams demonstrate the afferent and efferent vessels.

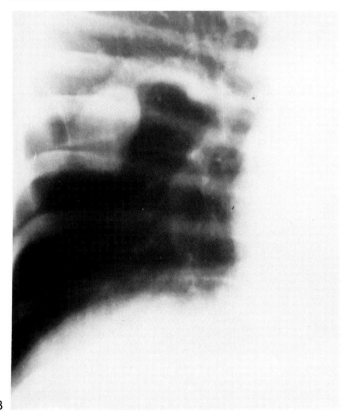

B

A

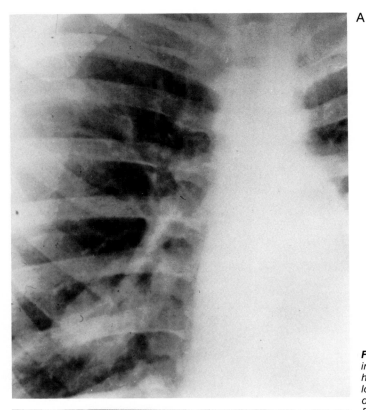

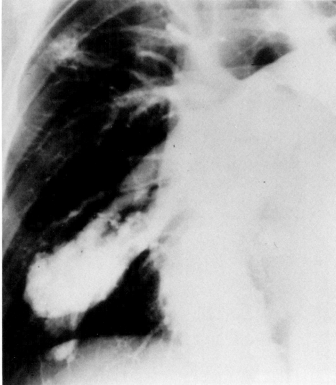

Figure 7–2. *Pulmonary arteriovenous fistula in a 6-year-old child whose pulmonary lesion had mistakenly been diagnosed as tuberculosis. A, Routine chest radiographs show discrete nodular lesion in the right base. B, Pulmonary arteriograms show the arteriovenous fistula in the right base, as well as a second unsuspected arteriovenous fistula in the right upper lobe.*

B

will show minute small fistulae scattered throughout the lungs (Fig. 7–3). This anomaly apparently results from persistence of fetal anastomotic capillaries.

There are various congenital anomalies associated with such problems as abnormal pulmonary venous return, anomalous pulmonary arterial supply, pulmonary sequestrations, and pulmonary artery atresia and agenesis.

Although agenesis or hypoplasia of one lung is rarely a cause of respiratory distress in the newborn or young infant, it should be considered, particularly when chest radiographs show diminished or absent aeration of a lung. In both conditions the affected hemithorax is smaller than the opposite side, and mediastinal structures are shifted to the involved side (Fig. 7–4). Bronchoscopy and bronchography are of no value, and in fact may produce serious complications. These anomalies are easily demonstrated, either by direct arteriography or by digital subtraction arteriography (Figs. 7–5, 7–6, 7–7, and 7–8). The "horseshoe" lung is a rare anomaly in which the posterobasal segments of the right and left lungs are fused behind the pericardial reflection. Cardiovascular anomalies similar to the hypogenetic right lung syndrome are commonly present. Angiography in such cases usually demonstrates the branch of the right pulmonary artery extending inferiorly and across the midline into the left lung.

PULMONARY LYMPHANGIECTASIA

The severe form of pulmonary lymphangiectasia is incompatible with life beyond the newborn period. The pulmonary lymphatics are markedly hyperplastic, and present as reticular nodular densities scattered throughout the lungs (Fig. 7–9). Less severe forms of pulmonary lymphangiectasia may be incidental findings in asymptomatic children or adults. Associated peripheral lymphangiomas or intestinal lymphangiectasia may be present.

Pathologically the condition consists of hyperplasia of the lymph vessels within the lung parenchyma, similar to but much less severe than that in the lethal form seen in the young infant.

Radiographically there are reticulolinear densities scattered throughout both lungs, the prominence of which depend on the severity of involvement. Horizontal linear densities above the costophrenic sulci (Kerley's B lines) are invariably present, and their identification in a patient without pulmonary venous obstruction or left-sided congestive failure is presumptive evidence of pulmonary lymphangiectasia (Fig. 7–10).

PULMONARY LYMPHANGIOMYOMATOSIS

Pulmonary lymphangiomyomatosis is probably a form of hamartoma that arises from the proliferation of smooth muscle in the walls of lymphatic vessels. The clinical features consist of chylothorax and progressive dyspnea, and it occurs almost exclusively in females. The radiographic features consist of pleural effusion and pulmonary reticulolinear densities, similar to those of lymphangiectasia, and multiple Kerley's B lines (Fig. 7–11).

VASCULITIS

In this age of antibiotic and chemotherapeutic drugs there is ample evidence of increased incidence of sensitivity reactions throughout the general population. Although sensitivity reactions in children occur less frequently than in adults, a significant number of reactions occur in childhood, particularly in patients receiving multiple cytotoxic and other agents for treatment of malignancy, immune defi-

Text continued on page 320

A

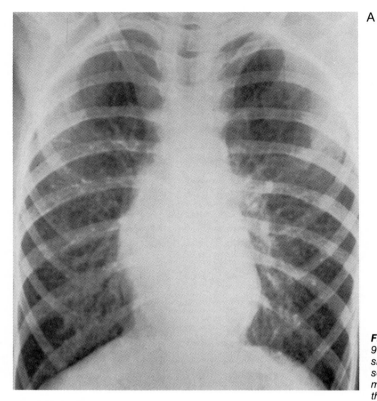

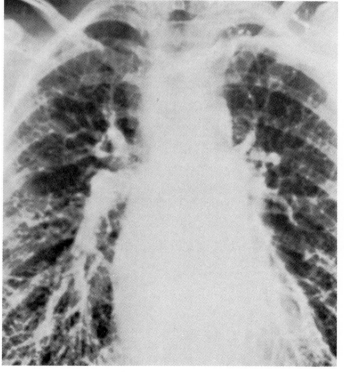

B

Figure 7–3. *Pulmonary telangiectasia in a 9-year-old girl. A, Routine chest radiograph shows ill-defined multiple small densities scattered throughout both lungs. B, Pulmonary arteriogram shows opacification of the minute densities, identifying them as multiple small arteriovenous fistulae. The patient also had multiple telangiectasias involving the buccal mucosa. (From Cooley DA, and McNamara DG: J Thorac Surg, 27:614, 1954.)*

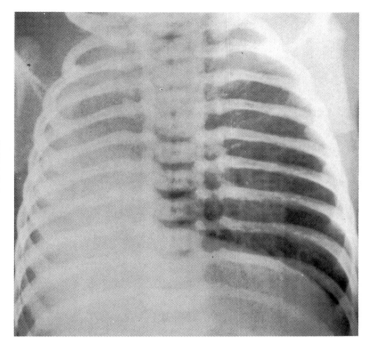

Figure 7–4. Pulmonary agenesis. The right lung is completely opacified and the right hemithorax is small. The left lung is hyper-expanded and the pulmonary artery is unusually prominent. Angiocardiography showed absence of right pulmonary artery.

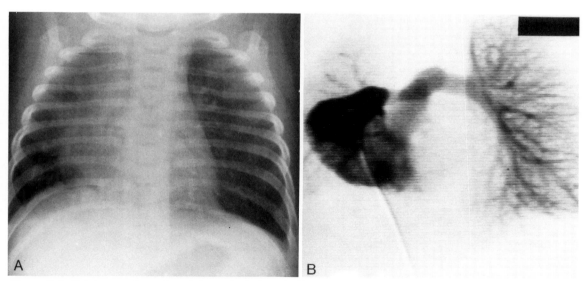

Figure 7–5. Scimitar syndrome in a 3½-month-old boy. A, Frontal view of chest at age 3 months. There is a shift of the heart and mediastinum to the right, with an ill-defined right heart border. B, Pulmonary digital subtraction angiography, dextro phase, shows cardiac shift to the right. The right pulmonary artery and peripheral branches are smaller than those on the left.

Illustration continued on following page

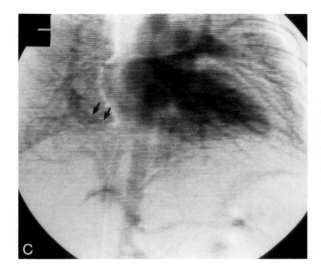

Figure 7–5. C, Levo phase reveals lack of veins entering the left atrium from the right lung. The pulmonary
veins drain to the inferior vena cava (arrow). Note the
vessels from the upper abdominal aorta supplying the
right lung base. (From Wagner ML, Singleton EB, and
Egan ME: The use of digital subtraction angiography in
evaluating pulmonary abnormalities in children. Texas
Heart Inst J, 12(1):73, 1985.)

Figure 7–6. Left pulmonary
agenesis in a 6-month-old girl.
A, Frontal chest radiograph
shows opacification of the left
hemithorax, shift of the heart
and mediastinum into the left
chest, and herniation of the right
lung into the left chest cavity. B,
Digital subtraction angiogram.
The frontal view shows marked
deviation of the heart into the
left hemithorax. There is filling
of only the right main and
peripheral pulmonary arteries.
(From Wagner ML, Singleton
EB, and Egan ME: The use of
digital subtraction angiography
in evaluating pulmonary abnormalities in children. Texas Heart
Inst J, 12(1):73, 1985.)

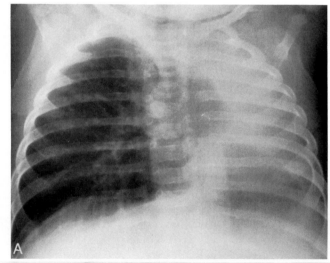

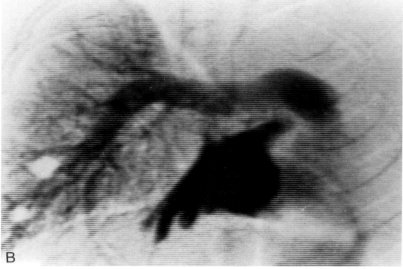

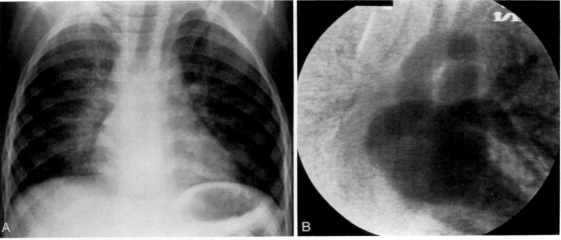

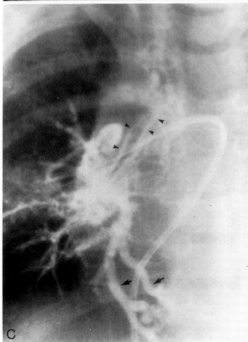

Figure 7–7. *Right pulmonary vein atresia in a 3-year-old boy. A, Frontal chest radiography shows prominent pulmonary markings on the right. B, In the levo phase, there is nonvisualization of the right pulmonary veins. C, Right wedge angiocardiogram shows nonopacification of pulmonary veins and collateral circulation about trachea and bronchi (arrowheads). Large veins course from central trunk to azygous system (arrows). (From Wagner ML, Singleton EB, and Egan ME: The use of digital subtraction angiography in evaluating pulmonary abnormalities in children. Texas Heart Inst J, 12(1):73, 1985.)*

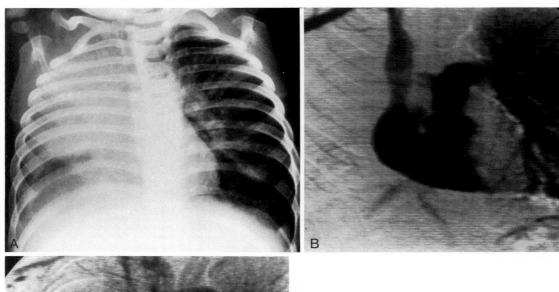

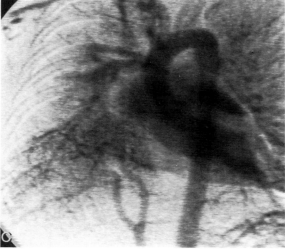

Figure 7–8. Absence of right pulmonary veins in a 9-month-old asymptomatic boy. A, Chest examination 7 months after respiratory infection. There is nearly complete opacification of right lung, with volume loss. B, Digital subtraction angiogram. There is lack of filling of the right pulmonary artery. C, Large vessel arising from below the diaphragm supplies the right lung base. A tortuous network of vessels extends from the upper abdominal aorta to a vascular structure in the right midlung field. (From Wagner ML, Singleton EB, and Egan ME: Digital subtraction angiography in children. Am J Roentgenol, 140:127, 1983.)

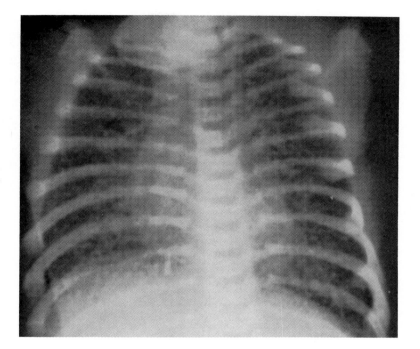

Figure 7–9. *Pulmonary lymphangiectasia. Small nodular and reticular densities are scattered throughout both lungs. (Courtesy of Dr. V. Mikity.)*

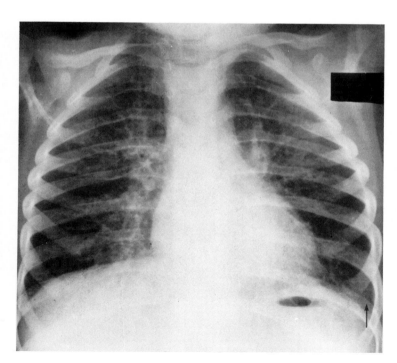

Figure 7–10. *Pulmonary lymphangiectasia in a 4-year-old girl who had an associated lymphangioma of her left arm. Abnormal reticular densities occupy both lungs, and associated septal B lines are identified above each costophrenic sulcus (arrow). (Courtesy of Dr. F. N. Silverman.)*

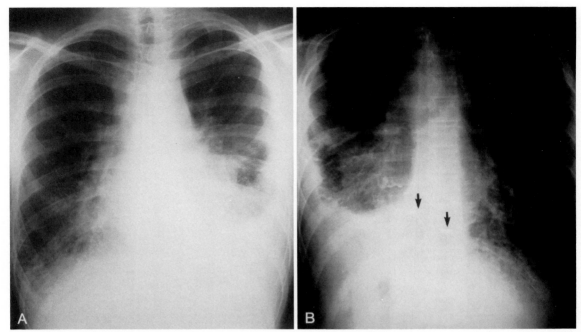

Figure 7–11. *Lymphangiomyomatosis proven by biopsy in a 14-year-old boy. A, Chest radiograph shows extensive left pleural effusion, dilated lymphatics, and interstitial lung disease. B, Postlymphangiogram radiograph of the chest demonstrates collection of contrast medium in dilated lymph channels (arrows). (From Singleton EB: Film Interpretation Session. Radiology, 137:7, 1980).*

ciency diseases, and collagen vascular diseases. Most drugs produce lung disease either by direct toxicity or by hypersensitivity reactions. Several of the chemotherapeutic drugs, including methotrexate, bleomycin, and nitrofurantoin, can be associated with both mechanisms. The host response to drug sensitivity is variable and unpredictable but not uncommon. Pulmonary changes are often nonspecific, but one pattern of vasculitis consists of prominent pulmonary vessels with indistinct boundaries confined mainly to the hilar and midlung areas (Figs. 7–12 and 7–13). Drug abuse, particularly of heroin and other narcotics, may be responsible for acute pulmonary edema or chronic vasculitis of multiple organs (Fig. 7–14). Other drug-related pulmonary patterns include acute diffuse alveolar, acute diffuse interstitial, chronic interstitial, pleuropulmonary, and hilar adenopathy.

Other diseases associated with vasculitis include Schistosoma, Pseudomonas, and Rickettsia infections. The vasculitis that accompanies Rocky Mountain spotted fever produces radiographic changes consisting of reticulolinear densities that usually involve the perihilar areas (Fig. 7–15). Areas of consolidation may also be present, simulating those of pulmonary edema. The radiographic findings are nonspecific, but the rash that usually accompanies the disease, as well as the appropriate complement fixation tests, establish the true nature of the pulmonary process.

Congenital heart diseases, particularly those with long-standing left-to-right shunts, produce medial muscular hypertrophy of the arterioles followed by endothelial proliferation, an end stage of vasculitis. Chronic obstructive disease of the left heart or pulmonary veins may also produce pulmonary vasculitis (Fig. 7–16). The vasculitis associated with the end stages of pulmonary hypertension is usually overshadowed by changes of congestive heart failure, and cannot be recognized as a specific vascular phenomenon.

Immunopathologic reactions such as Wegener's granulomatosis, periarteritis nodosa, lupus erythematosus, and other collagen diseases may also be responsible for pulmonary vasculitis.

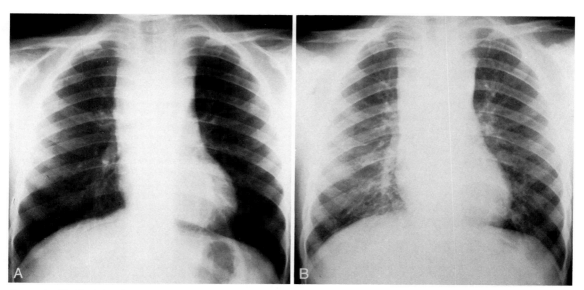

Figure 7–12. *Hodgkins' disease in a 12-year-old boy. A, Chest radiograph shows superior mediastinum mass. B, Chest radiograph 1 month following bleomycin therapy reveals parenchymal changes of vasculitis secondary to drug toxicity.*

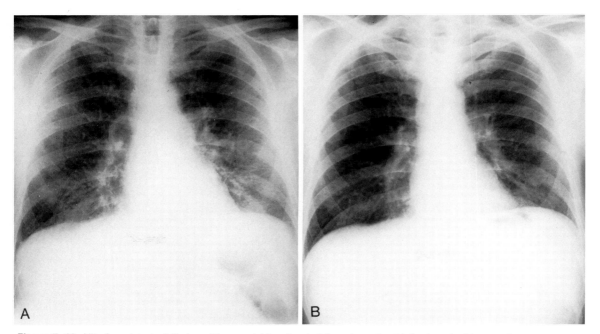

Figure 7–13. *Nitrofurantoin toxicity in a 16-year-old boy treated for urinary tract infection. A, Chest radiograph shows diffuse interstitial lung disease secondary to drug toxicity. B, Repeat radiograph 10 days following withdrawal of the medication. The lungs show nearly complete clearing.*

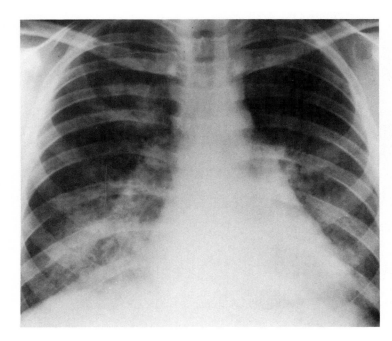

Figure 7–14. Heroin and amphetamine drug abuse in an 18-year-old boy. The chest radiograph shows moderate cardiac enlargement and interstitial pulmonary edema. (From Singleton EB: Radiologic case presentation—necrotizing angiitis associated with drug abuse. Cardiovasc Dis Bull Texas Heart Inst, 1:374, 1974.)

Figure 7–15. Pulmonary vasculitis in a 13-year-old boy with Rocky Mountain spotted fever. Chest radiograph shows bilateral perihilar densities extending peripherally into the lung parenchyma.

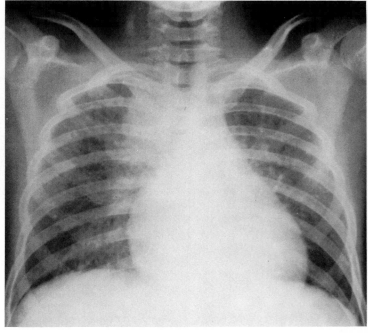

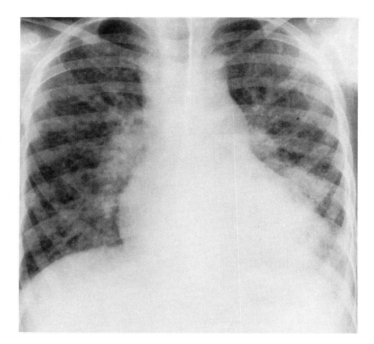

Figure 7–16. *Congestive heart failure and vasculitis secondary to congenital mitral stenosis in a 5-year-old Latin American boy. The diagnosis was confirmed by pulmonary biopsy and cardiac catheterization. Following insertion of mitral valve prosthesis, the pulmonary changes regressed.*

PULMONARY HEMOSIDEROSIS

Pulmonary hemorrhage in children is uncommon, but may result from primary pulmonary pathology or be secondary to heart disease or systemic abnormalities. Symptoms common to all these diseases are those of respiratory distress of varying severity and anemia of the iron deficiency type.

Idiopathic Pulmonary Hemosiderosis. This is the most striking form of pulmonary hemorrhage found in children. The onset of disease generally occurs after the first year and within the first decade of life. Symptomatology depends on the severity of the intra-alveolar hemorrhage, with the usual course being protracted and consisting of poor weight gain, fatigue, pallor, and mild to moderate respiratory distress. If the bleeding episode is severe, the clinical features consist of cough with hemoptysis and hematemesis. Severe dyspnea, tachycardia, and fever are also associated features. Some cases of hemosiderosis may be complications of sensitivity to cow's milk. These cases show high titers of precipitins to cow's milk and positive intradermal skin tests to milk proteins. The symptomatology improves when cow's milk is removed from the diet, and recurs when it is reintroduced. The relationship of cow's milk sensitivity to other forms of primary pulmonary hemosiderosis is uncertain.

Microcytic hypochromic anemia secondary to the blood loss is the most consistent laboratory finding, along with reticulocytosis and a frequent occurrence of unexplained eosinophilia.

The prognosis is poor, but steroid therapy has been successful in a number of cases. The patient's demise may be a result of severe pulmonary hemorrhage with respiratory insufficiency, or may be secondary to acute right heart failure. In long-standing cases cor pulmonale may develop.

The roentgenographic manifestations depend on the amount of hemorrhage present and on the duration of the disease. In acute cases, mottled, bilateral confluent perihilar infiltrations are seen, simulating those of pulmonary edema (Fig. 7–17). However, the more typical radiographic picture is that of multiple, small, discrete nodules uniformly distributed throughout both lungs, particularly in the perihilar areas. These probably occur as a result of the accumulation of

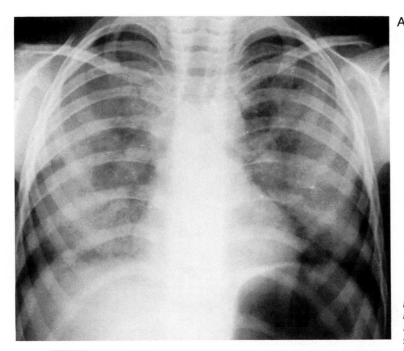

A

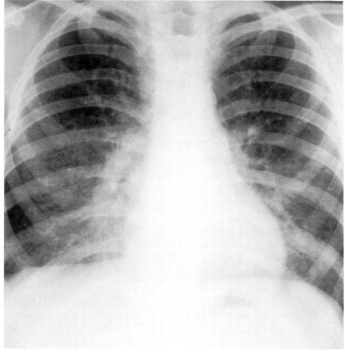

B

Figure 7–17. Idiopathic pulmonary hemosiderosis in a 4-year-old boy. A, In the acute phase, chest radiographs show consolidation of both lungs with relative sparing of the apical and basal areas. B, Follow-up radiograph 1 year later while the patient was on steroid therapy shows multiple small granular densities in the perihilar areas.

hemosiderin within the alveolar septa and the wall of the smaller blood vessels. Ultimately, pulmonary fibrosis and degeneration of elastic tissue develop.

Diagnosis is confirmed by the recovery of hemosiderin-laden macrophages, either from sputum or gastric contents. More often, however, needle aspiration of the lung or open lung biopsy is necessary.

Radionuclide studies of the lungs following injection of ^{51}Cr-labeled red cells or ^{99m}Tc-pertechnetate may be positive.

Pulmonary hemosiderosis may occur secondary to *advanced mitral stenosis or chronic left ventricular failure.* There is an increase in pulmonary venous pressure, with secondary diapedesis of red blood cells into the alveoli. This form of pulmonary hemosiderosis is most frequently encountered in the adult.

Systemic lupus erythematosus may also present with pulmonary hemorrhage, and must be excluded.

SUGGESTED READINGS

CONGENITAL PULMONARY VASCULAR ABNORMALITIES

1. Amundson GM et al.: Pediatric digital subtraction angiography. Radiology, 153:649, 1984.
2. Brant-Zawadzki M et al.: Digital subtraction cerebral angiography by intra-arterial injection: Comparison with conventional angiography. Am J Roentgenol, 140:347, 1983.
3. Chang R et al.: Digital subtraction angiography in interventional radiology. Am J Roentgenol, 142:363, 1984.
4. Cooley DA, and McNamara DG: Pulmonary telangiectasia: A report of a case proved by pulmonary biopsy. J Thorac Surg, 27:614, 1954.
5. Felman AH: Radiology of the Pediatric Chest. pp 52–53. New York, McGraw Hill, 1987.
6. Godwin JD, and Webb ER: Dynamic computed tomography in the evaluation of vascular lung lesions. Radiology, 138:629, 1981.
7. Higgins CB, and Wexler L: Clinical and angiographic features of pulmonary arteriovenous fistulas in children. Radiology, 119:171, 1976.
8. Jeresaty RN, Knight HF, and Hart WE: Pulmonary arteriovenous fistulas in children. Report of two cases and review of literature. Am J Dis Child, 111:256, 1966.
9. Mistretta CA: Development of digital subtraction angiography. In Mistretta CA et al. (eds): Digital Subtraction Arteriography: An Application of Computerized Fluoroscopy, pp 7–15. Chicago, Year Book Medical Publishers, 1982.
10. Rankin S, Faling LJ, and Pugatch RD: CT diagnosis of pulmonary arteriovenous malformations. J Comput Assist Tomogr, 6:746, 1982.
11. Reilley RF et al.: Digital subtraction angiography: Limitations for the detection of pulmonary embolism. Radiology, 183:379, 1983.
12. Sloan RD, and Cooley RN: Congenital pulmonary arteriovenous aneurysm. Am J Roentgenol, 70:183, 1953.
13. Wagner ML, Singleton EB, and Egan ME: Digital subtraction angiography in children. Am J Roentgenol, 140:127, 1983.
14. Wagner ML, Singleton EB, and Egan ME: The use of digital subtraction angiography in evaluating pulmonary abnormalities in children. Tex Heart Inst J 12:73, 1985.

PULMONARY LYMPHANGIECTASIA

1. Carter RW, and Vaughn HN: Congenital pulmonary lymphangiectasis. Report of a case with roentgen findings. Am J Roentgenol, 86:576, 1961.
2. Felman AH, Rhatigan R, and Pierson KK: Pulmonary lymphangiectasia. Observations in 17 patients and proposed classification. Am J Roentgenol, 116:548, 1972.
3. Fronstin NH et al.: Congenital pulmonary cystic lymphangiectasis. Case report and a review of 36 cases. Am J Dis Child, 114:330, 1967.
4. Laurence KM: Congenital pulmonary cystic lymphangiectasis. J Pathol Bacteriol, 70:325, 1970.
5. Rywlin AN, and Fojaco RN: Congenital pulmonary lymphangiectasis associated with a blind pulmonary vein. Pediatrics, 41:931, 1968.

PULMONARY LYMPHANGIOMYOMATOSIS

1. Cornog JL Jr, and Enterline HT: Lymphangiomyoma: A benign lesion of chyliferous lymphatics synonymous with lymphangiopericytoma. Cancer, 19:1909, 1966.
2. Frack MD, Simon L, and Dawson BH: The lymphangiomyomatosis syndrome. Cancer, 22:428, 1968.

3. Stocker JT, Drake RM, and Madewell JE: Cystic and congenital lung disease in the newborn. In Rosenberg HS, and Bolande RP (eds): Perspectives in Pediatric Pathology, Vol 4, pp 93–154. Chicago, Year Book Medical Publishers, 1978.

VASCULITIS

1. Brettner A, Heitzman ER, and Woodin WG: Pulmonary complications of drug therapy. Radiology, 96:31, 1970.
2. Churg J, and Strauss L: Allergic granulomatosis, allergic angiitis, and periarteritis nodosa. Am J Pathol, 27:277, 1951.
3. Claussen KP, and Geer JC: Hypertensive pulmonary arteritis. Am J Dis Child, 118:718, 1969.
4. Davies PDB: Drug-induced lung disease. Br J Dis Chest, 63:57, 1969.
5. Gefter WB: Drug-induced disorder of the chest. In Taveras JM, and Ferrucci JT (eds): Radiology, Diagnosis-Imaging-Intervention, Chap 52. Philadelphia, J.B. Lippincott, 1986.
6. Heitzman ER: The lung. Radiologic-Pathologic Correlations, 2nd ed., pp 334–344. St. Louis, CV Mosby, 1984
7. McCoombs RP, Patterson, JF, and MacMahon HE: Syndromes associated with allergic vasculitis. N Engl J Med, 255:251–261, 1956.
8. Morrison DA, and Goldman AL: Radiographic patterns of drug-induced lung disease. Radiology, 131:299, 1979.
9. Seltzer SE, and Herman PG: Pulmonary abnormalities associated with the administration of drugs. In Putman CE (ed): Pulmonary Diagnosis, Imaging and Other Techniques, pp 185–202. New York, Appleton-Century-Crofts, 1981.
10. Symmers WS: The occurrence of angiitis and of other generalized diseases of connective tissues as consequences of administration of drugs. Proc R Soc Med, 55:20, 1962.
11. Wagenvoort CA, Heath D, and Edwards JE: The Pathology of the Pulmonary Vasculature. Springfield, IL, Charles C Thomas, 1964.
12. Wechsler RJ et al.: Chest radiograph in lymphomatoid granulomatosis: Comparison with Wegener's granulomatosis. Am J Roentgenol, 142:79, 1984.

PULMONARY HEMOSIDEROSIS

1. Albelda SM et al.: Diffuse pulmonary hemorrhage: A review and classification. Radiology, 154:289, 1985.
2. Benoit FL et al.: Goodpasture's syndrome. Am J Med, 37:424, 1964.
3. Donald KJ, Edwards RL, and McEvoy JDS: Alveolar capillary basement membrane lesions in Goodpasture's syndrome and idiopathic pulmonary hemosiderosis. Am J Med, 59:642, 1975.
4. Elgenmark O, and Kjellberg SR: Hemosiderosis of the lungs—typical roentgenological findings. Acta Radiol, 29:32, 1947.
5. Gellis SS, Reinhold JLD, and Green S: Use of aspiration lung puncture in diagnosis of idiopathic pulmonary hemosiderosis. Am J Dis Child, 85:303, 1953.
6. Heiner DC: Pulmonary hemosiderosis. In Kendig EL Jr, and Chernick V (eds): Disorders of the Respiratory Tract in Children, 3rd ed, pp 538–550. Philadelphia, W.B. Saunders, 1977.
7. Heiner D, Sears J, and Kniker W: Multiple precipitins to cow's milk in chronic respiratory disease. Am J Dis Child, 103:634, 1962.
8. Hyatt RW et al.: Ultrastructure of the lung in idiopathic pulmonary hemosiderosis. Am J Med, 52:822, 1972.
9. Proskey AJ et al.: Goodpasture's syndrome. A report of five cases and review of the literature. Am J Med, 48:162, 1970.
10. Ramirez RE et al.: Pulmonary hemorrhage associated with systemic lupus erythematosus in children. Radiology, 152:409, 1984.
11. Repetto G et al.: Idiopathic pulmonary hemosiderosis. Clinical, radiologic and respiratory function studies. Pediatrics, 40:24, 1967.
12. Schwartz EE et al.: Pulmonary hemorrhage in renal disease: Goodpasture's syndrome and other causes. Radiology, 122:39, 1977.
13. Soergel KH, and Sommers SC: Idiopathic pulmonary hemosiderosis and related syndromes. Am J Med, 32:499, 1962.
14. Thomas HM: Classification of diffuse intrapulmonary hemorrhage. Chest, 68:483, 1975.

8

MISCELLANEOUS PULMONARY DISORDERS

TRAUMA
RADIATION FIBROSIS
END-STAGE PULMONARY FIBROSIS
COLLAGEN DISEASES
RHEUMATIC PNEUMONITIS

GLOMERULONEPHRITIS
PULMONARY ALVEOLAR
  PROTEINOSIS
PULMONARY ALVEOLAR
  MICROLITHIASIS

TRAUMA

Trauma has become the leading cause of death in children. Although motor vehicle and conventional accidents cause the vast majority of injuries, deliberate trauma (battered child syndrome) accounts for a significant number.

Rib fractures are more common in older children. They are frequently difficult to diagnose and may go unrecognized for 2 to 3 weeks, when callus formation is easily detected. This is of no great consequence in most instances, and diligent efforts to obtain multiple views of the chest to demonstrate rib fractures are usually counterproductive in the seriously injured patient. Multiple symmetric paraspinal or lateral midaxillary fractures in infants under 2 to 3 years of age should always suggest the possibility of occult trauma (Fig. 8–1).

Direct nonpenetrating forces may cause pulmonary injury resulting in lung contusion, hematoma, and pulmonary lacerations with subsequent pneumatocele, pneumothorax, and pneumomediastinum. Contusions may appear as diffuse hazy areas of density or as a large area of consolidation (Fig. 8–2). Recognizable hematomas are generally seen as sharply defined soft tissue masslike lesions (Fig. 8–3; also see Fig. 6–10), which may subsequently cavitate and develop fluid levels. Pulmonary lacerations are usually associated with atelectasis, pneumothorax, pneumomediastinum, or air entrapped in the lung parenchyma or adjacent pulmonary ligaments (Fig. 8–4).

A much more serious injury is that of tracheobronchial fracture, which may be very difficult to diagnose. This diagnosis should be considered when there is massive pneumothorax or pneumomediastinum that reoccurs or persists after evacuation measures (Fig. 8–5), or when there is massive atelectasis that does not respond to treatment. Other signs include lateral or inferior displacement of the lung away from the hilum. Bronchoscopy must be performed whenever this diagnosis is suspected.

Direct trauma may result in cardiac injury resulting in pericardial hemorrhage, myocardial damage, or aortic injury. Aortic injuries resulting in dissections or aneurysms are much more common in adults than in children.

Trauma to the lower chest and upper abdomen may result in diaphragmatic rupture, as well as injury to the liver and spleen. Such injuries require conventional radiographic studies of the chest and abdomen, upper gastrointestinal series (Fig.

Text continued on page 332

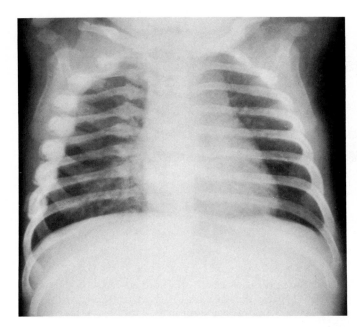

Figure 8–1. Multiple rib fractures of the right hemithorax in an infant who received a deliberate crush injury to the chest. Callus formation is identified at the lateral and paraspinal portions of the right second through seventh ribs.

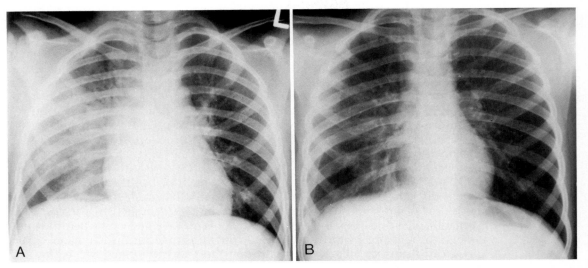

Figure 8–2. Lung trauma to the right hemithorax in an 8-year-old boy. A, Parenchymal density in the right lung represents pulmonary contusion and mild pleural effusion. B, Repeat examination 4 days later shows resolution of the pulmonary abnormality, with a small residual hemothorax.

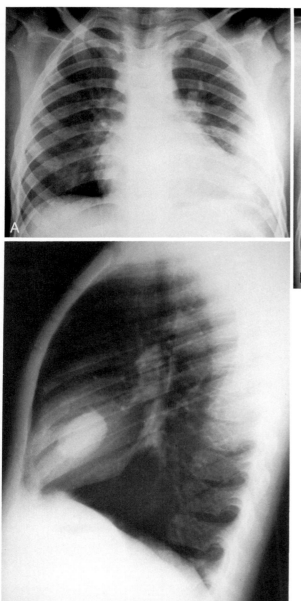

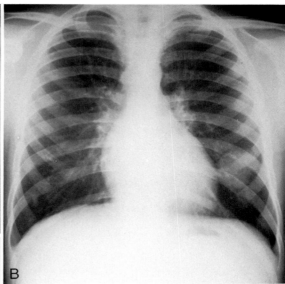

Figure 8–3. *Motor vehicle accident with resulting chest trauma in a 9-year-old boy. A, Parenchymal hemorrhage and pleural effusion are present in the left lower hemithorax, and poorly defined fractures involve the anterolateral portions of the left fifth, sixth, and seventh ribs. B, Repeat radiograph 7 weeks later shows resolution of the parenchymal and pleural hemorrhage, with a residual sharply demarcated round hematoma. C, Lateral radiograph shows the hematoma to lie either within the lingula or the interlobar fissure.*

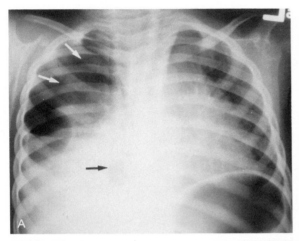

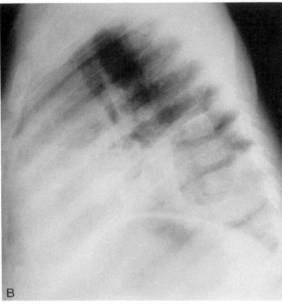

Figure 8–4. Traumatic hemopneumothorax in a 2-year-old boy. A, Chest radiographs show pneumothorax on the right (white arrowheads) with air also in the right inferior pulmonary ligament (black arrow). B, Lateral view reveals loculated air in the posterior portion of the left hemithorax.

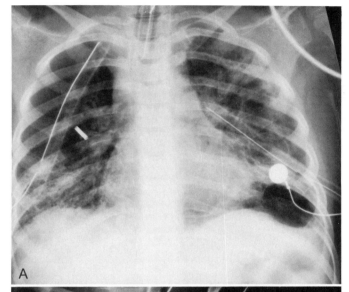

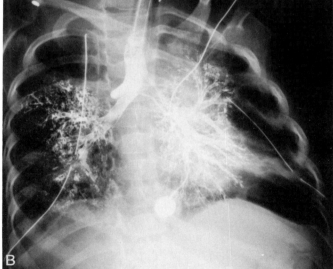

Figure 8–5. Young child who received a crushing injury to the chest. A, Chest tubes have been inserted for treatment of bilateral pneumothoraces. There is bilateral parenchymal abnormality secondary to lung contusion. B, Bronchogram demonstrates fracture and occlusion of the right upper lobe bronchus.

8–6), and nuclear scans for evaluation. Computerized tomography (CT) examination of the chest and abdomen is probably the diagnostic mode of choice for this type of injury. Rupture of the left hemidiaphragm is more reliably diagnosed than that of the right hemidiaphragm (Fig. 8–7). Penetrating injuries may produce almost any conceivable abnormality (Fig. 8–8).

RADIATION FIBROSIS

Radiation injury to the lungs may follow radiation therapy to the mediastinum or to the lungs. The increasing use of chemotherapeutic agents and the reduction in the use of radiation therapy for mediastinal and pulmonary malignancies in children has resulted in fewer cases of radiation fibrosis. Pulmonary function testing may be a more sensitive method of determining the extent of damage to the lungs following radiation therapy.

Radiographic changes are usually not evident until at least 4 weeks after cessation of treatment. The radiographic changes may consist of linear, patchy, or confluent areas of pulmonary alteration, and the areas of involvement are related to the radiation portals. Fibrotic changes result in loss of volume of the radiated area (Fig. 8–9). Pleural effusions are rare but pleural thickening is frequently evident.

END-STAGE PULMONARY FIBROSIS

Diffused end-stage pulmonary fibrosis may be secondary to fibrosing alveolitis, pulmonary injury secondary to unknown infectious agents, both viral and bacterial, various interstitial lung diseases that can be histologically distinguished in the early stages of the disease, pulmonary response to toxic inhalants, histiocytosis X, chronic vasculitis, and most of the collagen diseases. The pathologic changes of end-stage pulmonary fibrosis have usually progressed beyond histologic recognition of the etiology and pathogenesis, and can only be described as severe pulmonary fibrosis. Radiographically, the lungs show a reticular nodular pattern with pronounced "honeycombing," the pathognomonic finding of severe interstitial lung disease (Fig. 8–10).

COLLAGEN DISEASES

There are several clinical and radiographic features of the collagen diseases that overlap one another, making the differentiation often difficult. This is especially true when the more common lesions of rheumatic fever and rheumatoid arthritis are considered. Lupus erythematosus, dermatomyositis, scleroderma, and polyarteritis nodosa are uncommon in children. The radiographic findings are not diagnostic and, on many occasions, superimposed infectious pneumonia or aspiration may obscure the underlying process.

Dermatomyositis tends to produce less pulmonary abnormalities than the rest, but an occasional patient may present with densities indicative of pulmonary fibrosis. The findings may also simulate those of miliary tuberculosis.

Scleroderma in the pediatric patient usually occurs at puberty and, although the roentgenographic features are nonspecific, honeycombing and linear fibrotic densities in the lung bases may develop in advanced cases. On rare occasions blebs and pneumothorax occur, but this is more common in the adult. Primary pneumonitis or aspiration secondary to altered esophageal motility is not uncommon. Death, however, is usually a result of extrapulmonary causes.

Lupus erythematosus may present radiographically in many ways. Pneumonitis, with or without fibrosis, can be seen, along with pleural effusion or reaction.

Text continued on page 337

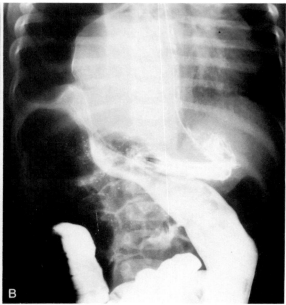

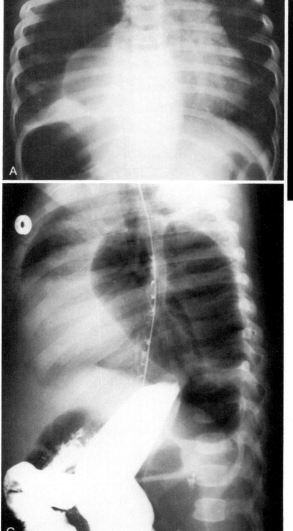

Figure 8–6. Blunt trauma to the upper abdomen of a 1½-year-old child and resulting rupture of the right hemidiaphragm. A, Chest radiograph shows herniation of bowel into the right hemithorax, with displacement of mediastinal structures to the left. B, Frontal projection following contrast study of the colon demonstrates the hepatic flexure extending into the right hemithorax. A small amount of contrast medium has been introduced into the stomach. C, Lateral view reveals contrast medium in the colon, with dilated hepatic flexure in the right hemithorax.

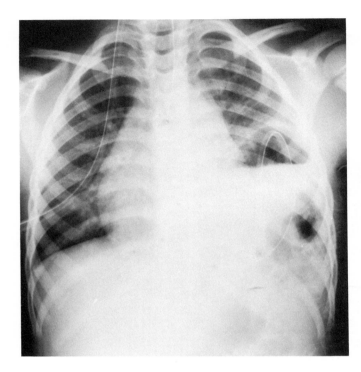

Figure 8–7. Rupture of the left hemidiaphragm in a 3-year-old boy who was run over by a car. Chest radiograph shows herniation of the stomach and the nasogastric tube into the left hemithorax.

Figure 8–8. Traumatic injury to the chest of a 9-year-old boy whose horse ran into a tree branch that pierced the anterior chest wall, and which by physical examination appeared only as a superficial abrasion. Chest radiograph outlines the branch, which measured 8 inches in length and 1 inch in diameter (arrow). The branch had passed posterior to the heart, but produced associated pleural and pulmonary hemorrhage.

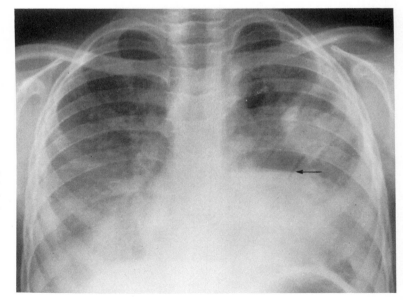

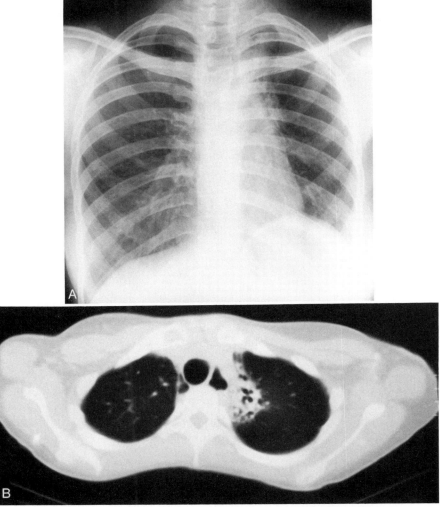

Figure 8–9. *Postradiation fibrosis in a 15-year-old girl with mediastinal Hodgkin's disease. A, Chest radiograph shows elevation of the left hemidiaphragm and mild retraction of the mediastinal structures to the left. The left superior mediastinum is poorly defined and irregular in outline. B, Computerized tomography demonstrates medial retraction of the left upper lobe, with associated bronchiectasis.*

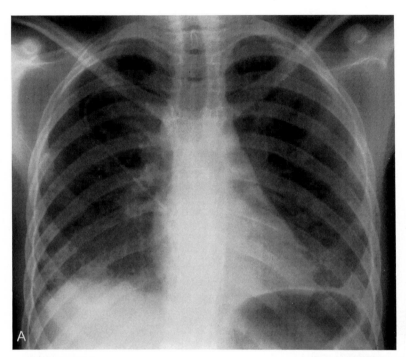

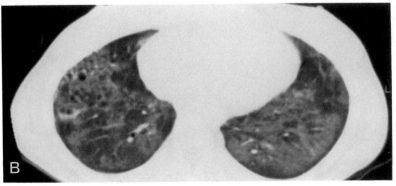

Figure 8–10. End-stage pulmonary fibrosis in a 13-year-old girl who had been treated with bleomycin for malignant teratoma. A, Chest radiograph shows reticulonodular pattern of both lungs, within which are several areas of "honeycombing." B, Computerized tomography shows the "honeycombed" and the linear fibrotic areas to better advantage.

Cardiac involvement is not unusual, nor is pericardial effusion. Inflammatory lesions of pulmonary vessels may produce patchy infiltration secondary to pulmonary hemorrhage.

Periarteritis nodosa may produce the most severe radiographic changes of all (Fig. 8–11). Because of the propensity for inflammatory changes of pulmonary arteries to occur, bilateral diffuse infiltrations may be found that may be severe enough to simulate pulmonary edema. On occasion there may be pulmonary necrosis, which simulates Wegener's granulomatosis. These infiltrates tend to persist for several weeks or longer. Although the disease may be suspected radiographically, hypertension, arthritis, neuritis, and renal disease are more helpful diagnostic features.

RHEUMATIC PNEUMONITIS

Although there has been some question as to whether or not rheumatic pneumonitis is a specific pulmonary disease, a considerable number of well-documented cases have been recorded to verify that it is a distinct entity. The pulmonary manifestations of rheumatic fever usually accompany the more common features of rheumatic fever—that is, arthritis and carditis. However, pneumonitis may be the initial abnormality. The incidence of rheumatic pneumonia is difficult to determine because many cases are subclinical.

The etiology is unknown but is assumed to be an allergic reaction to β-hemolytic streptococci, resulting in a loss of vascular integrity, edema, vasculitis, periadventitial collection of chronic inflammatory cells, and hyaline membrane formation.

There is no predominant roentgenographic pattern. However, the infiltrates change rapidly in extent and location, similar to those of Löffler's pneumonia. Generally, patchy infiltrates occur most frequently within the midlung zones, but it is not unusual to see prominent bronchopulmonary markings, or even small miliary-type infiltrations. Involvement of whole lobes is unusual, and the apices and bases are frequently spared. When perihilar infiltrations are severe and are accompanied by an enlarged cardiac silhouette of myocarditis or pericarditis, differentiation from pulmonary edema may be impossible. Small pleural effusions can be seen but are often fleeting. These pulmonary changes, developing in a child with rheumatic heart disease, should be considered as possibly being those of rheumatic pneumonitis but confirmation may be impossible (Fig. 8–12).

Other pulmonary manifestations of rheumatic disease are pulmonary fibrosis, pulmonary nodules and, rarely, spontaneous pneumothorax. These are all considerably more prominent in adults than in children.

Rheumatoid Nodules. Rheumatoid nodules of the lungs are rare in children and invariably develop after the clinical course of rheumatoid arthritis has been well established. Histologically, these nodules are similar to if not the same as subcutaneous nodules. Radiographically, they are usually multiple, smooth, round, or oval, and vary from a few millimeters to several centimeters in diameter (Fig. 8–13). They are frequently located in the subpleural parenchyma and may be lobulated. The lesions are generally solid but may later cavitate, producing a vague ringlike shadow with thick walls. New lesions may develop while other nodules are cavitating. Spontaneous regression may occur, but usually the nodules remain for many months or even years.

GLOMERULONEPHRITIS

Chest radiographs may be of considerable diagnostic assistance in clinically suspected or even unsuspected glomerulonephritis. The nature of the underlying

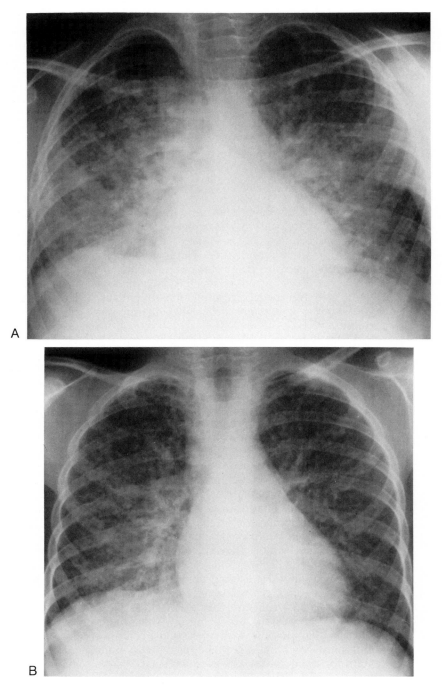

Figure 8–11. Periarteritis nodosa in an 11-year-old boy. A, Chest radiographs show extensive bilateral pulmonary abnormality consisting of nodular densities with areas of coalescence. B, Repeat radiograph 1 week later after introduction of steroid therapy shows improvement in the appearance of the chest.

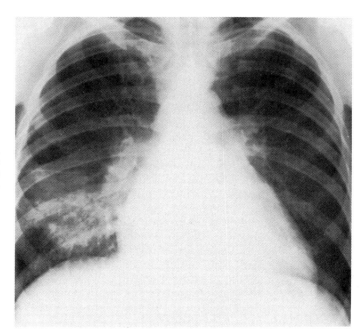

Figure 8–12. Rheumatic pneumonitis in a 14-year-old child with rheumatic carditis. Density in the right base disappeared in 4 days, and may have represented rheumatic pneumonitis (unproven).

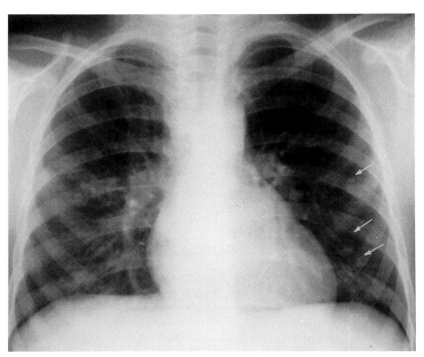

Figure 8–13. Rheumatoid nodules in a 9-year-old child with a long-standing history of rheumatoid arthritis. Chest radiograph shows multiple discrete nodular densities scattered throughout the lungs and several of these areas (arrows) show cavitation, which has persisted for months.

pathologic process that causes the radiographic manifestations is poorly under-stood. The overall appearance of the heart and lungs may provide very suggestive evidence of glomerulonephritis. Although any cause of pulmonary edema must be considered, the most frequently confused specific entities include viral and inhalation pneumonias, drug sensitivity, near drowning, neurogenic edema, and acute rheumatic disease. Differentiation can occasionally be suggested by intuitive radiographic gestalt, but more often it depends on the clinical circumstances.

Goodpasture's syndrome usually occurs in young men, and is rare or non-existent in children. It may be clinically and radiographically indistinguishable from acute glomerulonephritis. It is an autoimmune disease characterized by hemoptysis, anemia, pulmonary hemorrhage, and hematuria. The latter is caused by focal or diffuse glomerulonephritis. The course of the disease is usually rapid, ranging from several weeks to several months.

The radiographic features consist of cardiovascular as well as pulmonary changes. Generalized cardiac enlargement is usually present, and the hilar vessels are prominent. There may be an increase in the venous pattern, secondary to passive venous congestion, and Kerley's B lines are frequently prominent. Pulmonary edema, confined for the most part to the perihilar regions, occurs in advanced cases. Pleural effusion, usually bilateral, is a common finding, but may vary considerably in amount. Radiologically identifiable edema of the soft tissues of the chest wall and upper flank areas is frequently helpful in recognizing that the cardiac and pulmonary changes are secondary to glomerulonephritis (Fig. 8–14).

PULMONARY ALVEOLAR PROTEINOSIS

Pulmonary alveolar proteinosis is a rare pulmonary disease of unknown etiology usually found in men, but it may occur in infants and children.

The clinical findings are variable and consist of dyspnea, cough, and fatigue. The physical findings in the adult are often minimal compared to the severity of the chest radiography, but in the pediatric patient respiratory symptoms are severe and the prognosis is poor. Complicating infections such as cryptococcosis, mucor-mycosis, aspergillosis, and nocardiosis may develop in the terminal phase of the disease.

Although chest radiographs may show involvement of a localized pulmonary segment, the usual appearance is a bilateral symmetric pattern of ill-defined, diffuse, perihilar, fluffy, or feathery radiodensities radiating from the hilar regions. These findings simulate the "butterfly" pattern of pulmonary edema (Fig. 8–15), but the heart is normal in size and there is no associated pleural effusion. Overaeration or atelectasis may be present, and Kerley's B lines are occasionally seen. There is no evidence of calcification or adenopathy. Terminally the lungs may appear to be completely airless.

PULMONARY ALVEOLAR MICROLITHIASIS

Pulmonary alveolar microlithiasis is a chronic lung disease in which there is a strong familial predisposition, and it has been reported in premature twins. The etiology and pathogenesis are unknown, but most hypotheses incriminate some form of pulmonary metabolic or enzymatic deficiency, resulting in deposition of calcium in the alveoli. It is not known at what point in life the disease begins, but it is more common in young adults and may occur in pediatric patients. In the early stages the patients are usually asymptomatic, and the diagnosis is made when the patient receives a chest x-ray examination during a routine physical examination or for some other reason. When symptoms occur they consist of slow, progressive respiratory insufficiency, with ultimate development of pulmo-

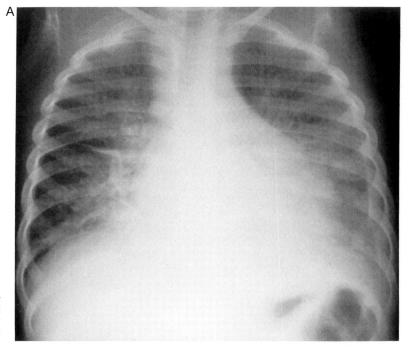

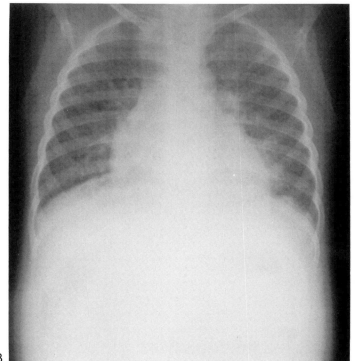

Figure 8–14. Acute glomerulonephritis. A, Chest radiograph in a 2-year-old girl shows cardiac enlargement and evidence of passive venous congestion, with associated pleural effusion. B, Chest radiograph in a 3-year-old girl shows similar changes of cardiac enlargement and passive venous congestion, with associated edema of the chest and abdominal wall.

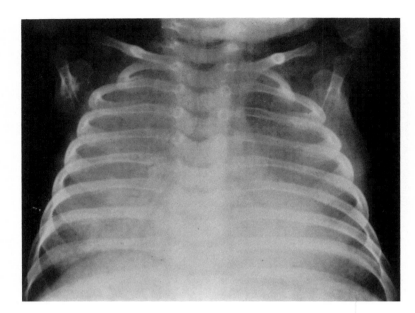

Figure 8–15. Pulmonary alveolar proteinosis in a 10-week-old boy whose symptoms of poor weight gain and cyanosis began at 4 weeks of age. Chest radiograph shows diffuse opacification involving both lungs, with relative sparing of the apical and costophrenic areas. The pulmonary biopsy was diagnostic of pulmonary alveolar proteinosis.

Figure 8–16. Pulmonary alveolar microlithiasis in a 6-year-old asymptomatic girl. Chest radiographs show multiple small punctate areas of calcific density scattered throughout both lungs.

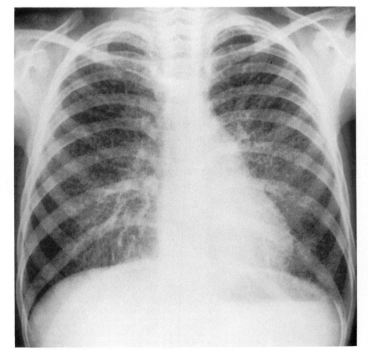

nary hypertension. Occasionally the patients describe their sputum as containing sand-sized particles. Laboratory findings are not helpful in the diagnosis.

The radiographic features are usually strikingly abnormal and out of proportion to the relatively asymptomatic clinical findings. There are myriads of tiny microcalcifications scattered diffusely throughout both lungs (Fig. 8–16). These tiny calcific densities can be more readily appreciated by viewing the film through a magnifying glass. Occasionally the total effect of the many nodules gives the impression that coalescence of the calcific deposits has occurred, producing larger lesions. With progression of the disease the cardiac borders and outlines of the diaphragm may become partially obliterated. The apices appear to be less involved than the remaining portions of the lungs. There is a fine rim of calcification in the subpleural areas, which can best be seen on overpenetrated films. There is no involvement of the pleura, and consequently a fine line of radiolucency may be seen about this calcific rim. In the late stages of the disease pulmonary emphysema and fibrosis develop and, as a result of the pulmonary hypertension, cardiac enlargement may be a terminal finding. Pleural effusion is uncommon. The course is extremely protracted, and the patients usually live for many years with only a gradual slow deterioration in their physical condition.

SUGGESTED READINGS

TRAUMA

Armstrong JD II, and Tocino I: Trauma to the lung. In Taveras JM, and Ferrucci JT (eds): Radiology, Diagnosis-Imaging-Intervention, Chap 50. Philadelphia, J.B. Lippincott, 1986.
Ball T et al.: Traumatic diaphragmatic hernia: Errors in diagnosis. Am J Roentgenol, 138:633, 1982.
Burke JF: Early diagnosis of traumatic rupture of the bronchus. JAMA, 181:682, 1962.
Burney RE et al.: Chest roentgenograms in diagnosis of traumatic rupture of the aorta. Observer variation in interpretation. Chest, 85:5, 1984.
Cochlin DL, and Shaw MRP: Traumatic lung cysts following minor blunt chest trauma. Clin Radiol, 29:151, 1978.
De Luca SA, Rhea JT, and O'Malley T: Radiographic evaluation of rib fractures. Am J Roentgenol, 138:91, 1982.
Fagan CJ, and Swischuk LE: Traumatic lung and paramediastinal pneumatoceles. Radiology, 120:11, 1976.
Lotz PR et al.: Significance of pneumomediastinum in blunt trauma to the thorax. Am J Roentgenol, 132:819, 1979.
Meller JL, Little AG, and Shermeta DW: Major thoracic trauma in children. Pediatr Clin North Am, 22:341, 1975.
Ravin C et al.: Post-traumatic pneumatocele in the inferior pulmonary ligament. Radiology, 121:39, 1976.
Sefczek DM, Sefczek RJ, and Deeb ZL: Radiographic signs of acute rupture of the thoracic aorta. Am J Roentgenol, 141:1259, 1983.
Shulman HS, and Samuels TH: The radiology of blunt trauma. J Can Assoc Radiol, 34:204, 1985.
Silberger ML, and Kushner LN: Tracheobronchial perforation: Its diagnosis and treatment. Radiology, 85:242, 1965.
Specht DE: Pulmonary hematoma. Am J Dis Child, 111:559, 1966.
Stevens E, and Templeton AW: Traumatic nonpenetrating lung contusion. Radiology, 85:247, 1965.
Wiot JF: The radiologic manifestations of blunt trauma. JAMA, 231:500, 1975.

RADIATION FIBROSIS

Paré JAP, and Fraser RG: Synopsis of Diseases of the Chest. Philadelphia, W.B. Saunders, 1983.

END-STAGE PULMONARY FIBROSIS

McLoud TC: Chronic infiltrative lung disorders. In Taveras JM, and Ferrucci JT (eds): Radiology, Diagnosis-Imaging-Intervention, Chap 55. Philadelphia, J.B. Lippincott, 1986.
Paré JAP, and Fraser RG: Synopsis of Diseases of the Chest. Philadelphia, W.B. Saunders, 1983.

COLLAGEN DISEASES

Burrows FGO: Pulmonary nodules in rheumatoid disease: A report of 2 cases. Br J Radiol, 40:256, 1967.

Gamsu G, and Webb WR: Pulmonary hemorrhage in systemic lupus erythematosus. J Can Assoc Radiol, 29:66, 1978.

Gondos B: Roentgen manifestations in progressive systemic sclerosis (diffuse scleroderma). Am J Roentgenol, 84:235, 1960.

Hunninghake GW, and Fauci AS: Pulmonary involvement in the collagen vascular diseases. Am Rev Respir Dis, 119:471, 1979.

Jordan JD: Cardiopulmonary manifestations of rheumatoid disease in childhood. South Med J, 57:1273, 1964.

Kirkpatrick JA Jr, and Fleisher DS: The roentgen appearance of the chest in acute glomerulonephritis in children. J Pediatr, 64:492, 1964.

Levin DC: Proper interpretation of pulmonary roentgen changes in systemic lupus erythematosus. Am J Roentgenol, 111:510, 1971.

Martel W et al.: Pulmonary and pleural lesions in rheumatoid disease. Radiology, 90:641, 1968.

Morgan WKC, and Wolfel DA: Lungs and pleura in rheumatoid arthritis. Am J Roentgenol, 98:334, 1966.

Ochsner SF, Hatch HB, and Leonard GL: Hypersensitivity and the lung. Am J Roentgenol, 107:290, 1969.

PULMONARY ALVEOLAR PROTEINOSIS

Carlsen ET, Hill RB Jr, and Rolands DT Jr: Nocardiosis and pulmonary alveolar proteinosis. Ann Intern Med, 60:275, 1964.

McCook TA et al.: Pulmonary alveolar proteinosis in children. Am J Roentgenol, 137:1023, 1981.

Ramirez-Rivera J: Pulmonary alveolar proteinosis, a roentgenographic analysis. Am J Roentgenol, 92:571, 1964.

Rosen SH, Castleman B, and Liebow AA: Pulmonary alveolar proteinosis. N Engl J Med 258:1123, 1958.

Sunderland WA, Campbell RA, and Edwards MJ: Pulmonary alveolar proteinosis and pulmonary cryptococcosis in an adolescent boy. J Pediatr, 80:450, 1972.

Wilkinson RH, Blanc WA, and Hagstrom JW: Pulmonary alveolar proteinosis in three infants. Pediatrics, 41:510, 1968.

PULMONARY ALVEOLAR MICROLITHIASIS

Balikian JP, Fulehan FJB, and Necho CN: Pulmonary alveolar microlithiasis: Report of five cases with special reference to roentgen manifestations. Am J Roentgenol, 103:509, 1968.

Caffre PR, and Altman RS: Pulmonary alveolar microlithiasis occurring in premature twins. J Pediatr, 66:758, 1965.

Sosman MC et al.: The familial occurrence of pulmonary alveolar microlithiasis. Am J Roentgenol, 77:947, 1957.

Index

Note: Page numbers in *italics* refer to illustrations; page numbers followed by (t) refer to tables.